dumb

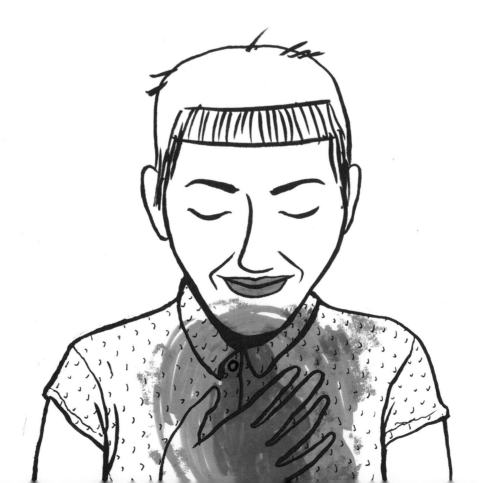

There is a river of gratitude, whose waters flow: to my parents and siblings, for unconditional support; to Stephen Wei, for teaching me the inner workings of comics; to Peter B, Meags F, Sophie Y, Bryn R-M, and Maisie J for essential reading and feedback; to Alonso G, Tereza J, Sophia K, Elizabeth E and Naada Yoga, the MEBG, La Maison de la BD de Montréal, and the whole Mile End community for allowing silence and space to exist around me; to the staff of the Toronto Comic Arts Festival for letting me (quietly) crash the party; to Carmen Y, and D Alex Meeks for a presence so pure. Long live the river!

Editor: Gary Groth
Design: Keeli McCarthy and Georgia Webber
Production: Paul Baresh
Promotion: Jacq Cohen
Editorial Assistance: Conrad Groth
Associate Publisher: Eric Reynolds
Publisher: Gary Groth

Fantagraphics Books, Inc.
7563 Lake City Way NE
Seattle, WA 98115
www.fantagraphics.com

First Printing: June 2018
ISBN 978-1-68396-116-1
Library of Congress Control Number: 2017957018
Printed in China

DUMB

LIVING WITHOUT A VOICE

A GRAPHIC MEMOIR BY
georgia webber

FANTAGRAPHICS BOOKS

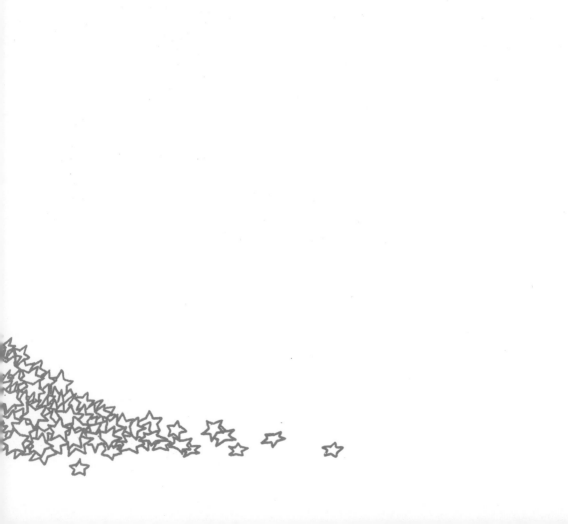

For those of us lost in a constant journey of self-discovery that borders on self-deprecation and melodrama, the search for our "true" voice is something way too familiar and, at times, tiring. Have you ever wondered what would happen if one day you woke up without a limb? What would you do if you were suddenly unable to see, or speak?...

Dumb is a story that answers just that. We take something valuable for granted, and then learn to live without it when inexplicably it is gone. The human voice has such packed connotations. If we really think about it, the "voice inside" is nothing more than our own selves in the form of thoughts and emotions. We spend all our time worrying about being liked and accepted by others, we forget the importance of figuring out who we are, and being content with what we find.

The story exposes a particular contrast between healthcare and self-care. Through Georgia Webber's story, we notice how young people are supposed to be healthy — and that they are less concerned with their health until something stops working properly.

There is no prescribed way, physically or emotionally, to get our voice back once it's lost. What we have do to is figure out a way to survive without it, and in the process, learn to go through the frustration, isolation, and pain of not knowing when it will come back.

A quiet woman is better than a loud one, as far as the patriarchy is concerned. "Saviour"-types love to fend for folks with different abilities and advantages, who are often able to fend for themselves just fine. But we cannot allow those who do not have our best interests at heart to speak on our behalf.

—Lido Pimienta
Dec 2017
Toronto

Lido Pimienta is a Columbian Canadian electronic musician, singer, and fine artist. Pimienta won the prestigious Polaris Music Prize for their album La Papessa *in 2017.*

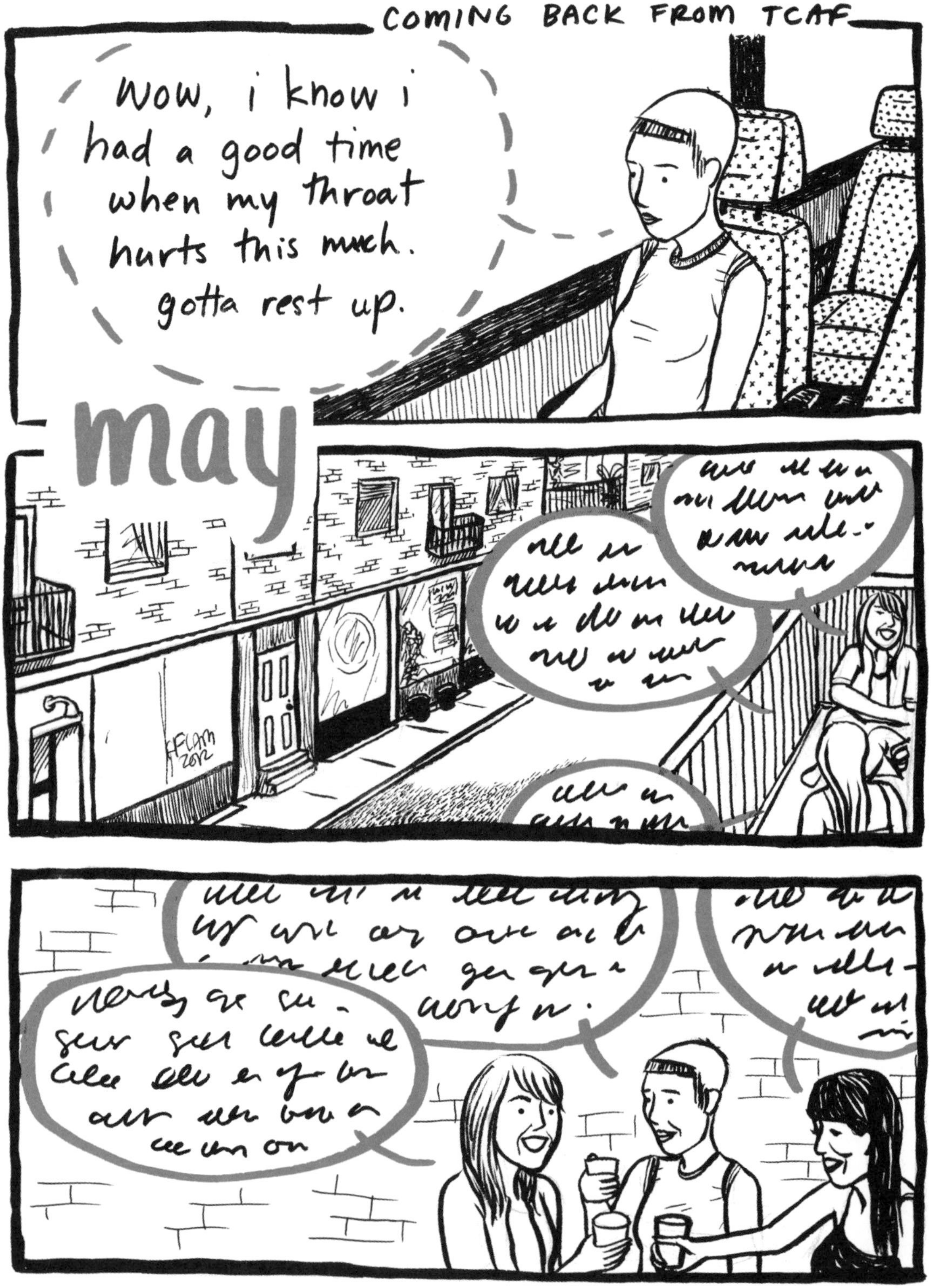
COMING BACK FROM TCAF
Wow, i know i had a good time when my throat hurts this much. gotta rest up.
may
KFLAM 2012

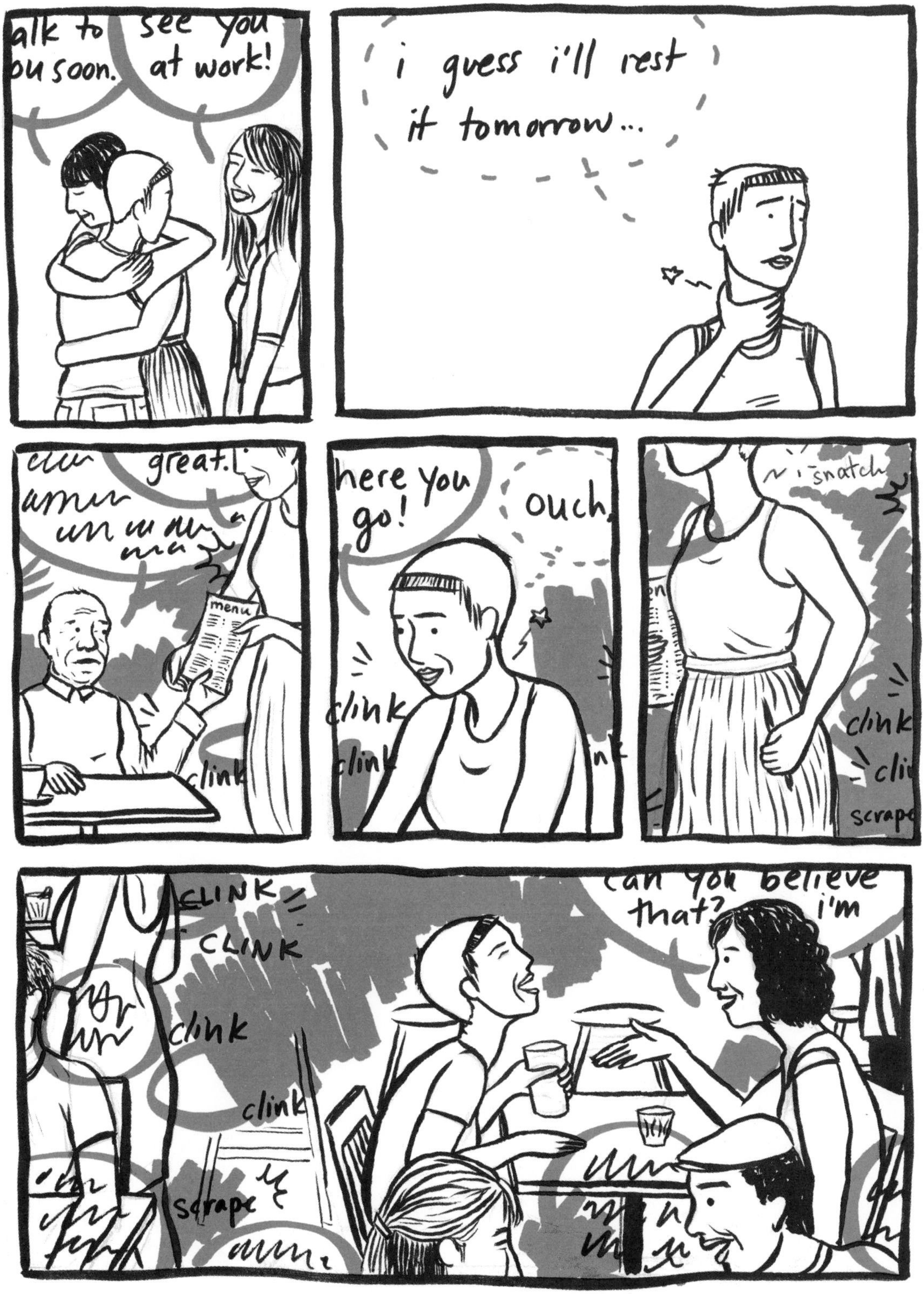
alk to
ou soon.
see you
at work!
i guess i'll rest
it tomorrow...
great.
menu
clink
here you
go!
ouch.
clink
clink
snatch
clink
cli
scrape
CLINK
CLINK
clink
clink
scrape
can you believe
that? i'm

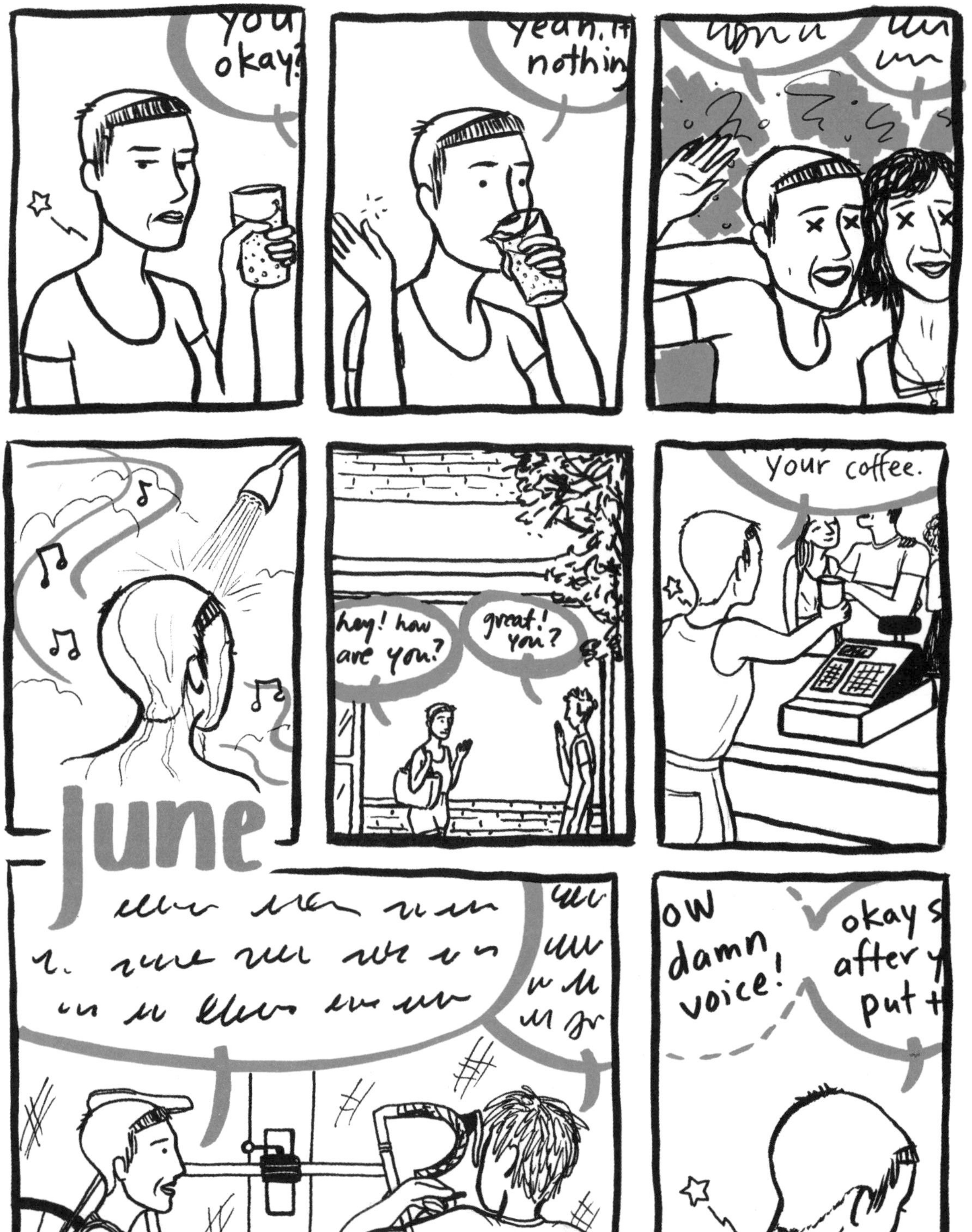
you okay?
yeah. it's nothing
your coffee.
hey! how are you?
great! you?
june
ow damn voice!
okay s after y put t

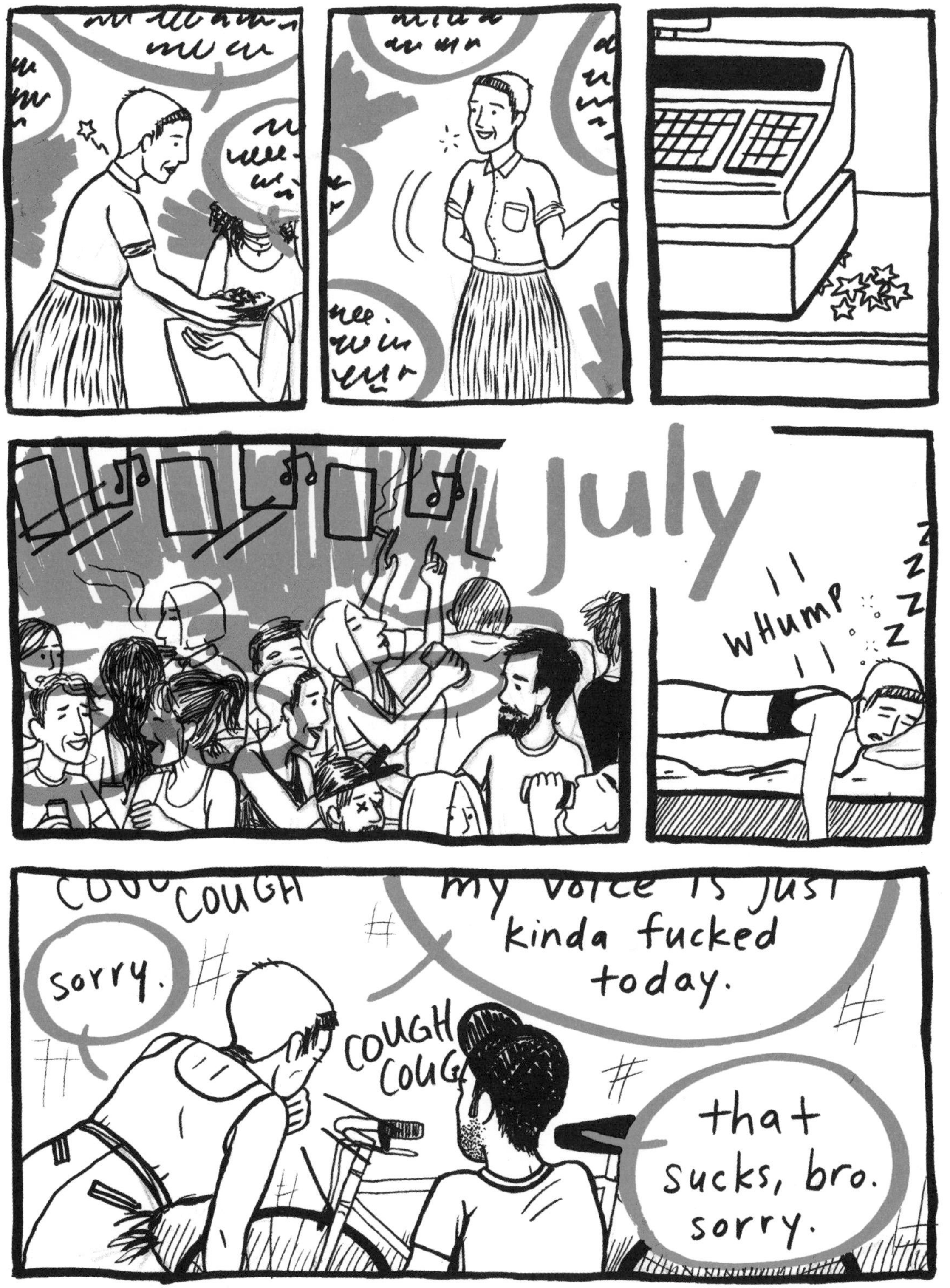
july
WHUMP
Z Z Z Z
COUG COUGH
my voice is just kinda fucked today.
sorry.
COUGH COUG
that sucks, bro. sorry.

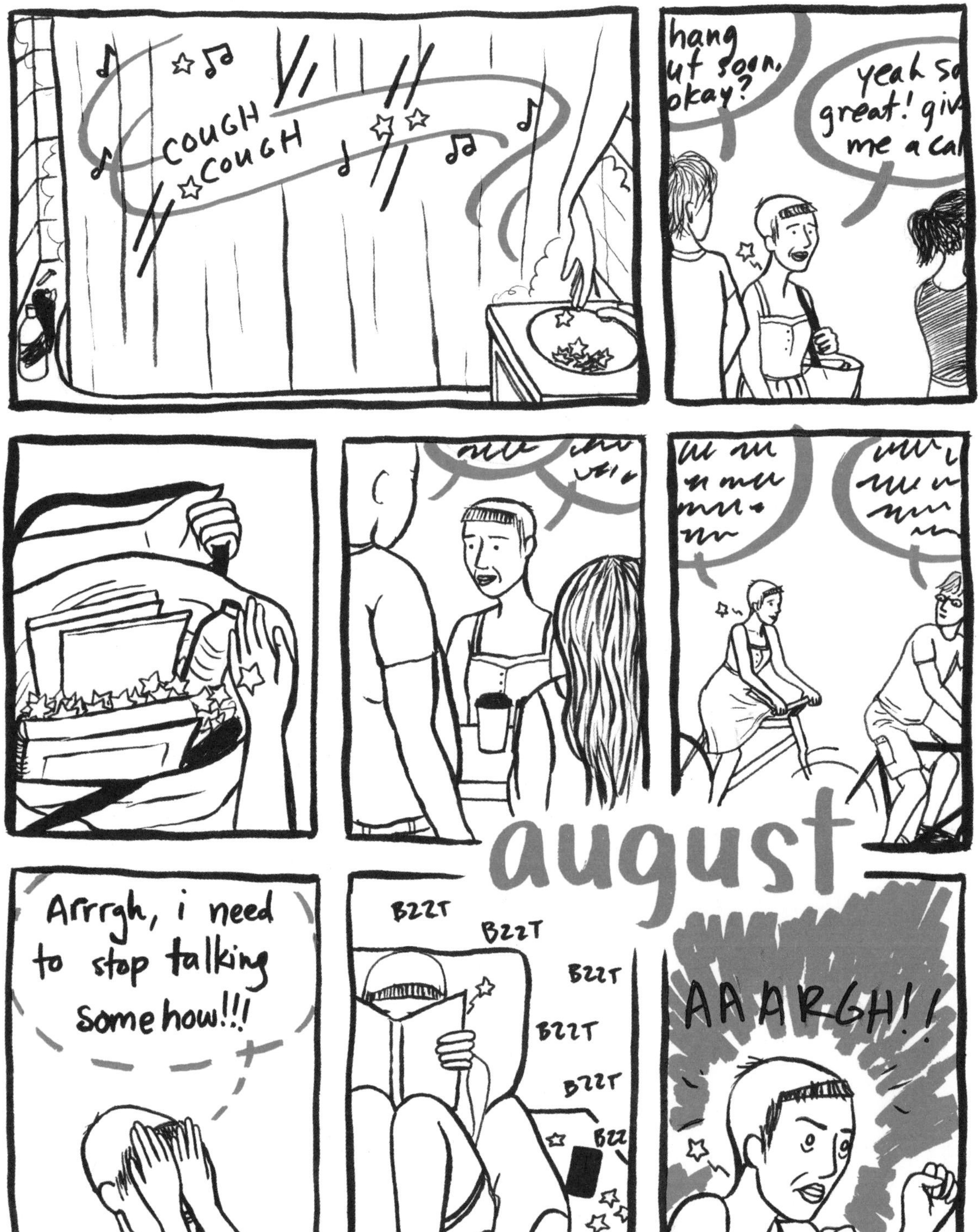
COUGH
COUGH
hang
up soon,
okay?
yeah so
great! give
me a cal
august
Arrrgh, i need
to stop talking
somehow!!!
BZZT
BZZT
BZZT
BZZT
BZZT
BZZ
AAARGH!!

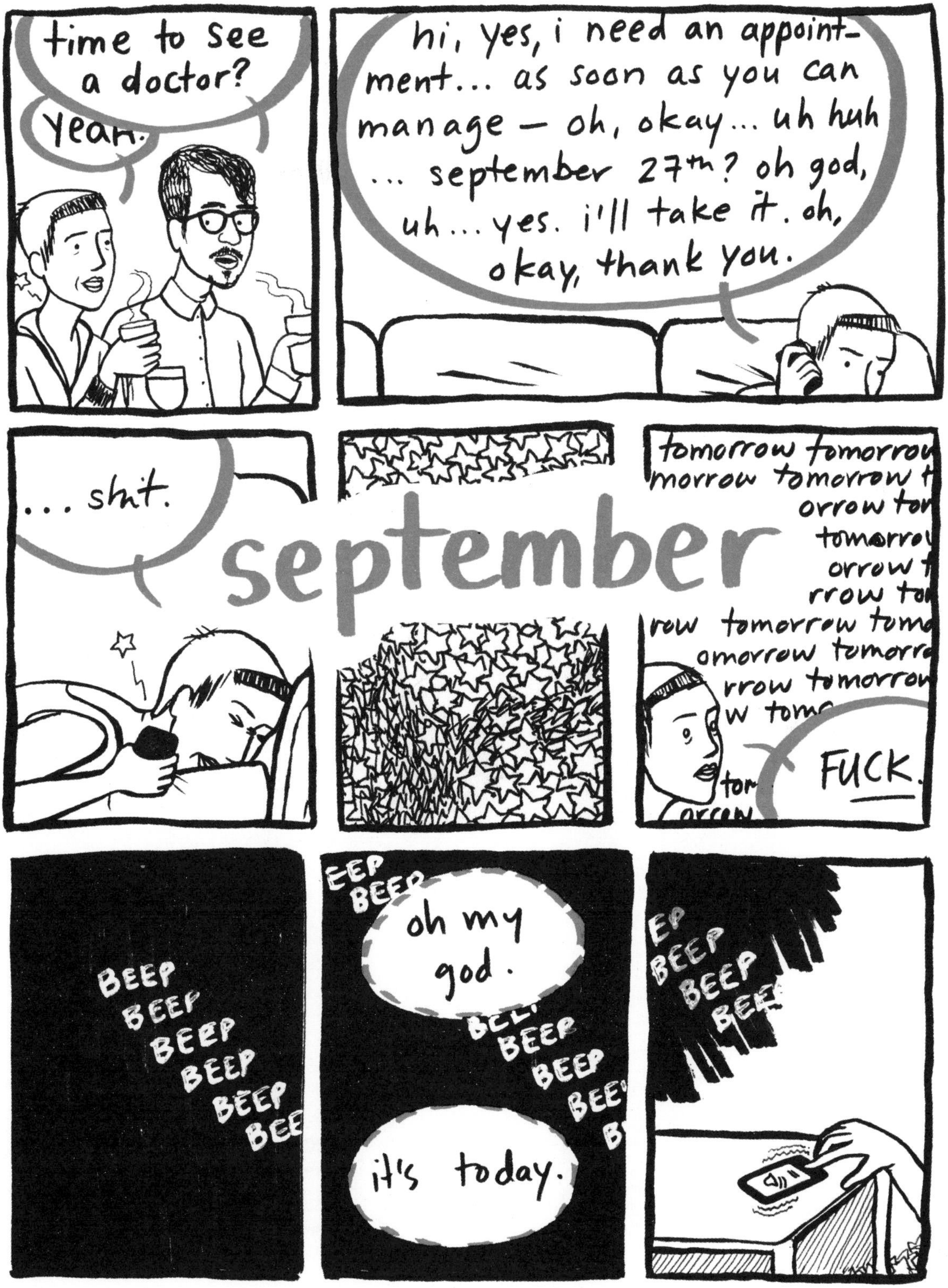

time to see a doctor?
yeah.
hi, yes, i need an appointment... as soon as you can manage — oh, okay... uh huh ... september 27th? oh god, uh... yes. i'll take it. oh, okay, thank you.
... shit.
september
tomorrow tomorrow
FUCK.
BEEP BEEP BEEP BEEP BEEP
oh my god.
it's today.
BEEP BEEP BEEP

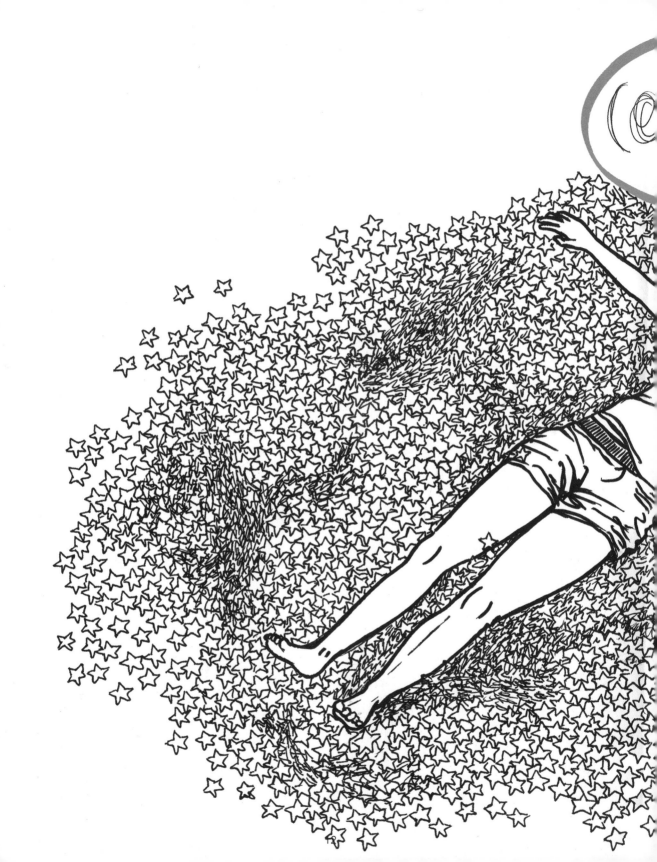

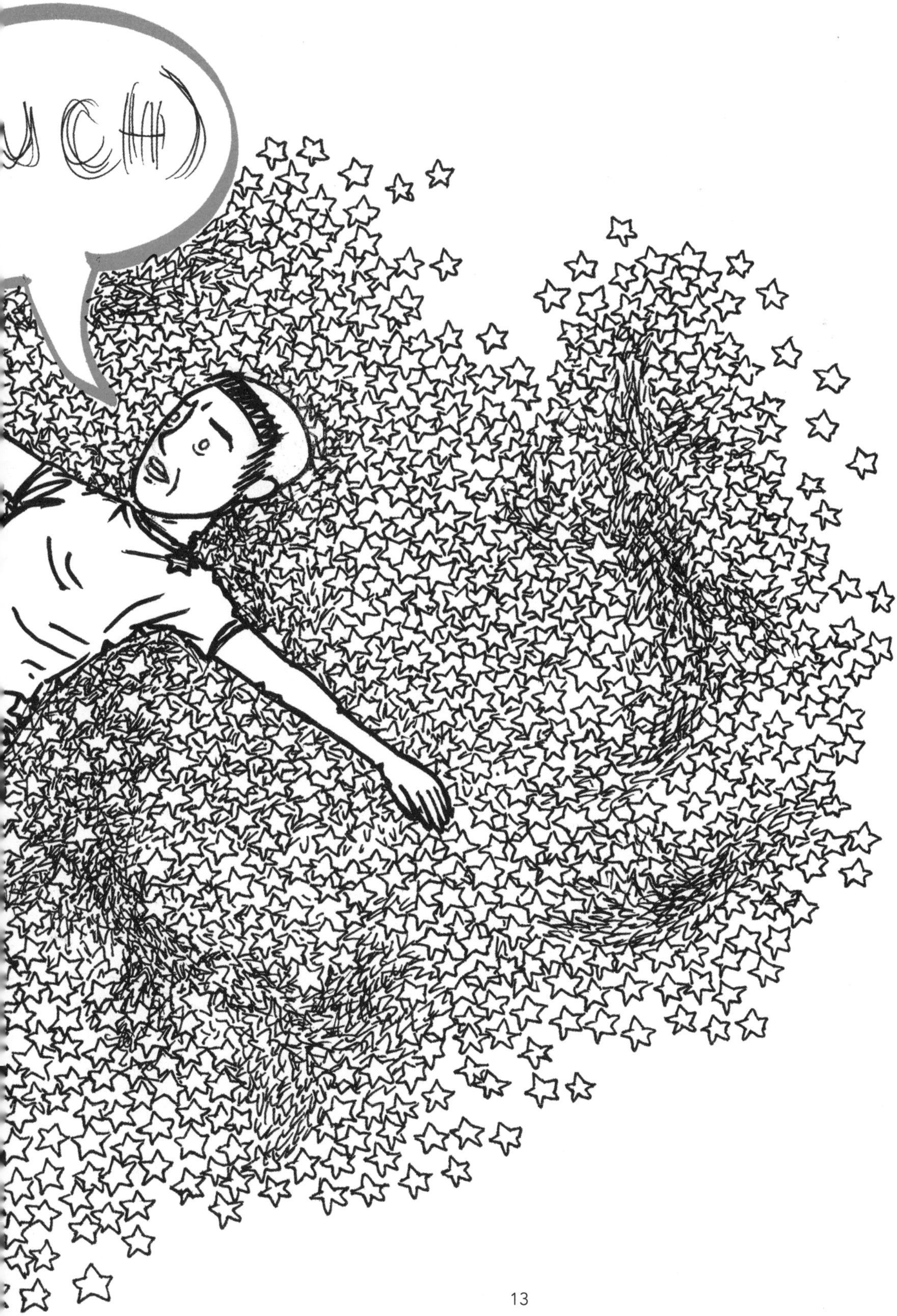

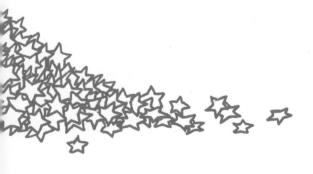

diagnosis

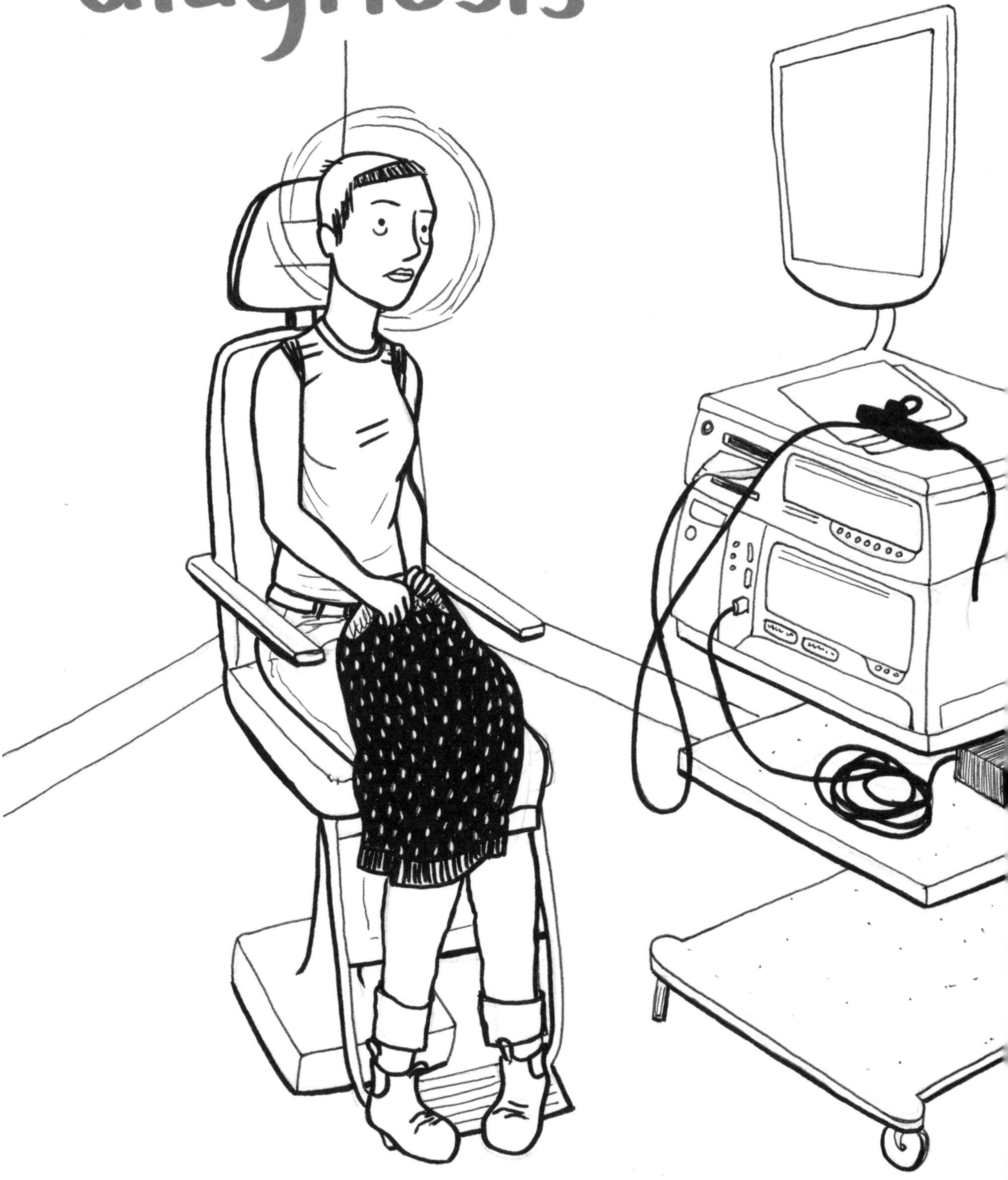

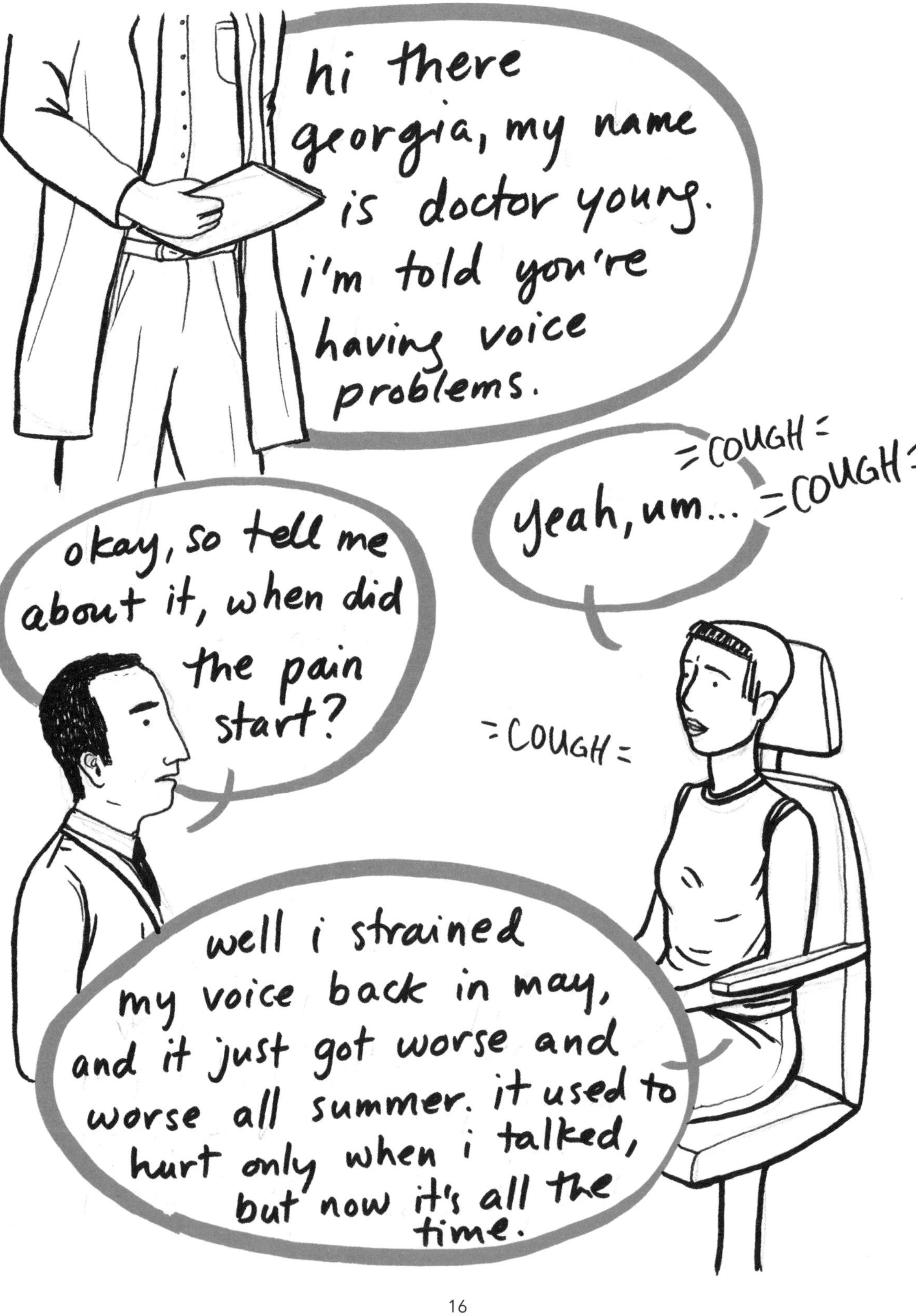
hi there georgia, my name is doctor young. i'm told you're having voice problems.
okay, so tell me about it, when did the pain start?
yeah, um...
=COUGH=
=COUGH=
=COUGH=
well i strained my voice back in may, and it just got worse and worse all summer. it used to hurt only when i talked, but now it's all the time.

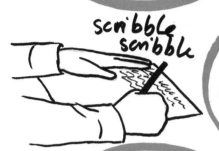
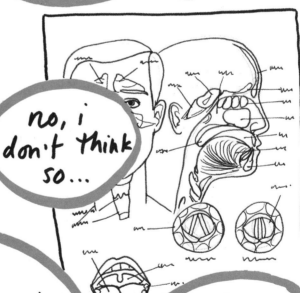
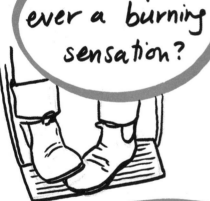
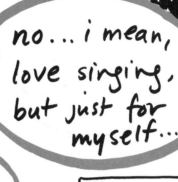

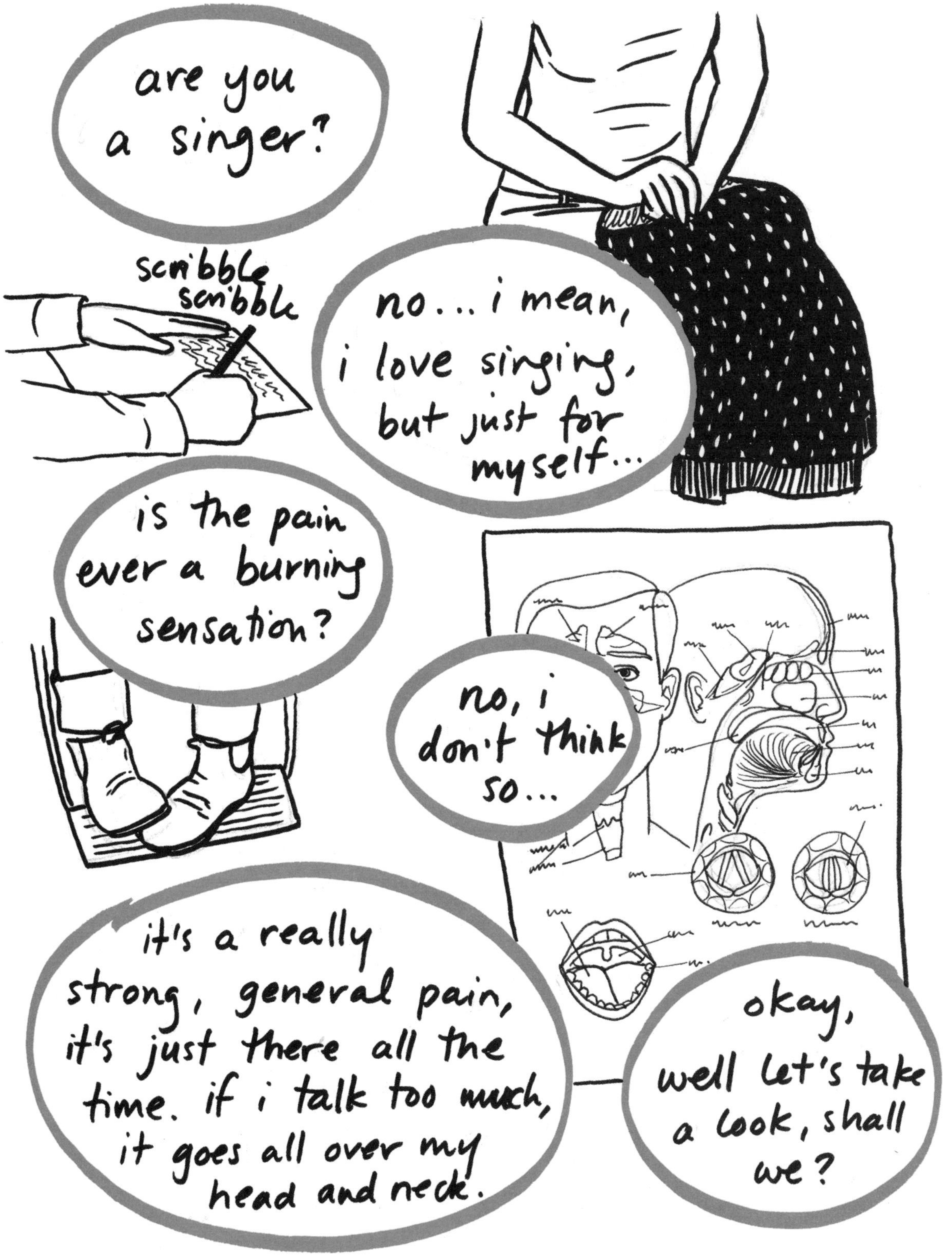

are you a singer?

scribble scribble

no... i mean, i love singing, but just for myself...

is the pain ever a burning sensation?

no, i don't think so...

it's a really strong, general pain, it's just there all the time. if i talk too much, it goes all over my head and neck.

okay, well let's take a look, shall we?

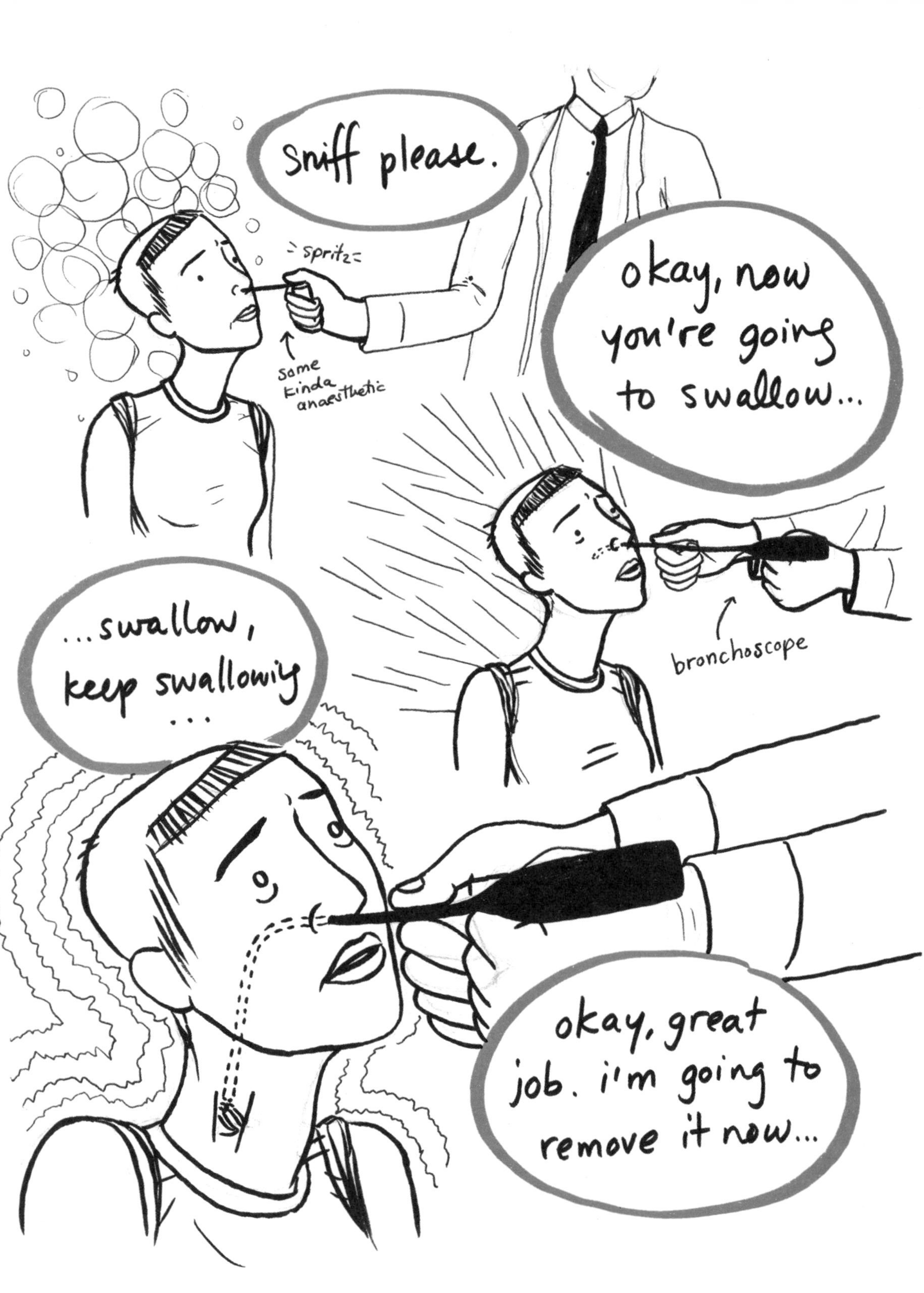
Sniff please.
spritz
some kinda anaesthetic
okay, now you're going to swallow...
bronchoscope
...swallow, keep swallowing ...
okay, great job. i'm going to remove it now...

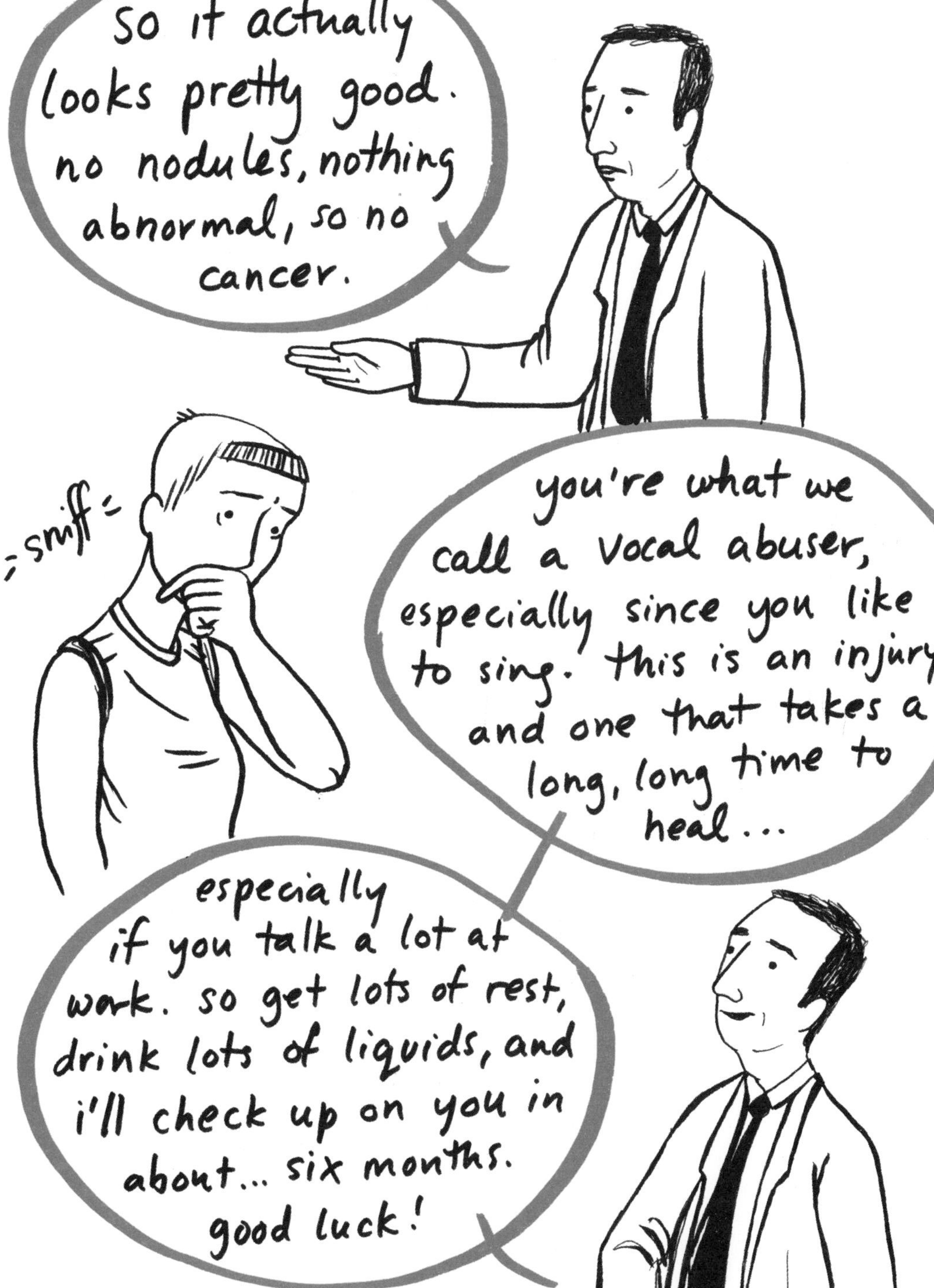
so it actually looks pretty good. no nodules, nothing abnormal, so no cancer.
sniff
you're what we call a vocal abuser, especially since you like to sing. this is an injury, and one that takes a long, long time to heal...
especially if you talk a lot at work. so get lots of rest, drink lots of liquids, and i'll check up on you in about... six months. good luck!

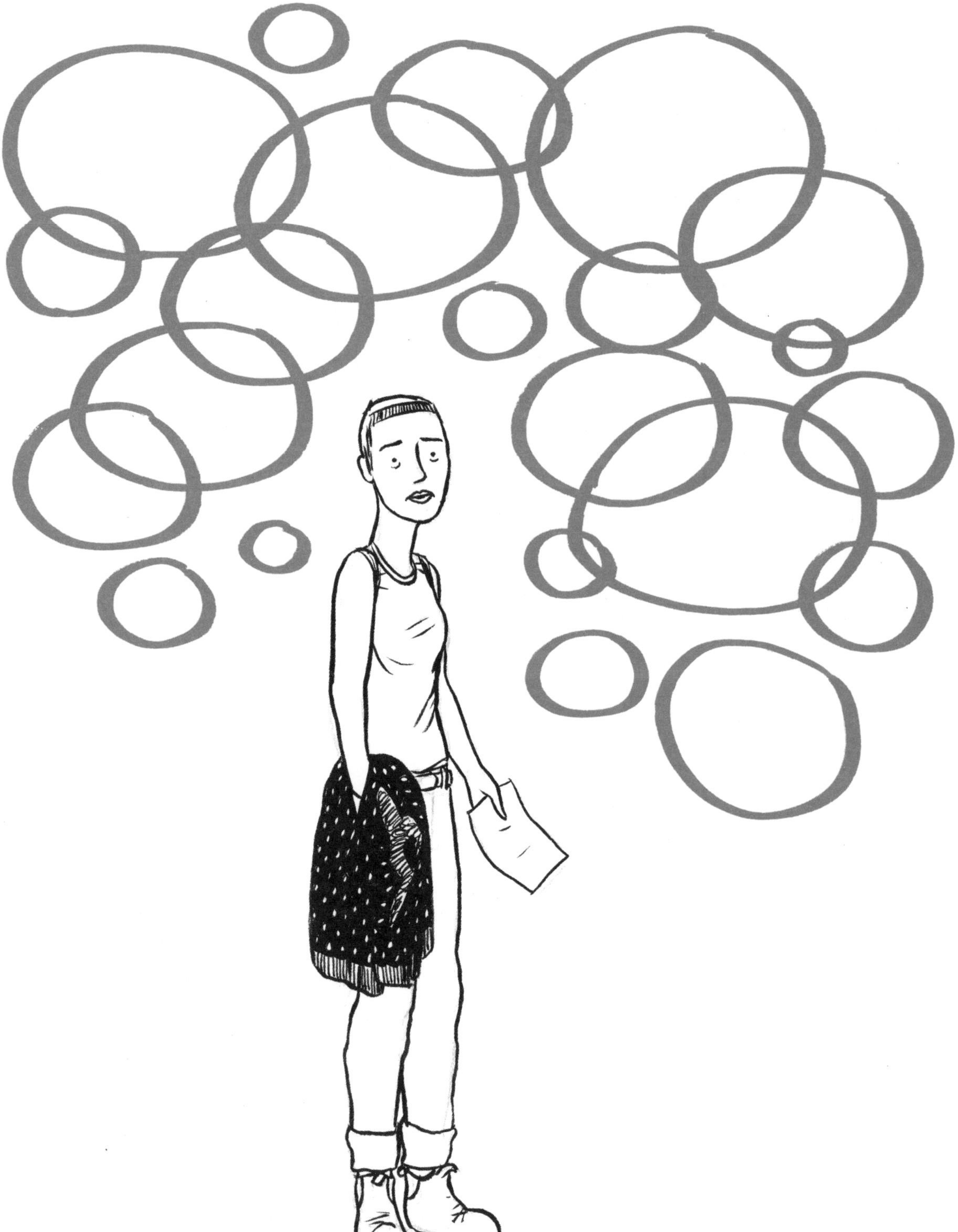

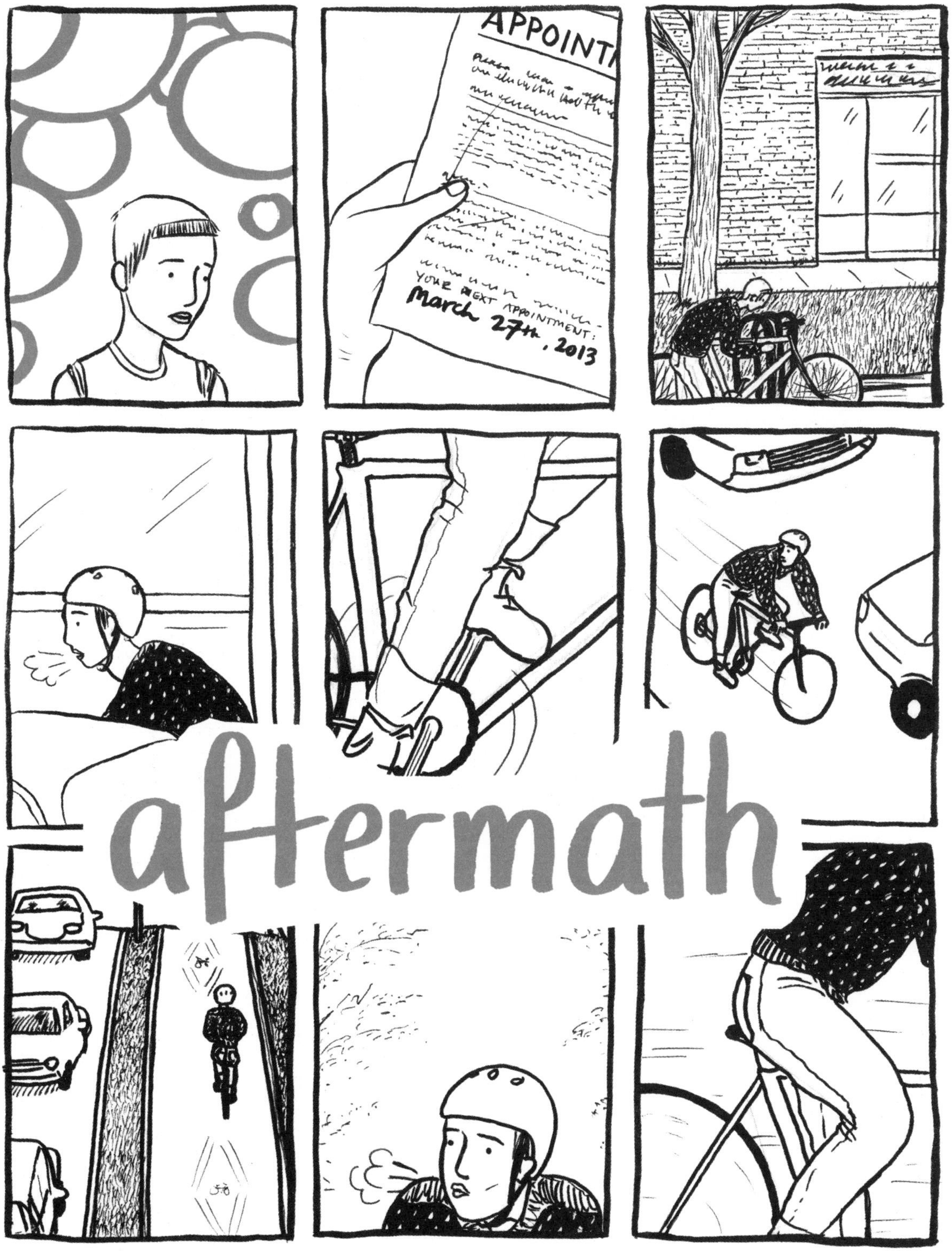
APPOINT
YOUR NEXT APPOINTMENT:
March 27th, 2013
aftermath

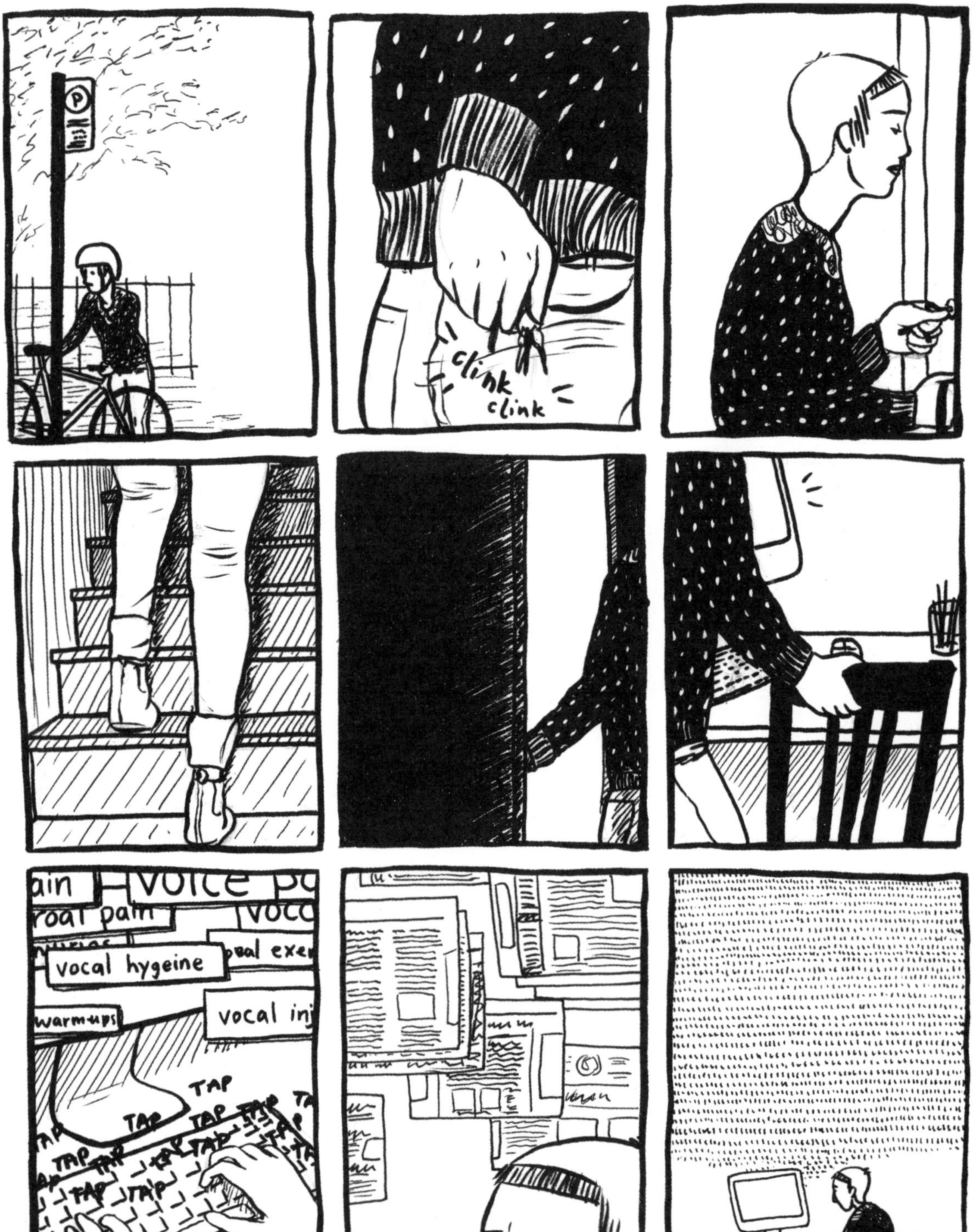
clink
clink
voice p
roat pain
vocal hygeine
warmups
vocal inj
TAP
TAP
TAP
TAP
TAP
TAP
TAP
TAP

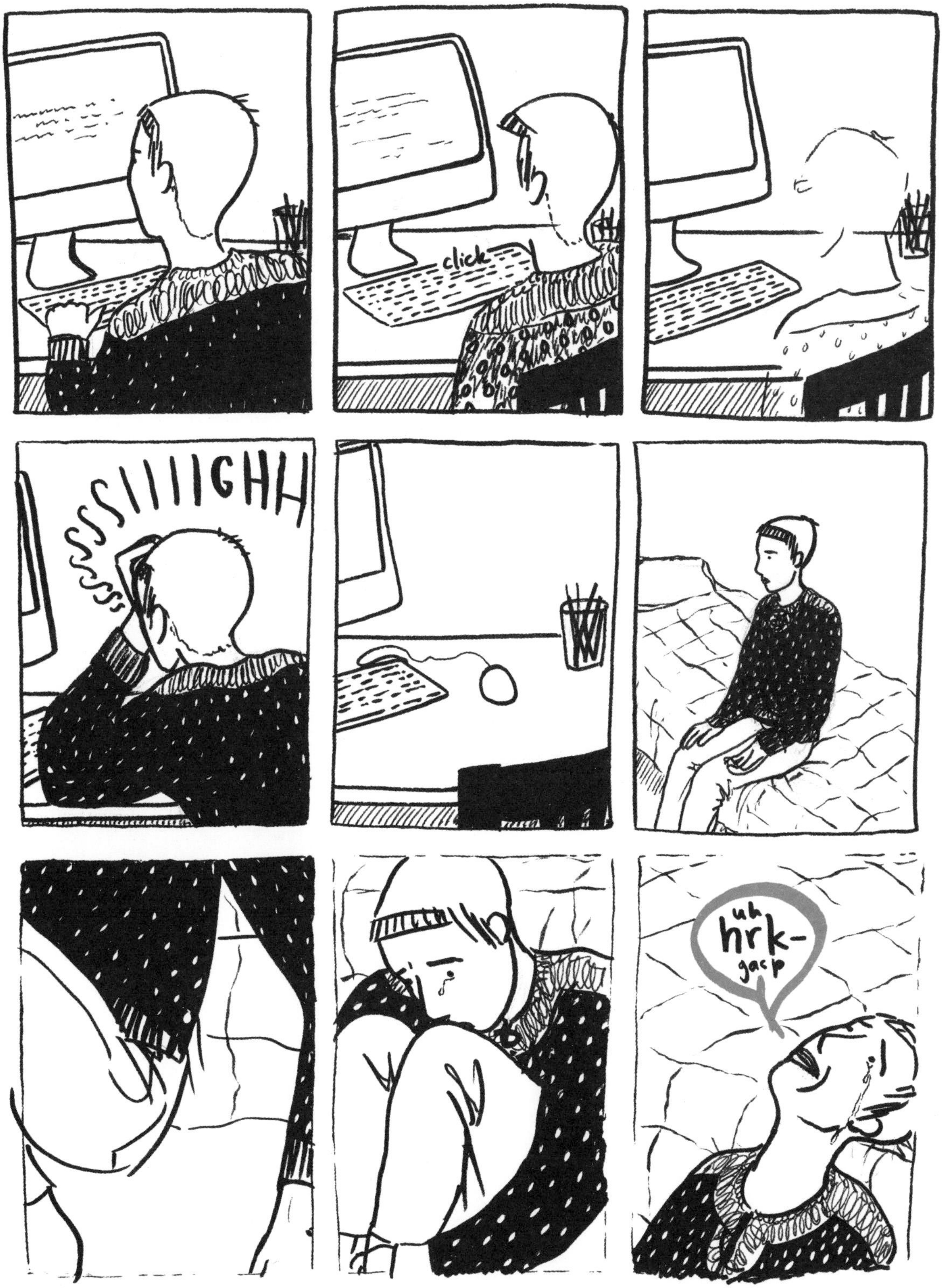
click
SSSIIIIIGHH
uh
hrk-
gasp

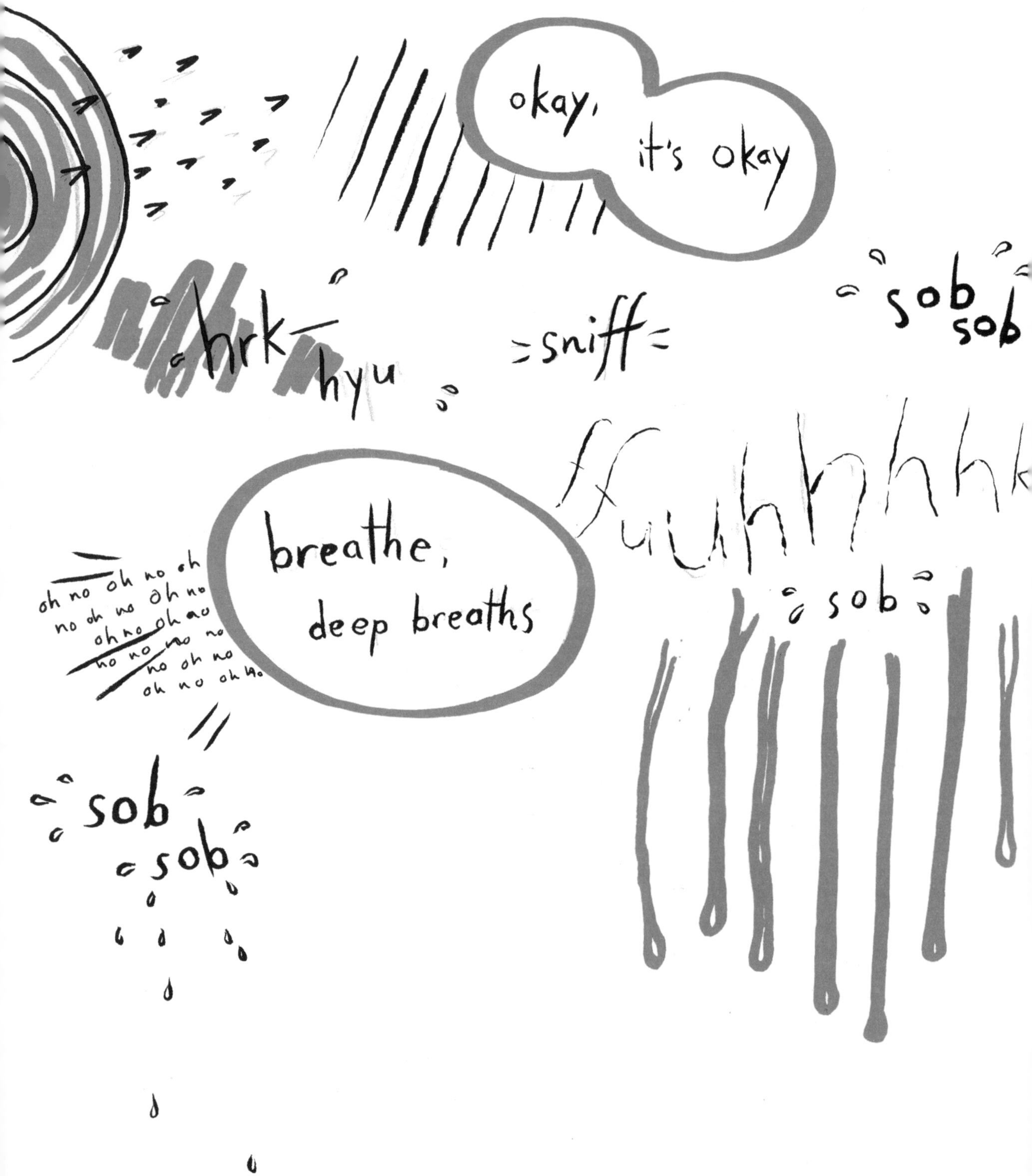
okay, it's okay
hrk hyu
sniff
sob sob
fuuhhhhh
breathe, deep breaths
oh no oh no oh
oh no oh no oh no
no oh no oh no
oh no oh no
no no no no
no oh no
oh no oh no
sob
sob sob
sob

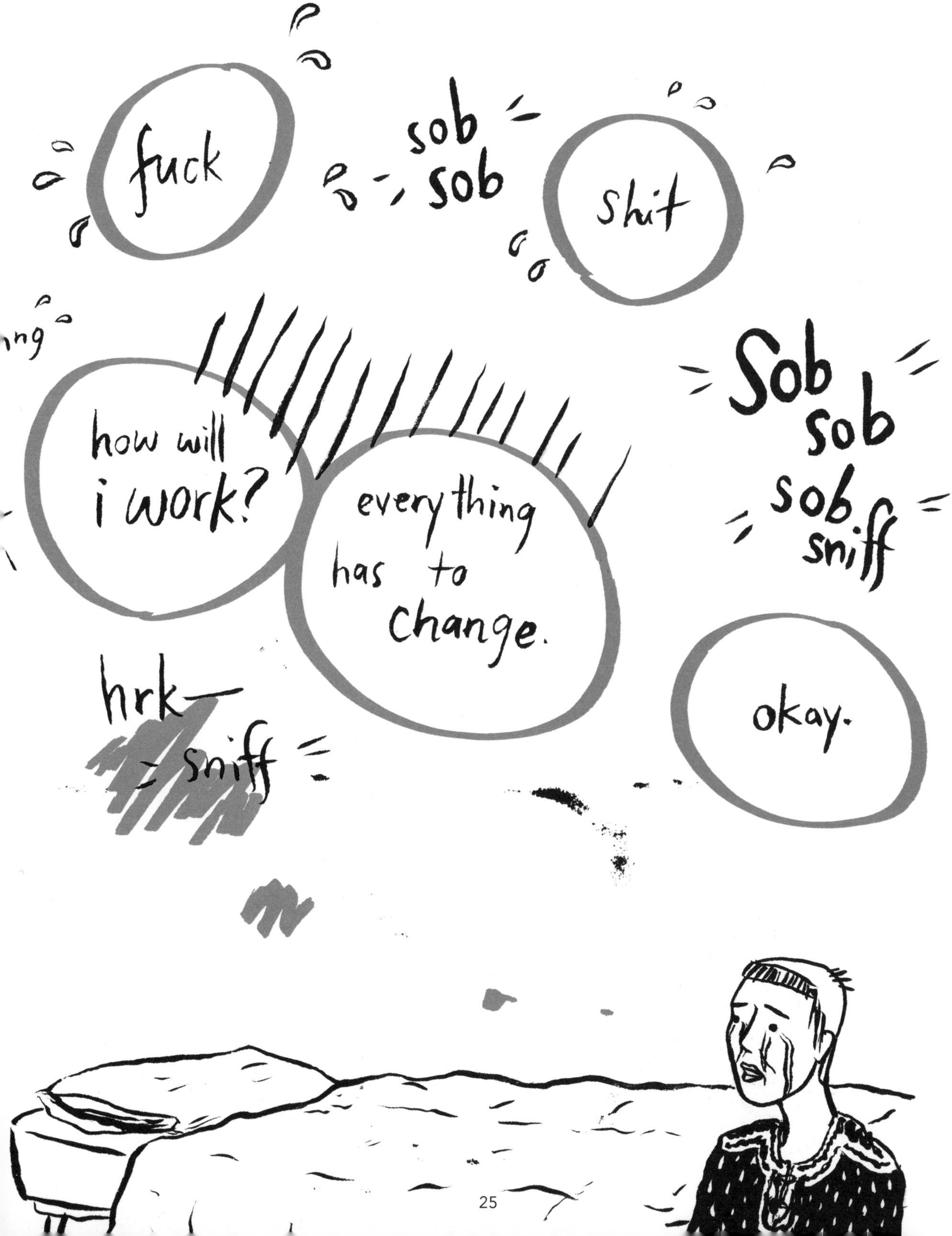
fuck
sob sob
shit
how will i work?
everything has to change.
Sob sob sob sniff
hrk—
sniff
okay.

splitting
Slip
fwump

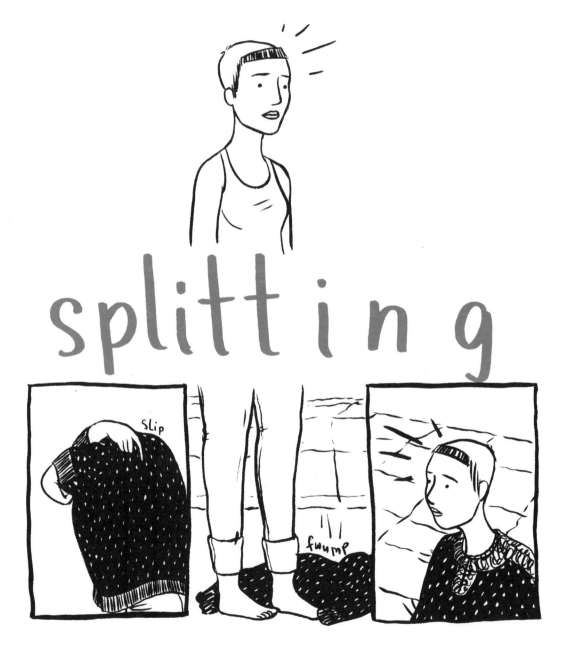

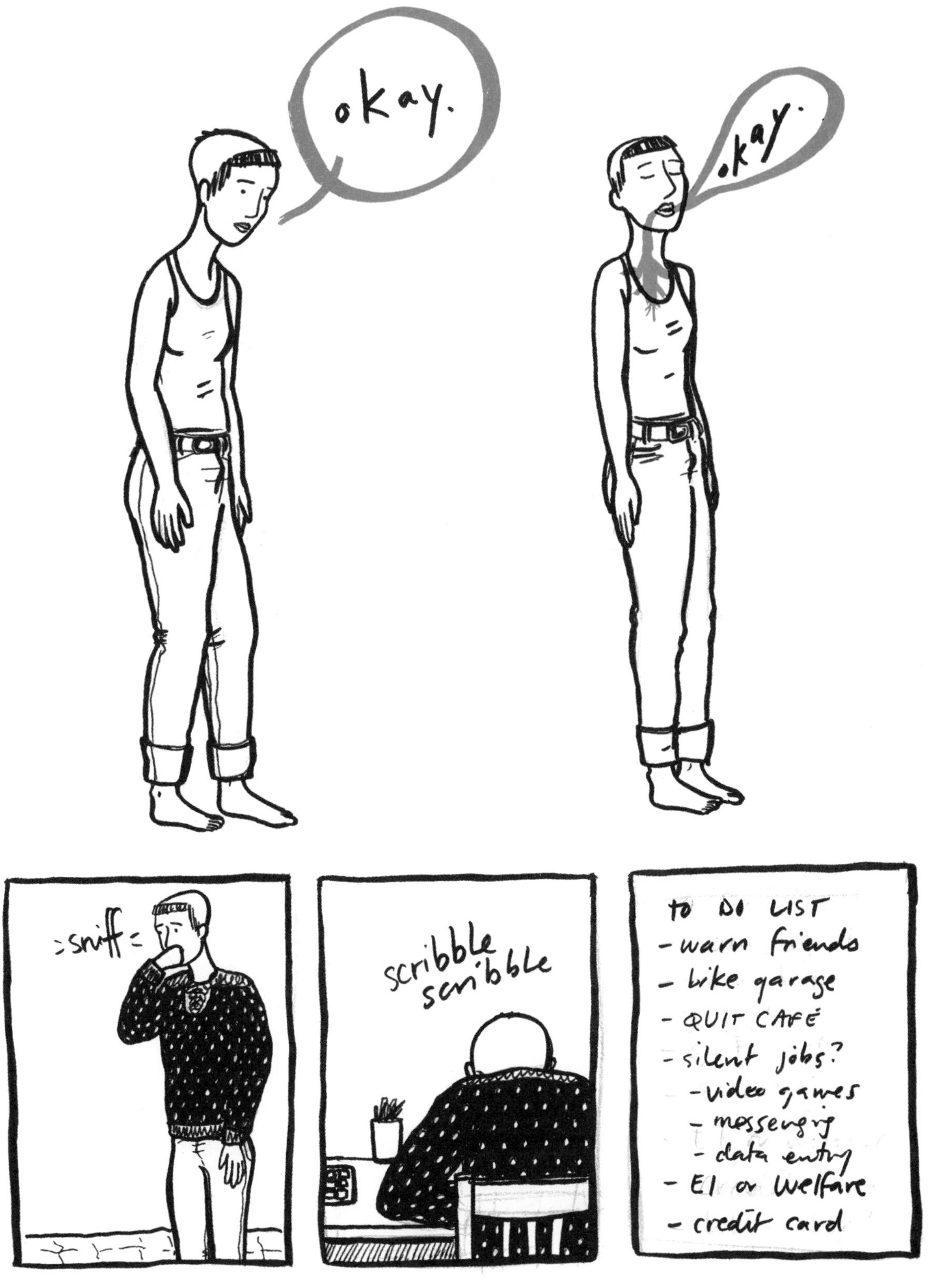
okay.
okay.
=sniff=
scribble scribble
TO DO LIST
- warn friends
- bike garage
- QUIT CAFÉ
- silent jobs?
- video games
- messenging
- data entry
- EI or Welfare
- credit card

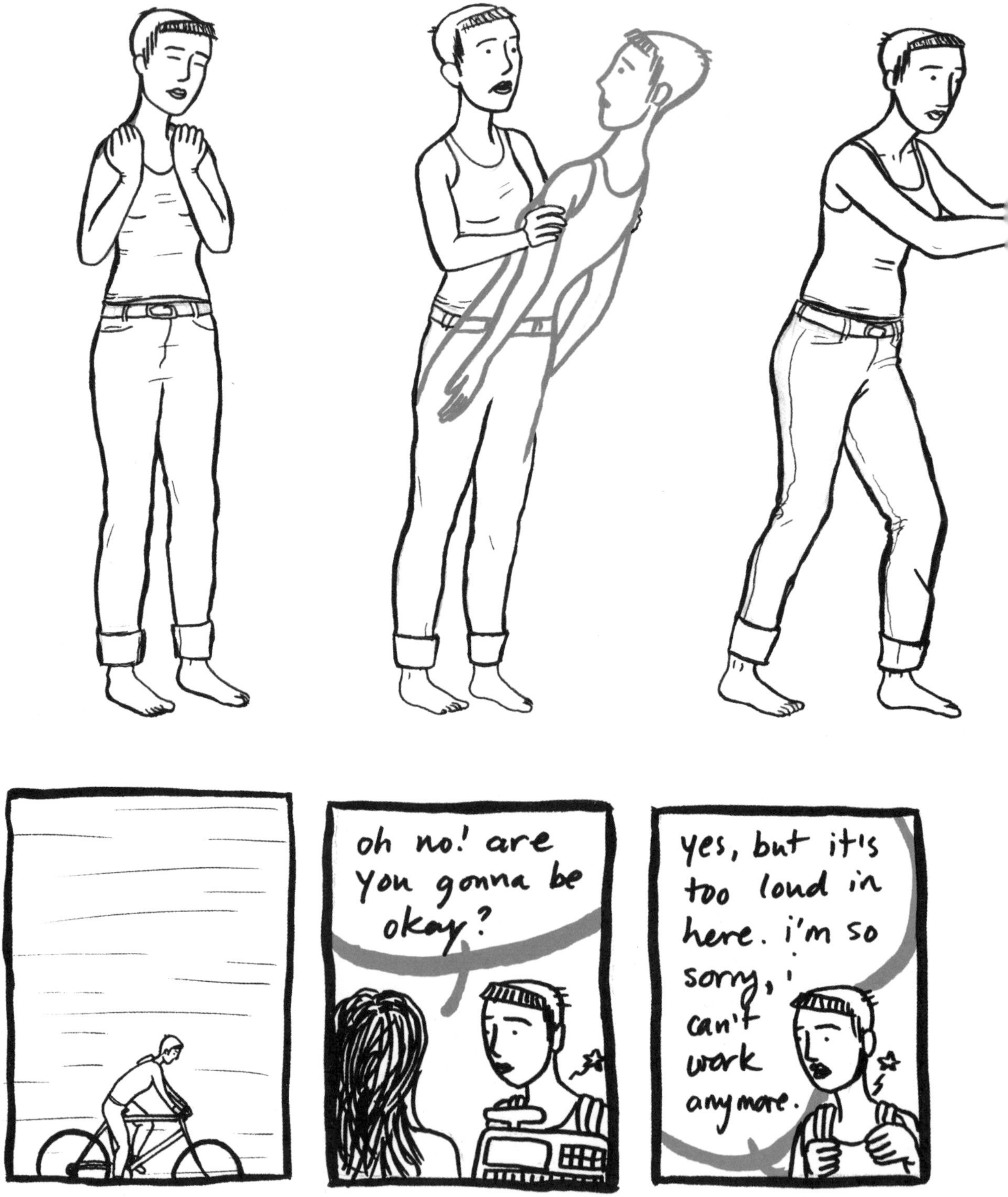
oh no! are you gonna be okay?
yes, but it's too loud in here. i'm so sorry, i can't work anymore.

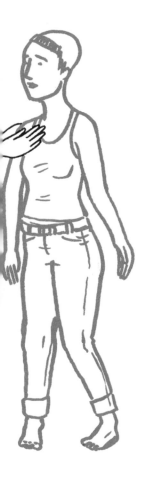
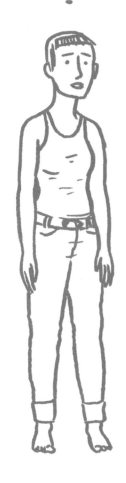
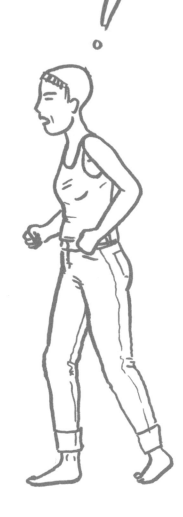
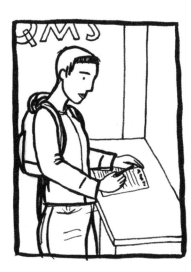
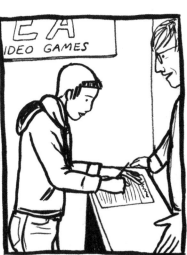

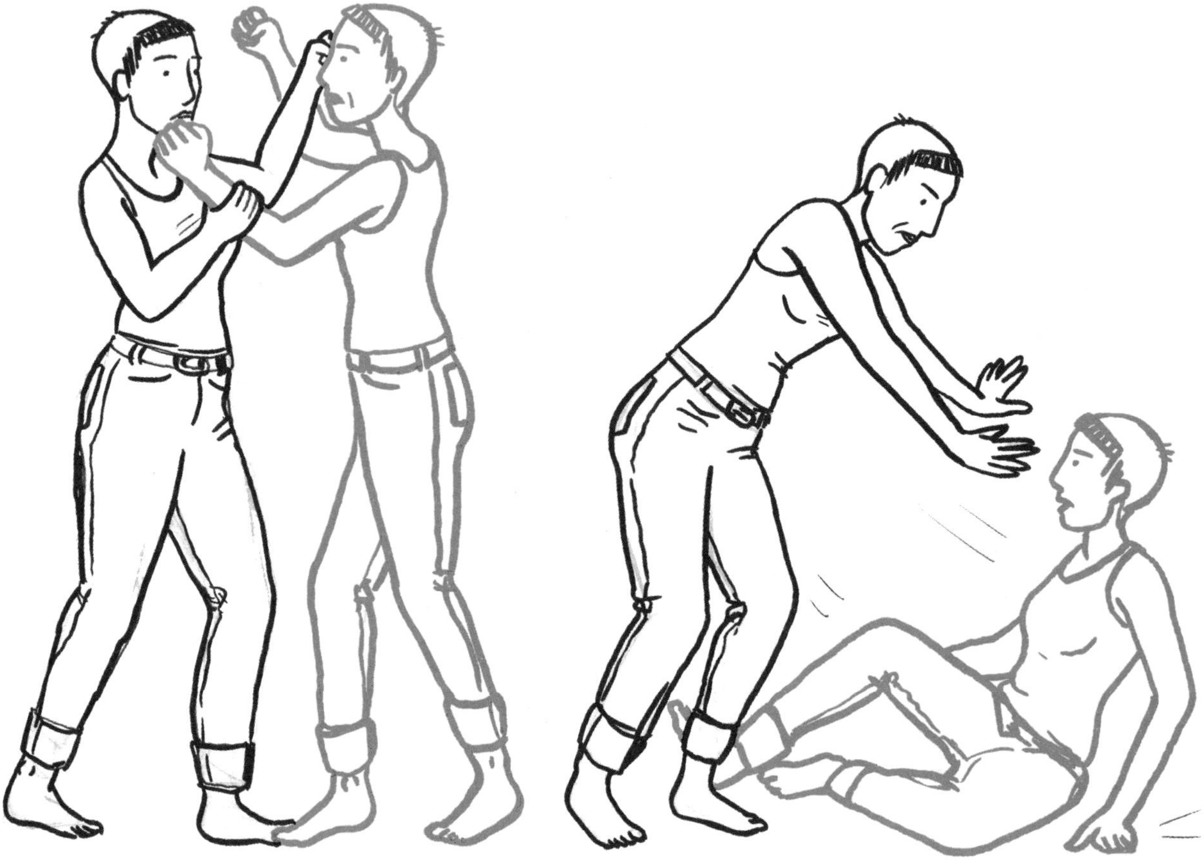

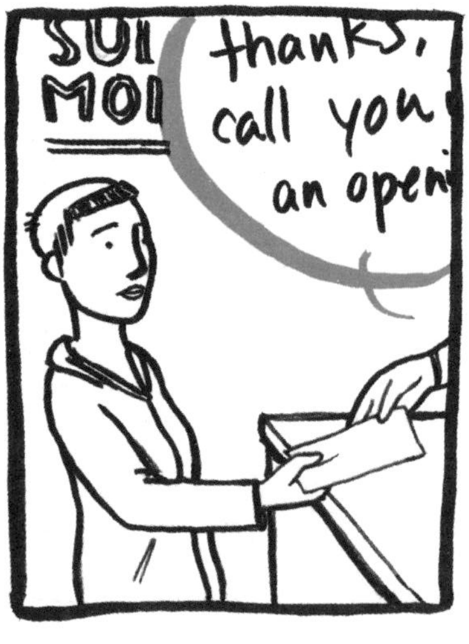
SUI
MO
thanks,
call you
an open

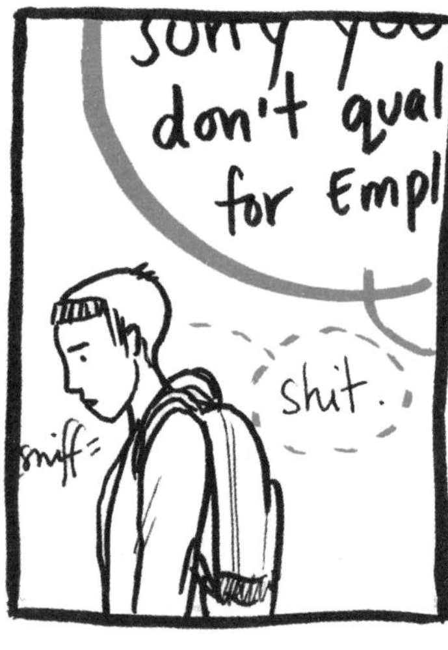
sorry you
don't qual
for Empl
sniff
shit.

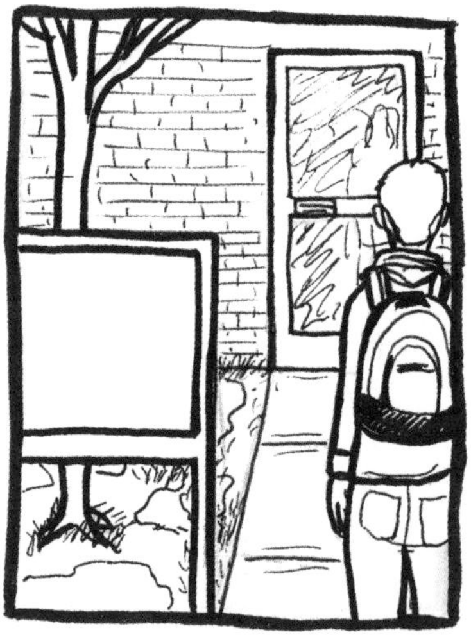

LAST RESOR
FINANCIAL
GULP
4

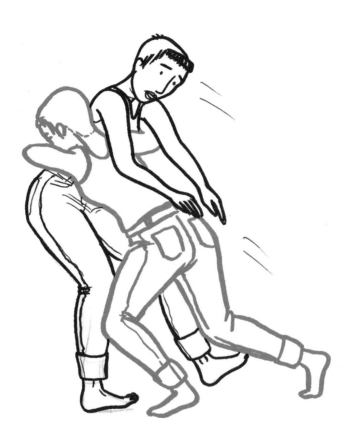

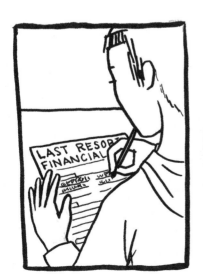

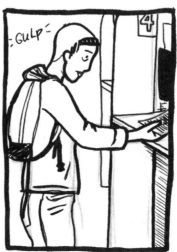

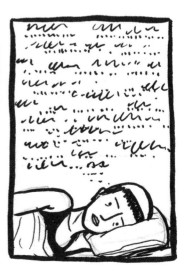

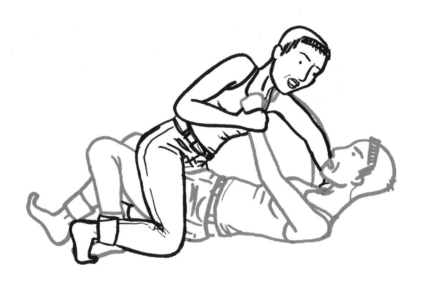

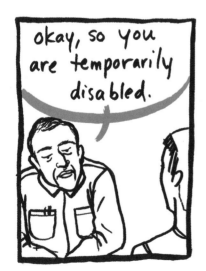

okay, so you are temporarily disabled.

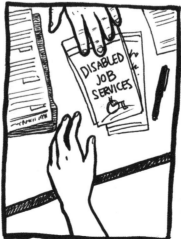

DISABLED JOB SERVICES

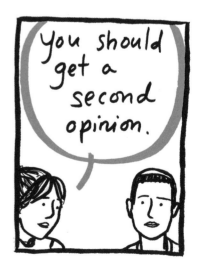

you should get a second opinion.

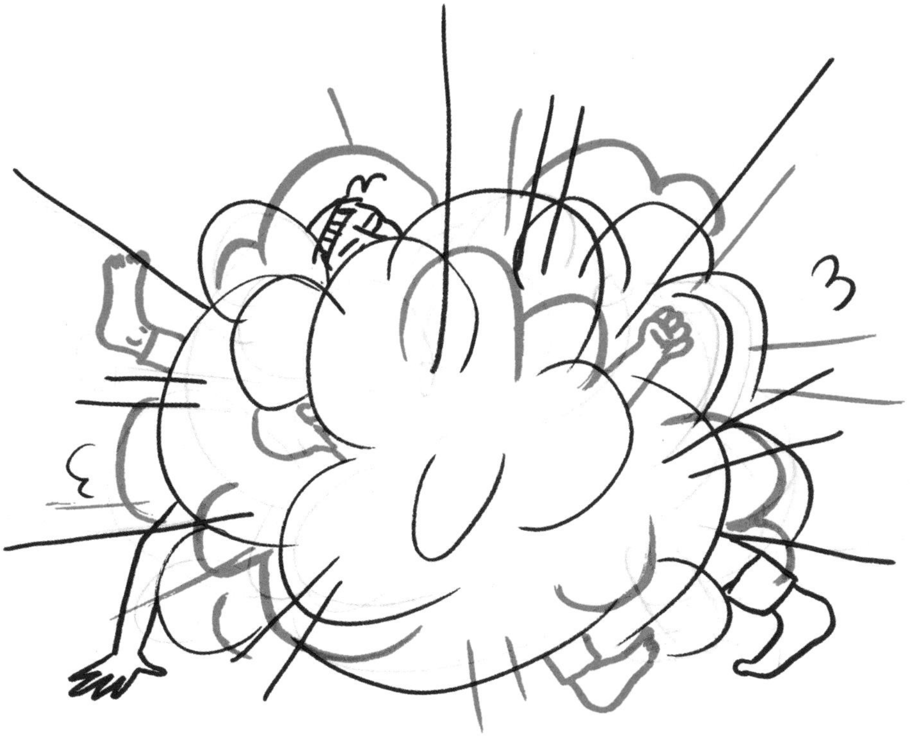

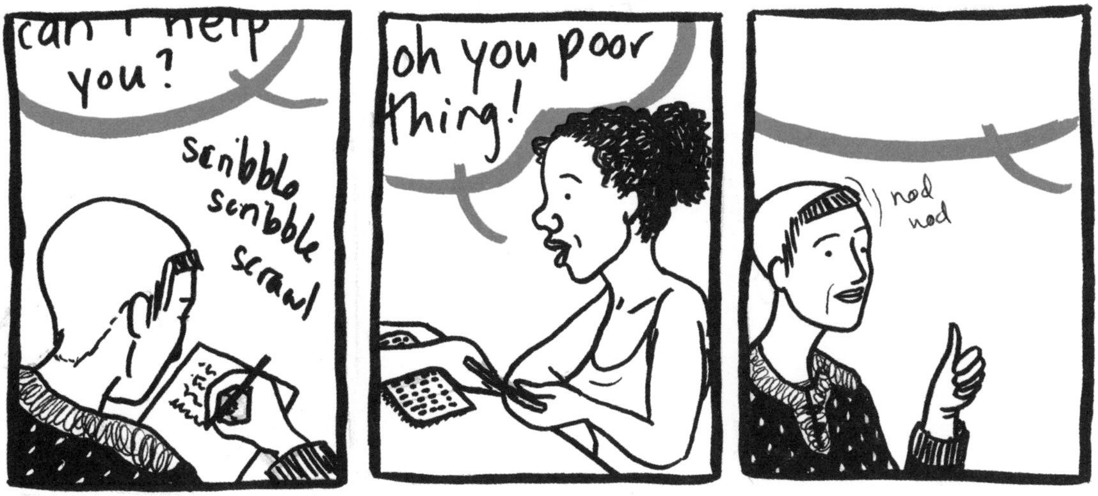
can I help you?
scribble scribble scrawl
oh you poor thing!
nod nod

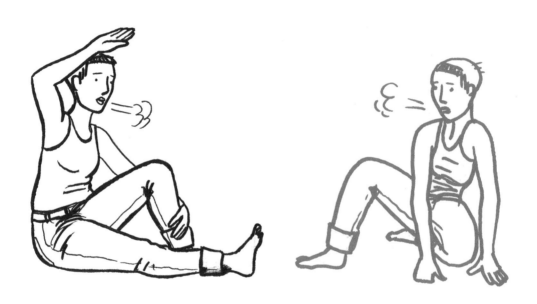

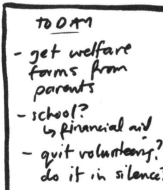

to DO AM
- get welfare
  forms from
  parents
- school?
  ↳ financial aid
- quit volunteering?
  do it in silence?

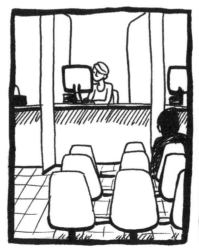

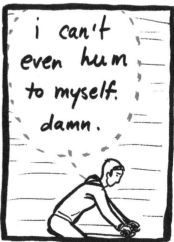

i can't
even hum
to myself.
damn.

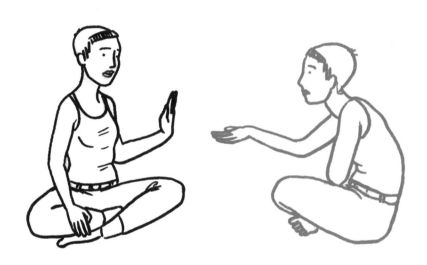

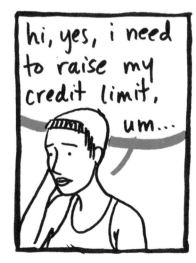

hi, yes, i need to raise my credit limit, um...

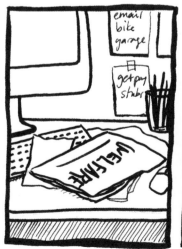

email
bike
garage

get pay
stubs

WELFARE

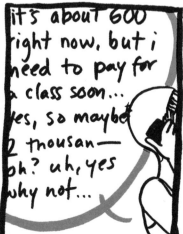

it's about 600 right now, but i need to pay for a class soon... yes, so maybe 2 thousan— oh? uh, yes why not...

SSSIICHH
email
bike
$$?
get pay stubs
SLAP
it's going to be okay
email
bike
$$?

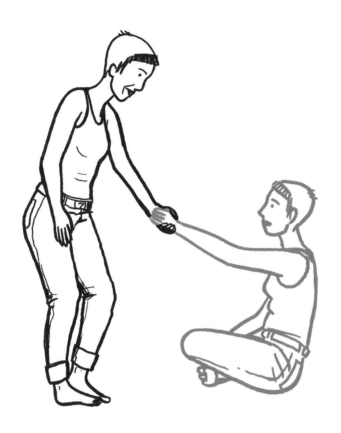

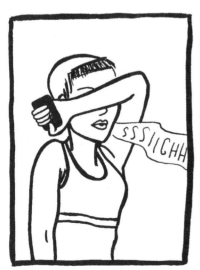

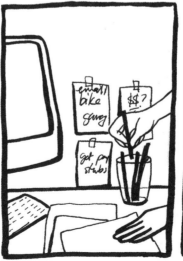

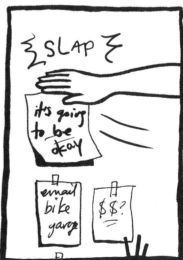

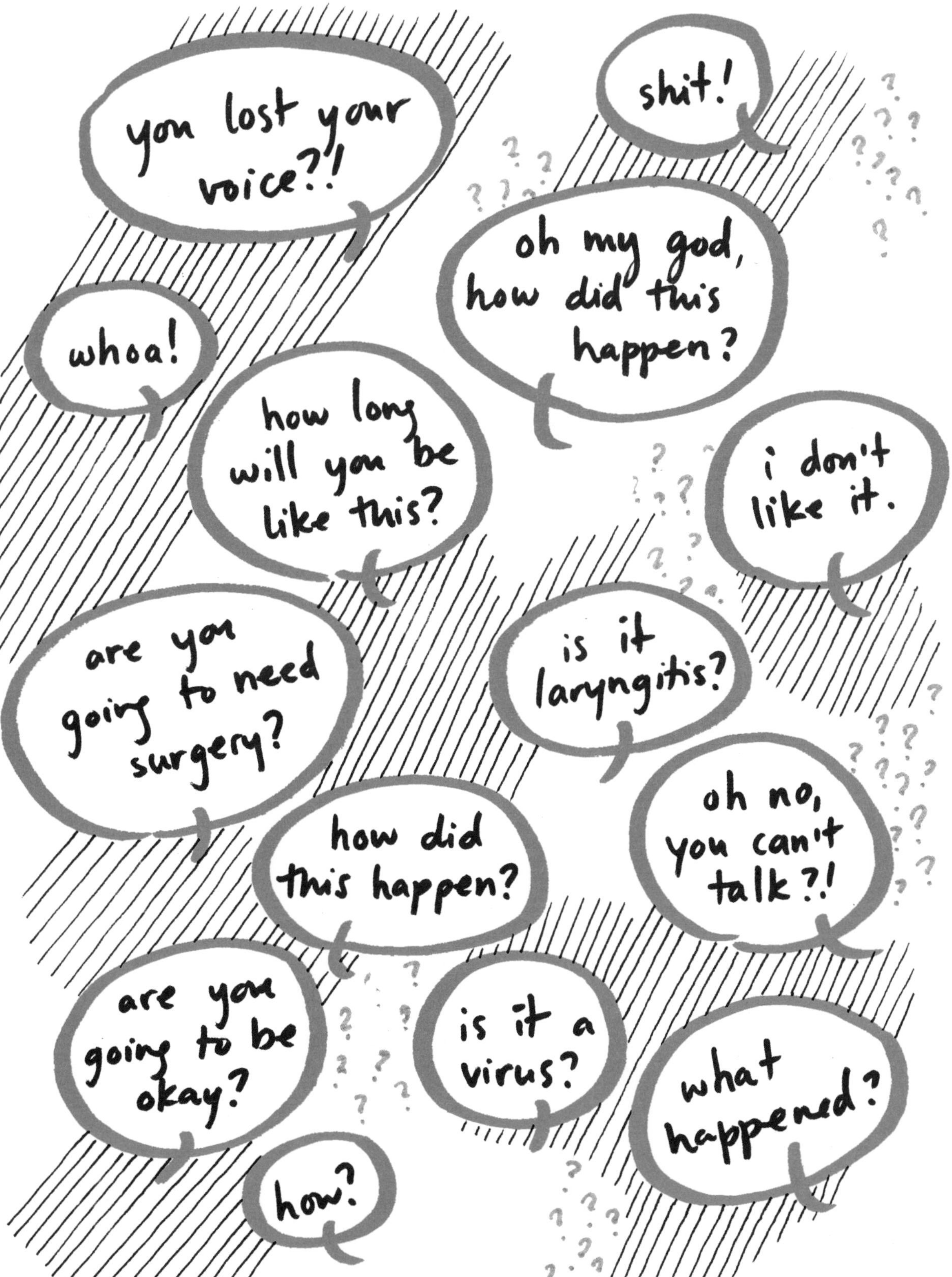
you lost your voice?!
shit!
oh my god, how did this happen?
whoa!
how long will you be like this?
i don't like it.
are you going to need surgery?
is it laryngitis?
oh no, you can't talk?!
how did this happen?
are you going to be okay?
is it a virus?
what happened?
how?

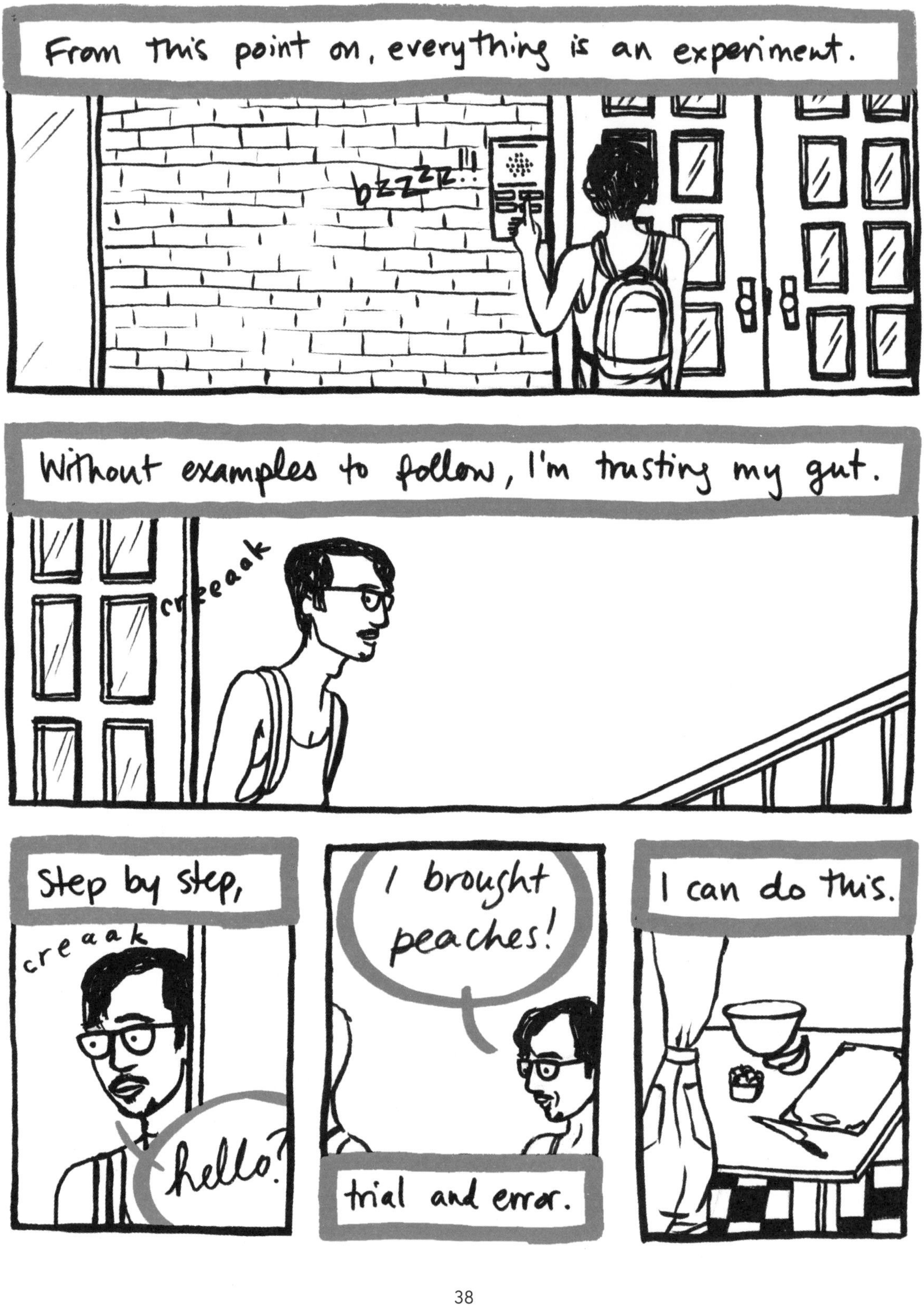
From this point on, everything is an experiment.
bzzzz!!
Without examples to follow, I'm trusting my gut.
creeaak
Step by step,
creaak
hello?
I brought peaches!
trial and error.
I can do this.

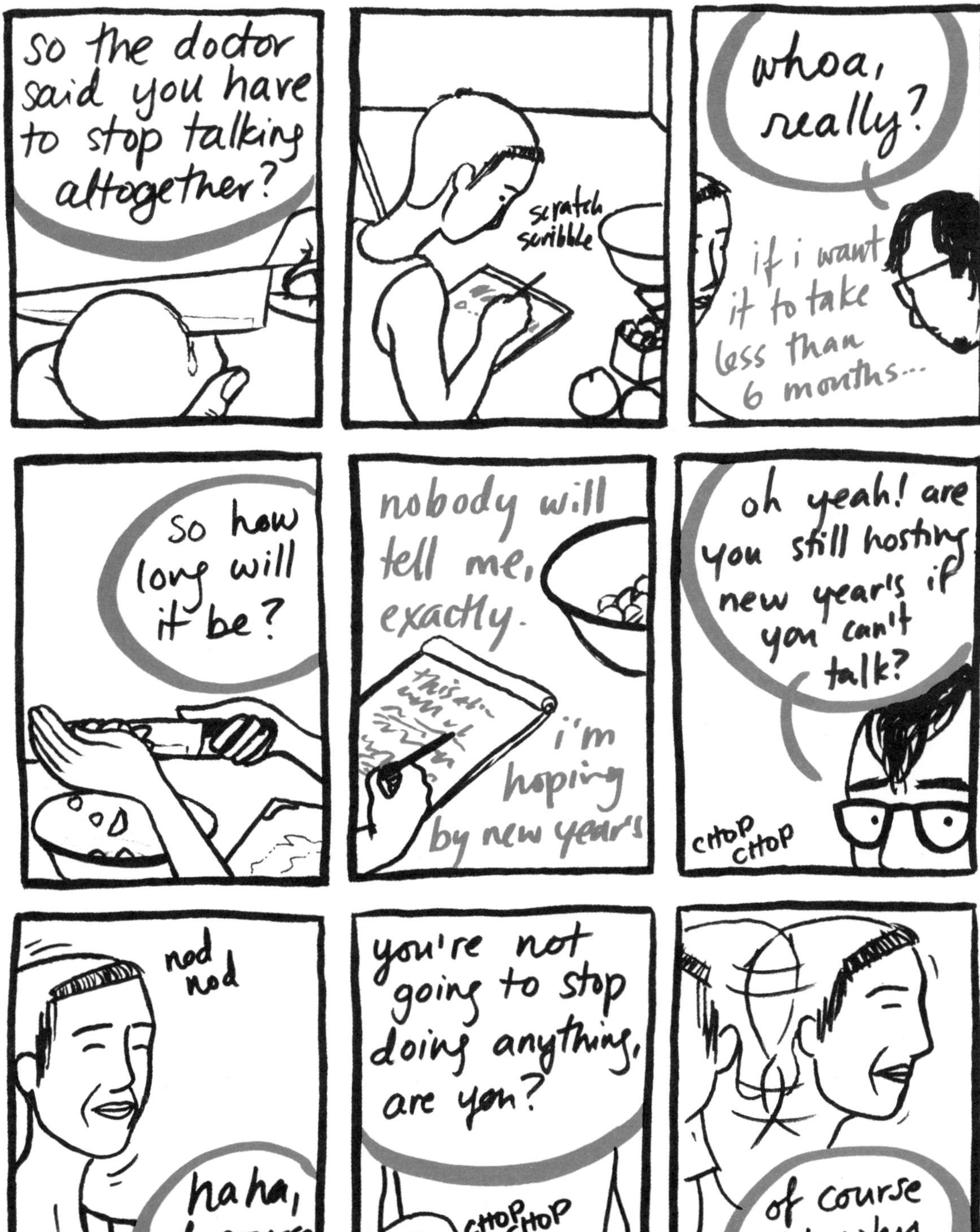
so the doctor said you have to stop talking altogether?
scratch scribble
whoa, really?
if i want it to take less than 6 months...
so how long will it be?
nobody will tell me, exactly.
i'm hoping by new year's
oh yeah! are you still hosting new year's if you can't talk?
CHOP CHOP
nod nod
haha, of course you are
you're not going to stop doing anything, are you?
CHOP CHOP
of course not! why would you?

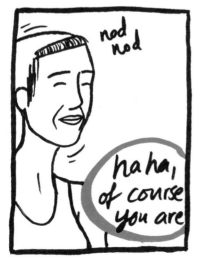

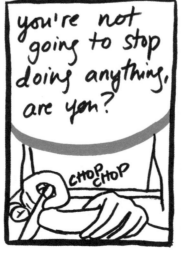

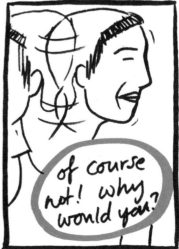

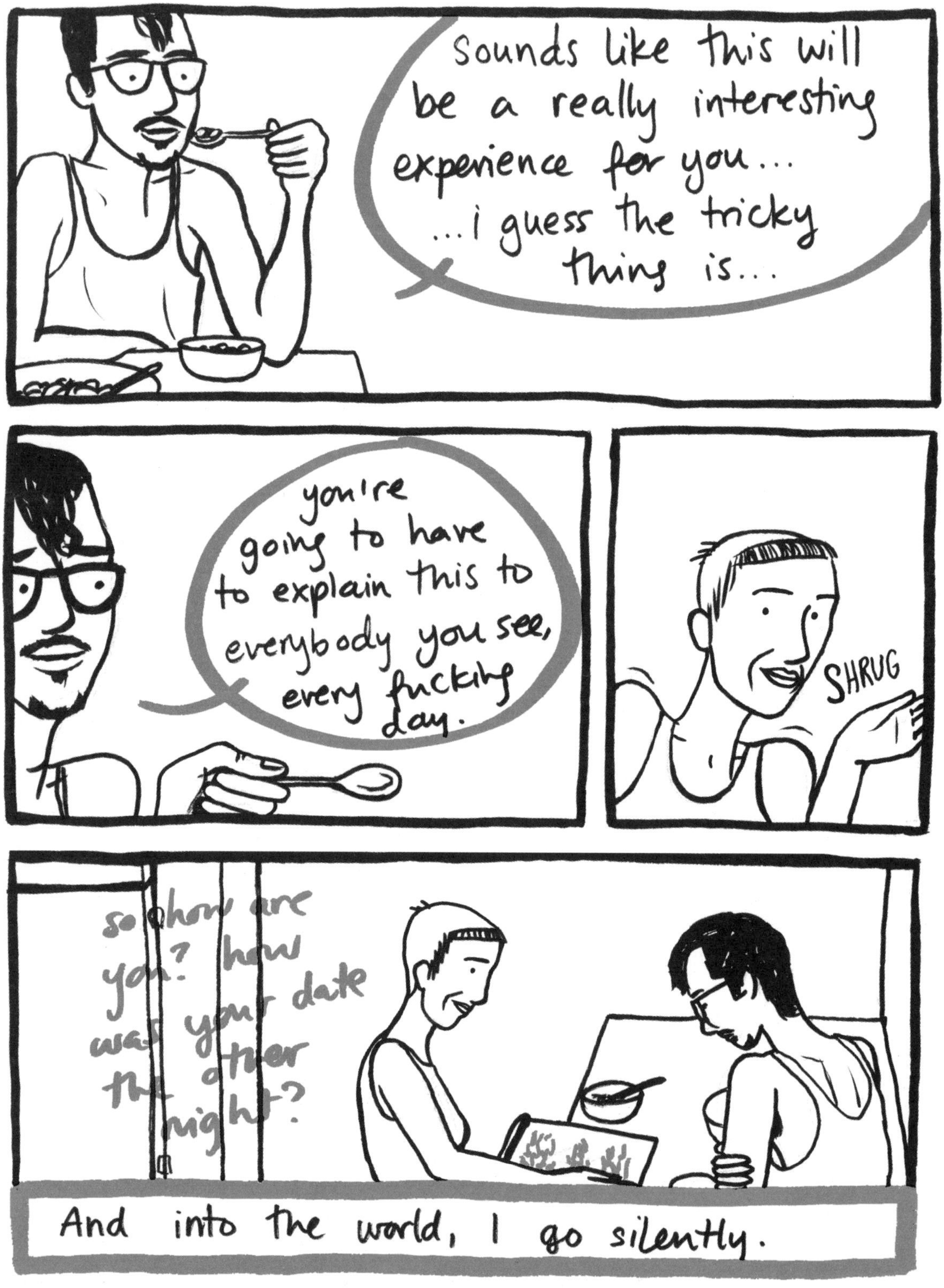
sounds like this will be a really interesting experience for you... ...i guess the tricky thing is...
you're going to have to explain this to everybody you see, every fucking day.
SHRUG
so how are you? how was your date the other night?
And into the world, I go silently.

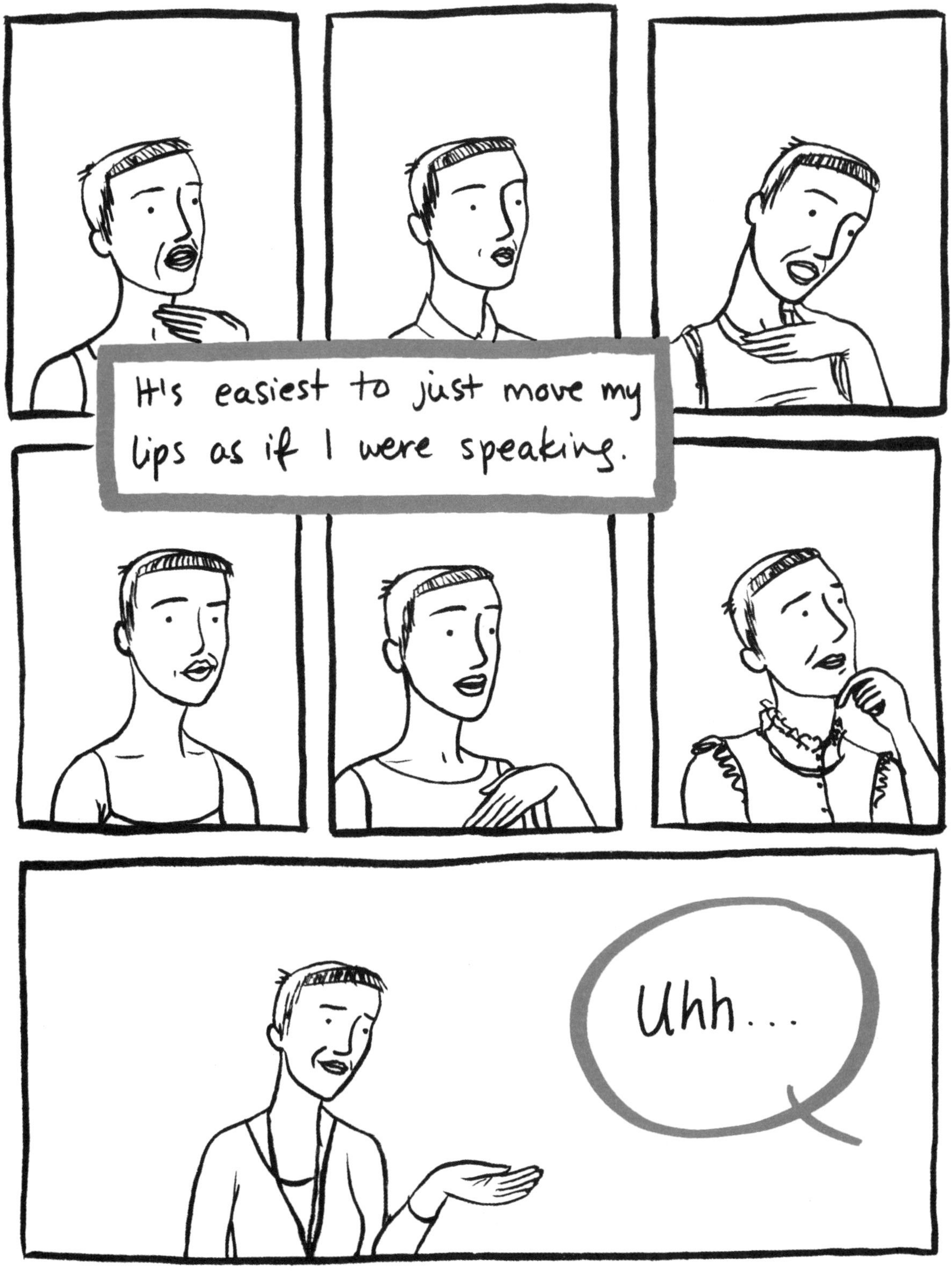
It's easiest to just move my lips as if I were speaking.
Uhh...

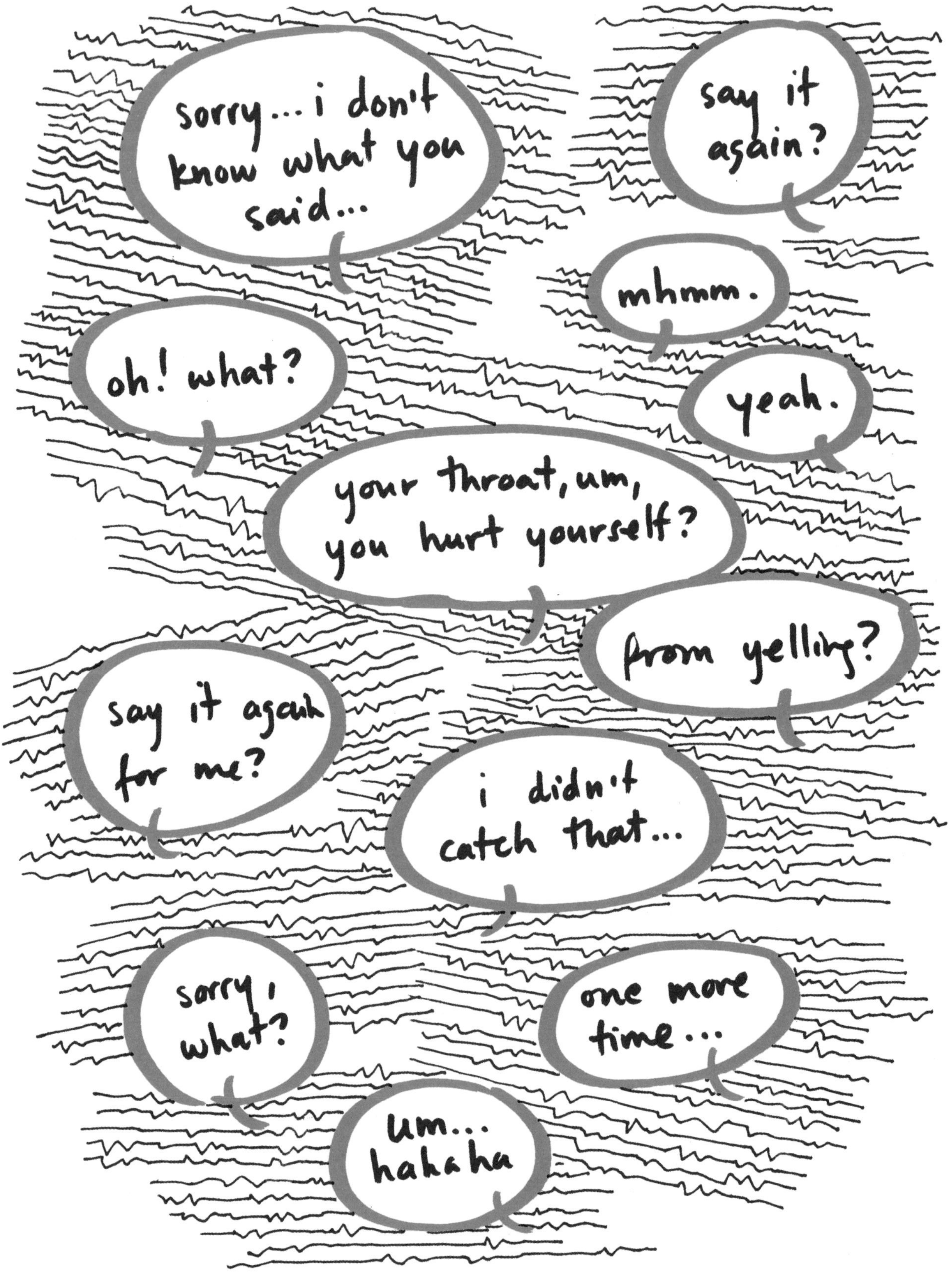
sorry... i don't know what you said...
say it again?
mhmm.
oh! what?
yeah.
your throat, um, you hurt yourself?
from yelling?
say it again for me?
i didn't catch that...
sorry, what?
one more time...
um... hahaha

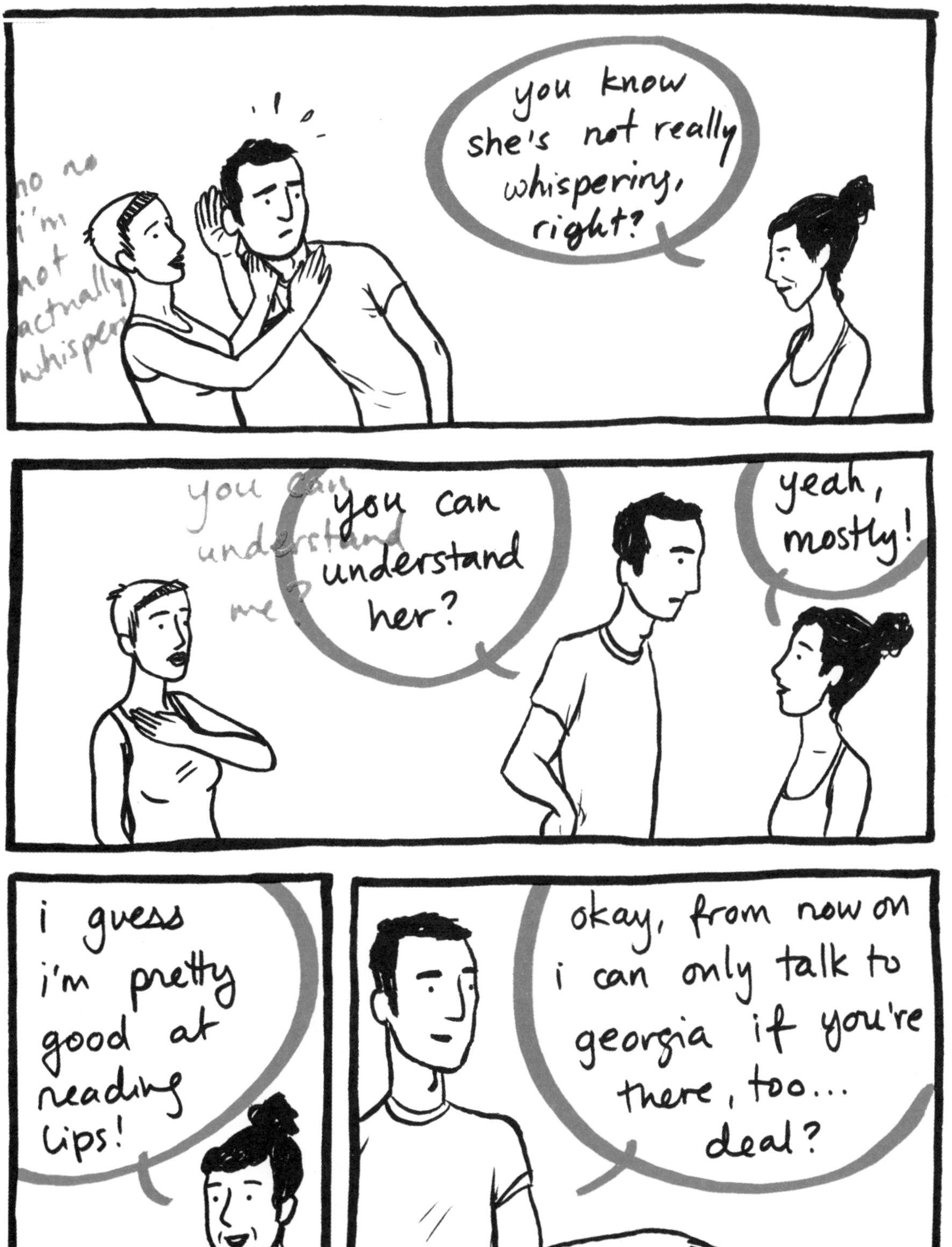
no no i'm not actnally whisper
you know she's not really whispering, right?
you can understand me?
you can understand her?
yeah, mostly!
i guess i'm pretty good at reading lips!
okay, from now on i can only talk to georgia if you're there, too... deal?

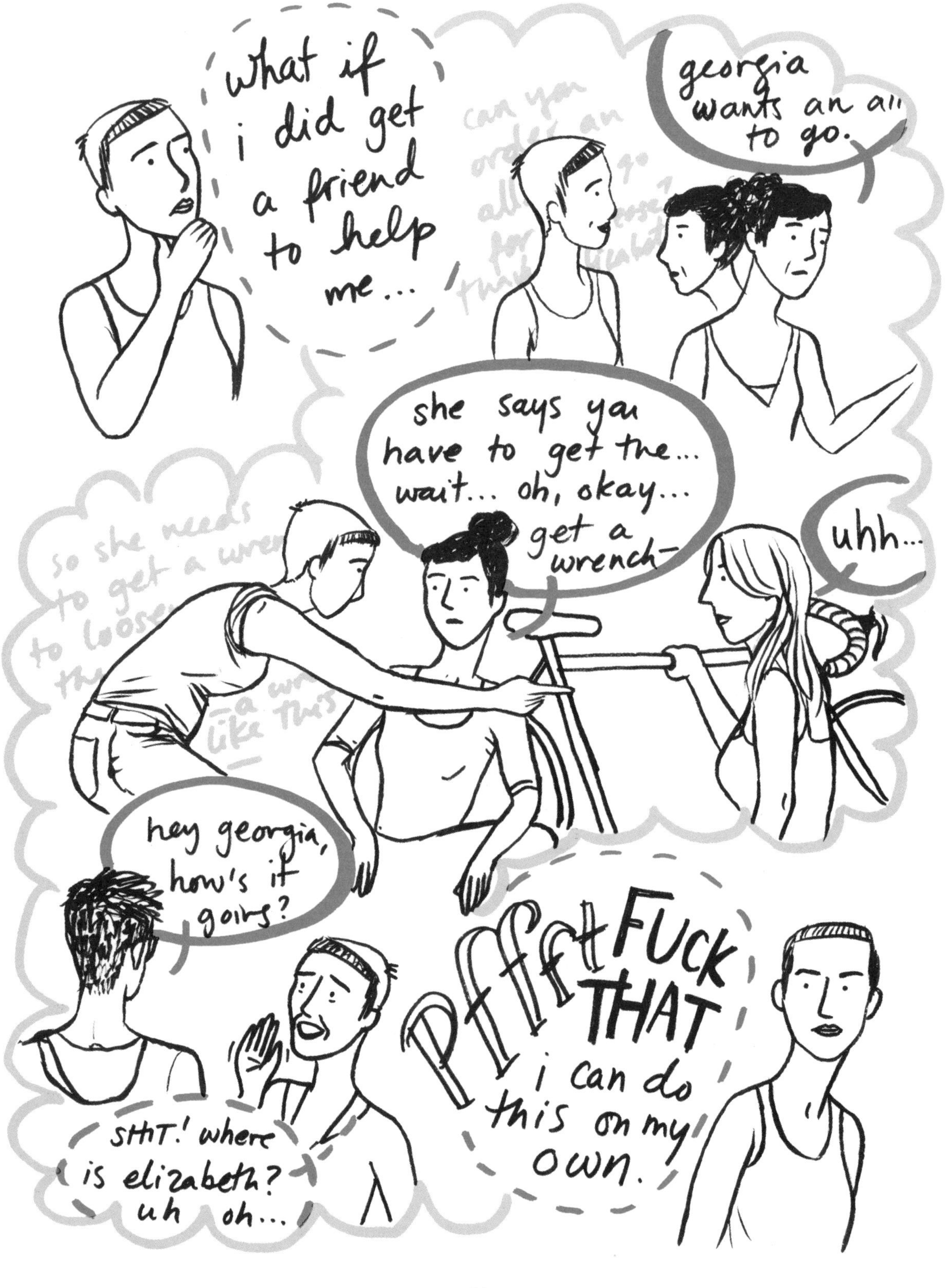

what if i did get a friend to help me...
georgia wants an all to go.
she says you have to get the... wait... oh, okay... get a wrench-
uhh...
hey georgia, how's it going?
SHIT! where is elizabeth? uh oh...
Pffft FUCK THAT i can do this on my own.

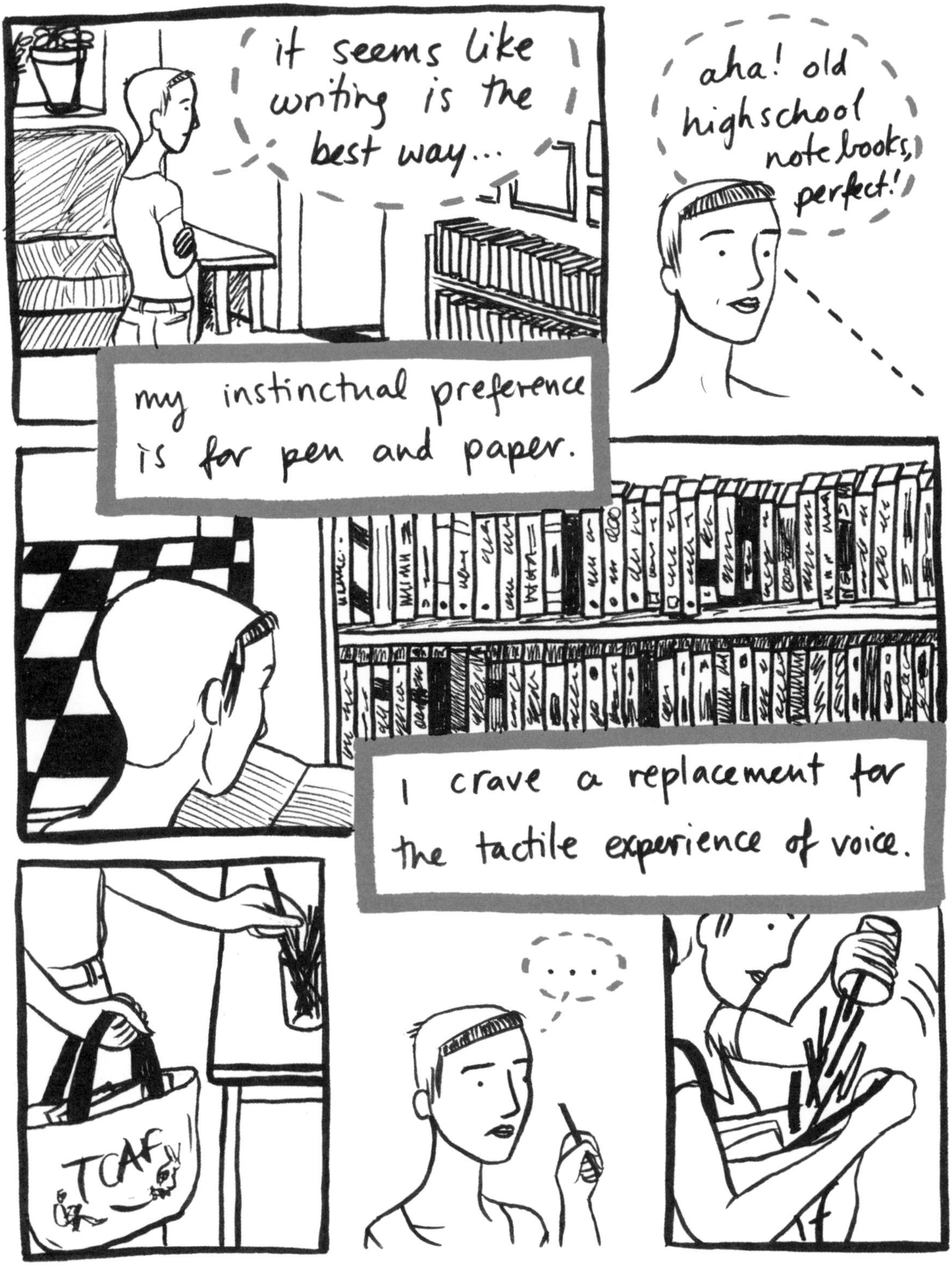
it seems like writing is the best way...
aha! old highschool notebooks, perfect!
my instinctual preference is for pen and paper.
I crave a replacement for the tactile experience of voice.
...
TCAF

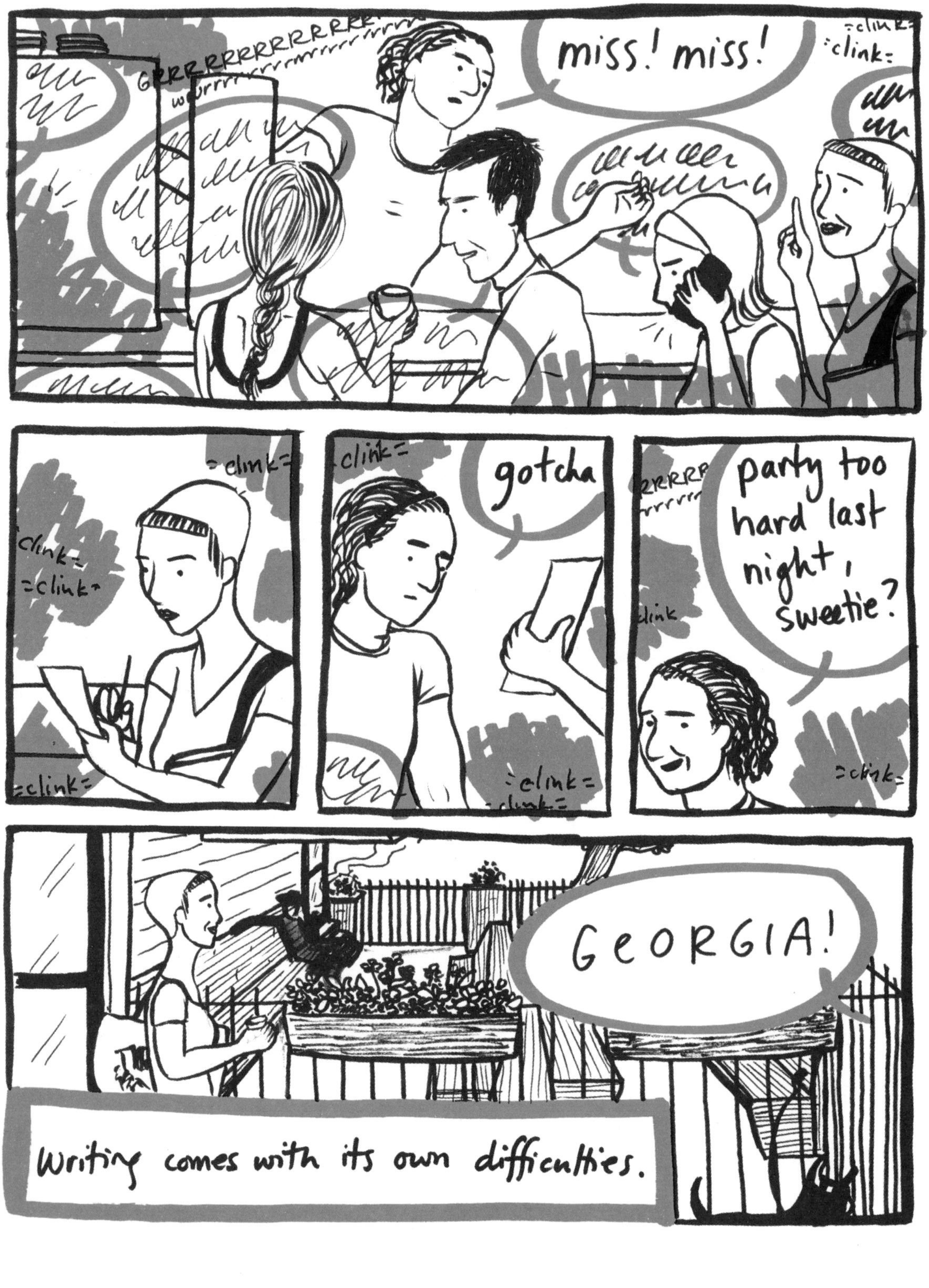
GRRRRRRRRRRRRRRR wurrrrrrrrrrrrrrrr
miss! miss!
=clink=
=clink=
=clink=
clink=
=clink=
=clink=
=clink=
gotcha
=clink=
RRRRR
party too hard last night, sweetie?
clink
=clink=
GEORGIA!
Writing comes with its own difficulties.

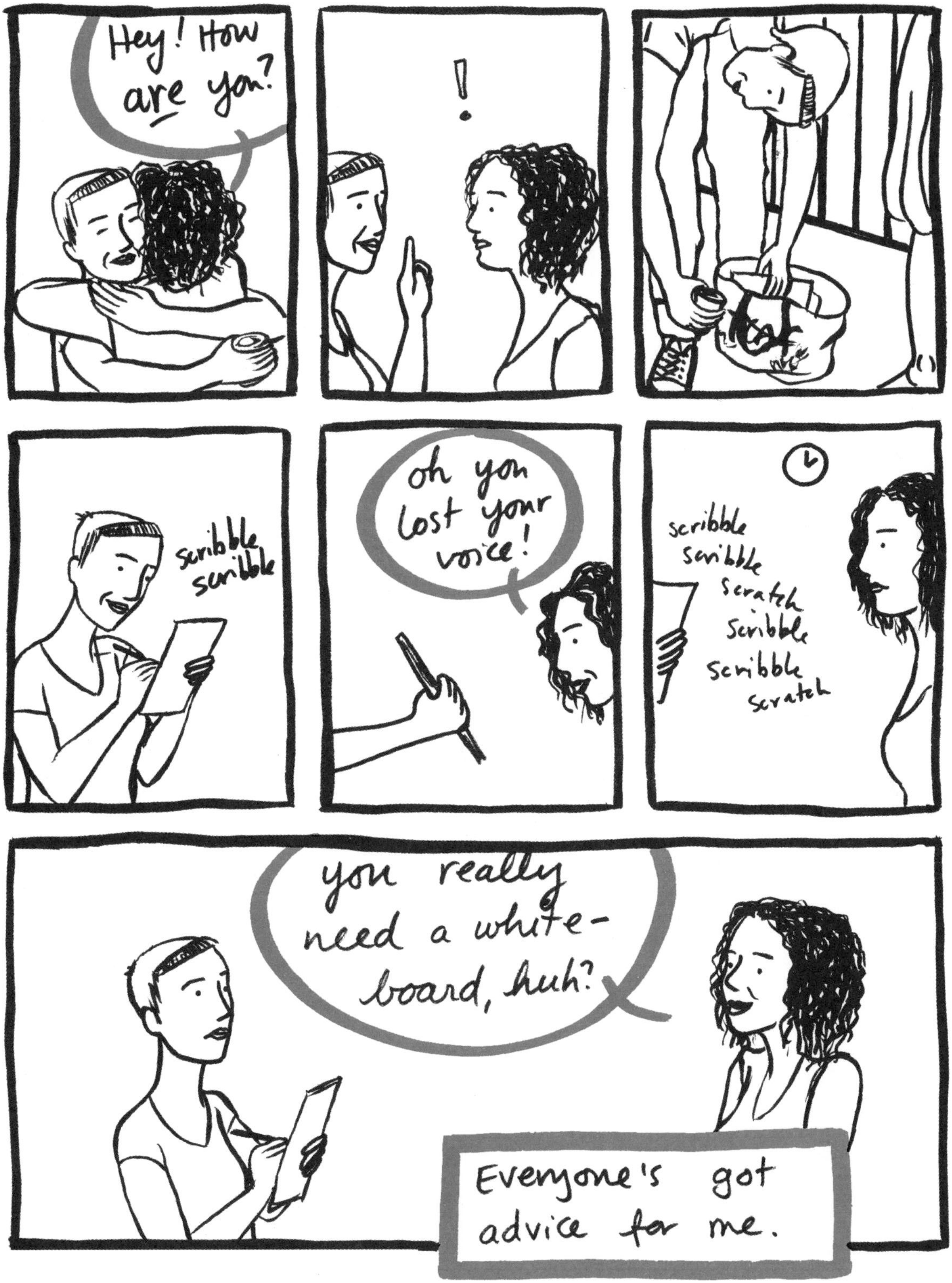
Hey! How are you?
!
scribble scribble
oh you lost your voice!
scribble scribble scratch scribble scribble scratch
you really need a white-board, huh?
Everyone's got advice for me.

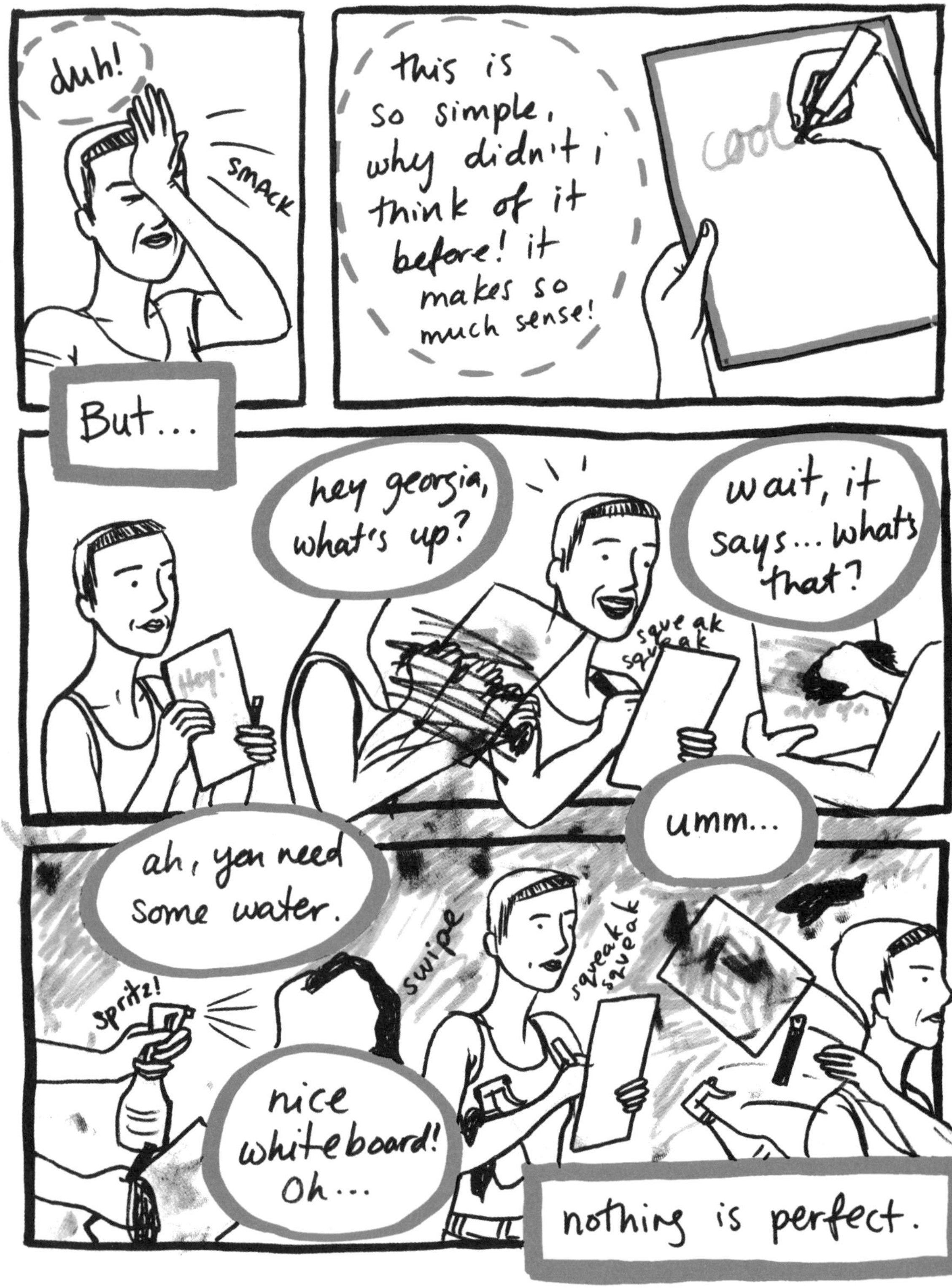
duh!
SMACK
this is so simple, why didn't i think of it before! it makes so much sense!
cool
But...
hey georgia, what's up?
Hey!
squeak squeak
wait, it says... what's that?
umm...
ah, you need some water.
spritz!
swipe
squeak squeak
nice whiteboard! Oh...
nothing is perfect.

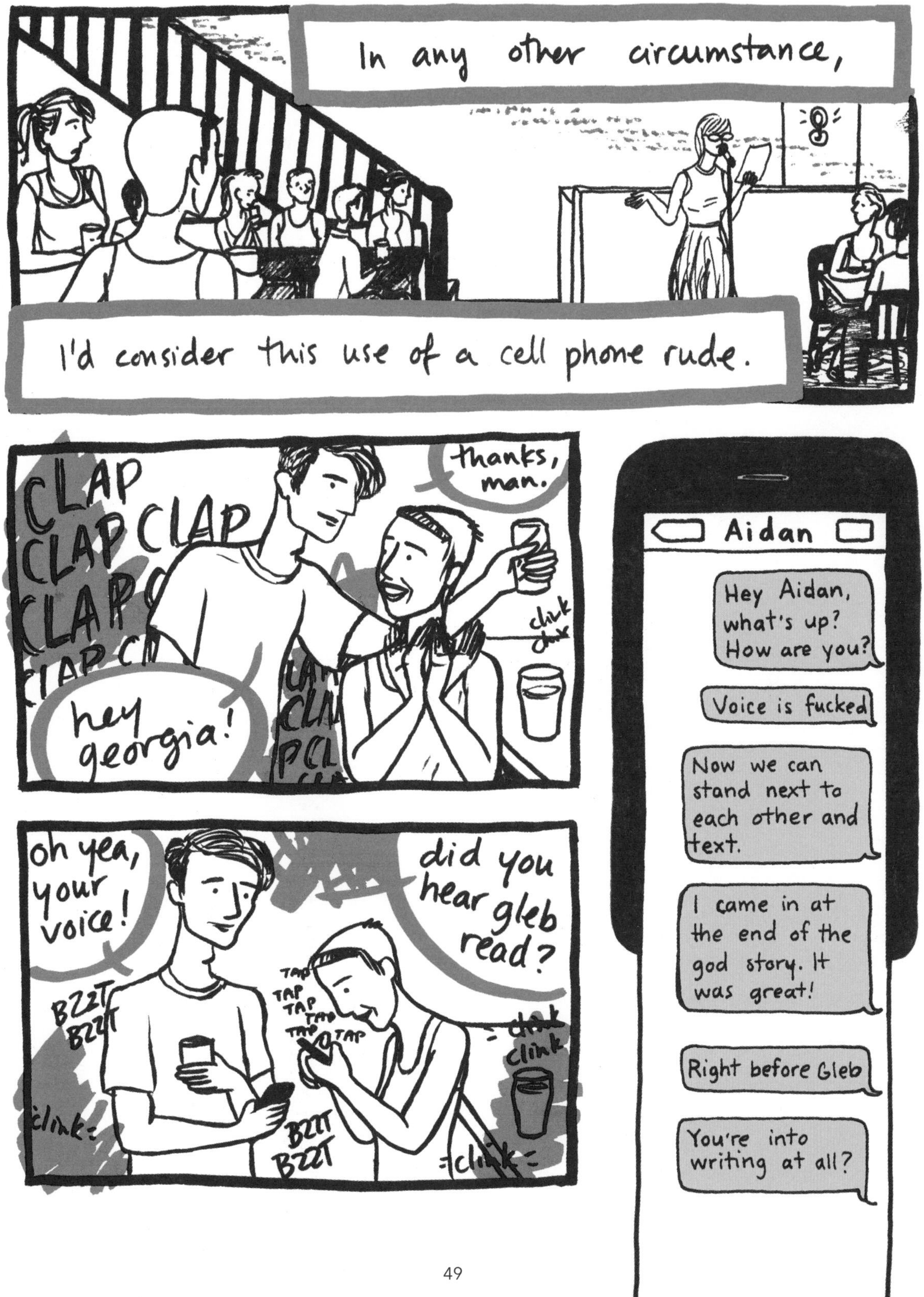
In any other circumstance,
I'd consider this use of a cell phone rude.
CLAP CLAP CLAP CLAP CLAP
thanks, man.
hey georgia!
clink clink
Aidan
Hey Aidan, what's up? How are you?
Voice is fucked
Now we can stand next to each other and text.
I came in at the end of the god story. It was great!
Right before Gleb
You're into writing at all?
oh yea, your voice!
did you hear gleb read?
BZZT BZZT
TAP TAP TAP TAP TAP TAP
clink clink
clink
clink

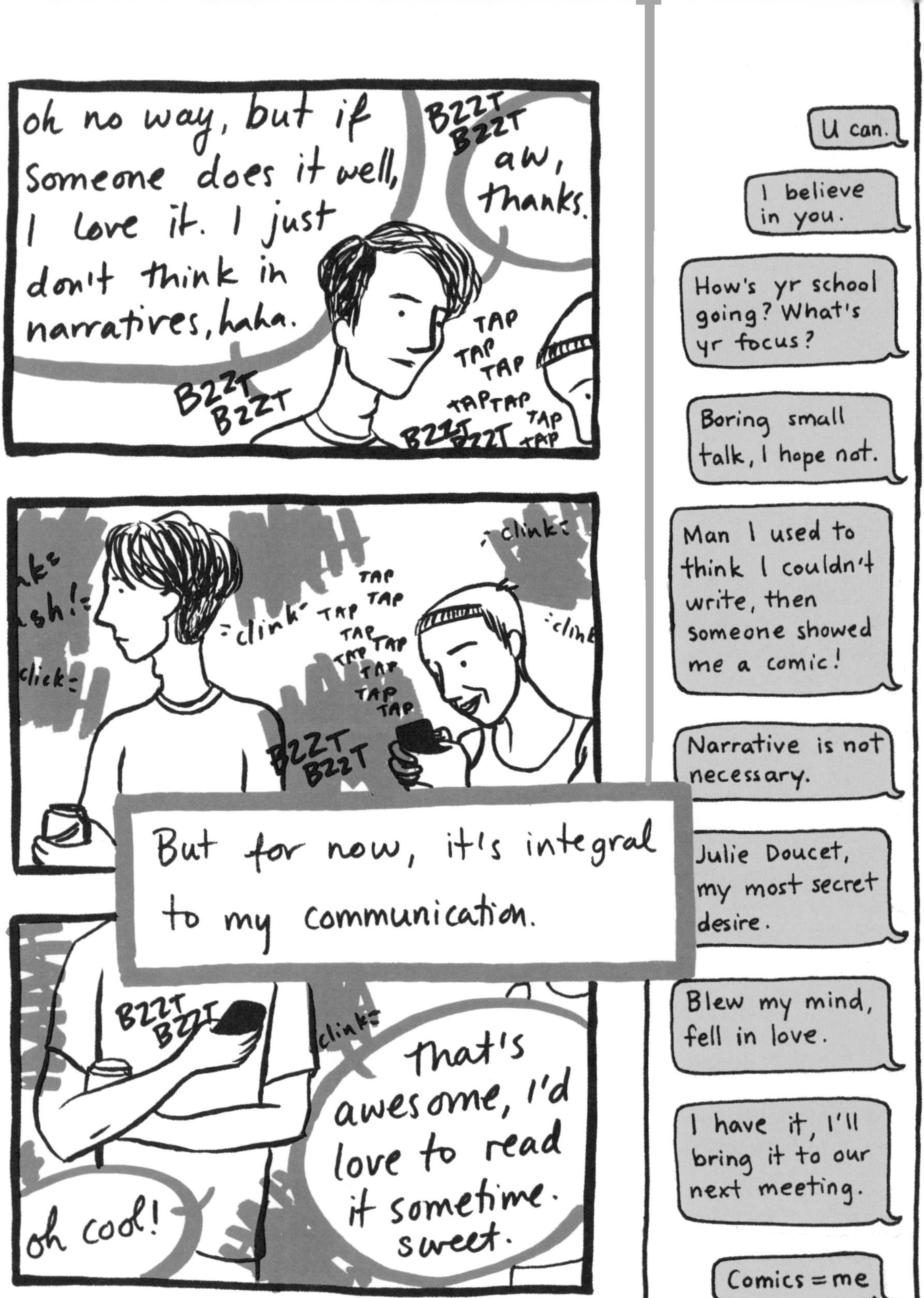

oh no way, but if someone does it well, I love it. I just don't think in narratives, haha.
BZZT BZZT
aw, thanks.
TAP TAP TAP
BZZT BZZT
TAP TAP TAP TAP
BZZT BZZT
click
clink
TAP TAP TAP TAP TAP TAP TAP TAP
clink
clink
BZZT BZZT
But for now, it's integral to my communication.
BZZT BZZT
clink
That's awesome, I'd love to read it sometime. sweet.
oh cool!
U can.
I believe in you.
How's yr school going? What's yr focus?
Boring small talk, I hope not.
Man I used to think I couldn't write, then someone showed me a comic!
Narrative is not necessary.
Julie Doucet, my most secret desire.
Blew my mind, fell in love.
I have it, I'll bring it to our next meeting.
Comics = me

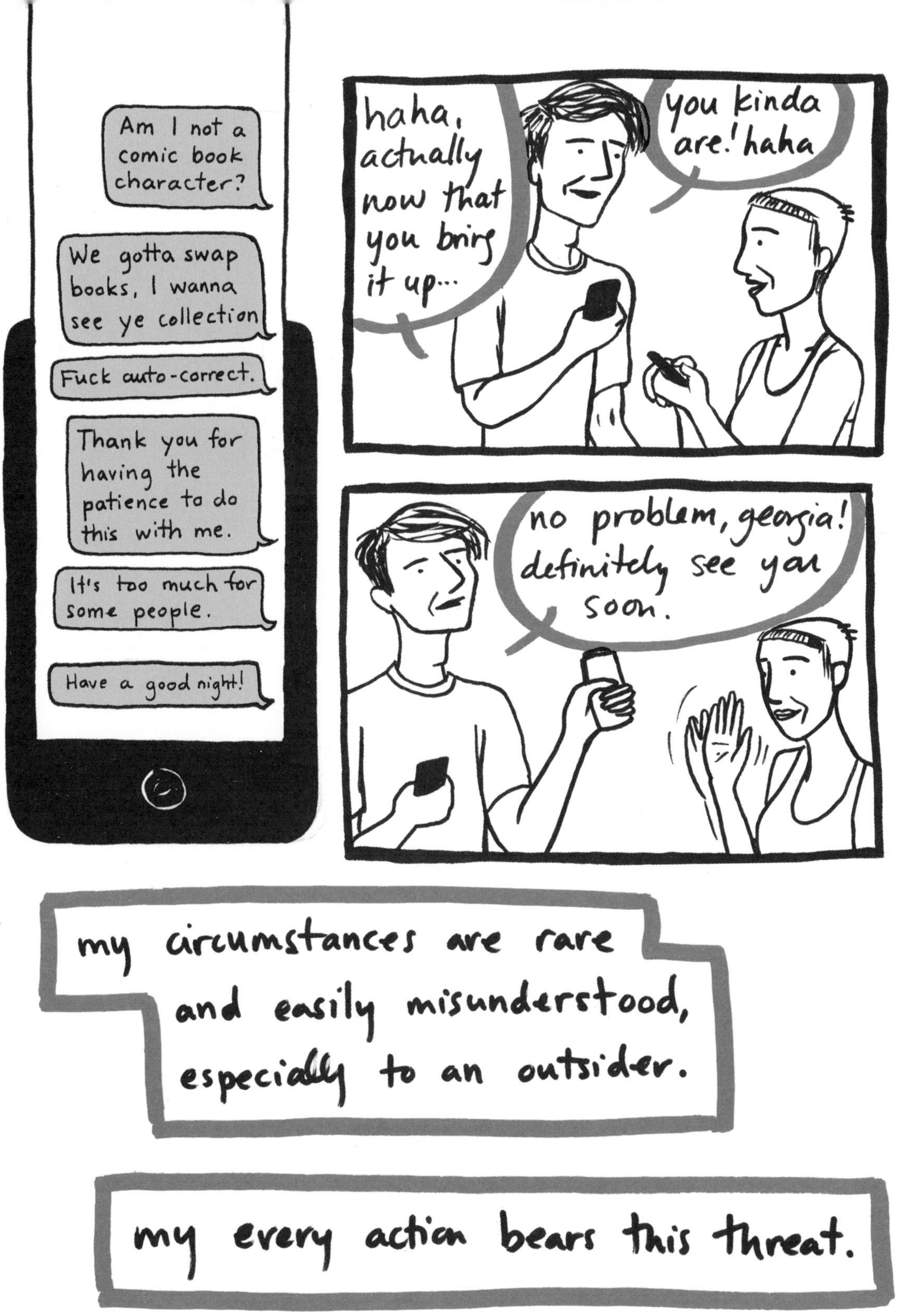
Am I not a comic book character?
We gotta swap books, I wanna see ye collection
Fuck auto-correct.
Thank you for having the patience to do this with me.
It's too much for some people.
Have a good night!
haha, actually now that you bring it up...
you kinda are! haha
no problem, georgia! definitely see you soon.
my circumstances are rare and easily misunderstood, especially to an outsider.
my every action bears this threat.

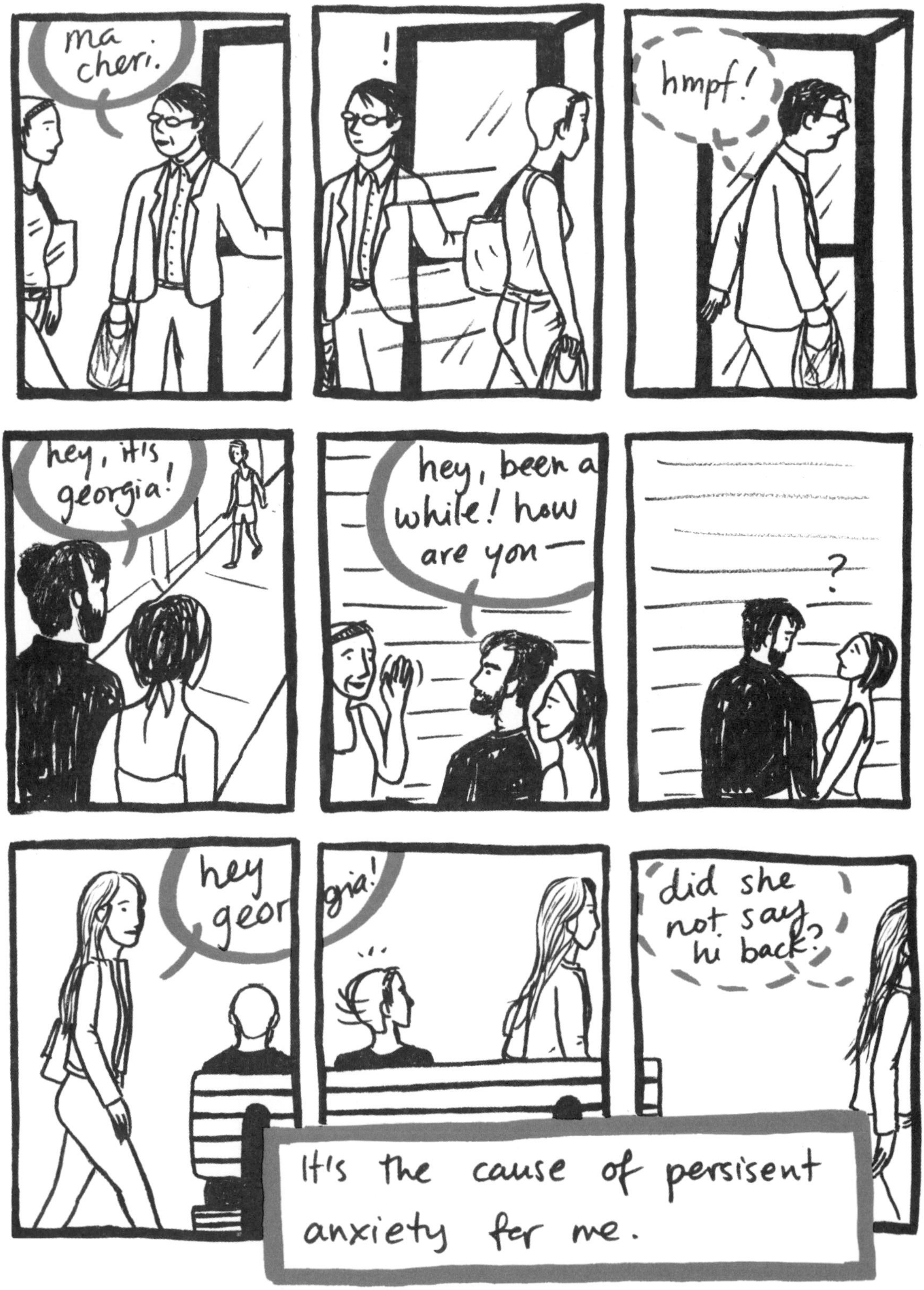
ma cheri.
!
hmpf!
hey, it's georgia!
hey, been a while! how are you—
?
hey georgia!
did she not say hi back?
It's the cause of persisent anxiety for me.

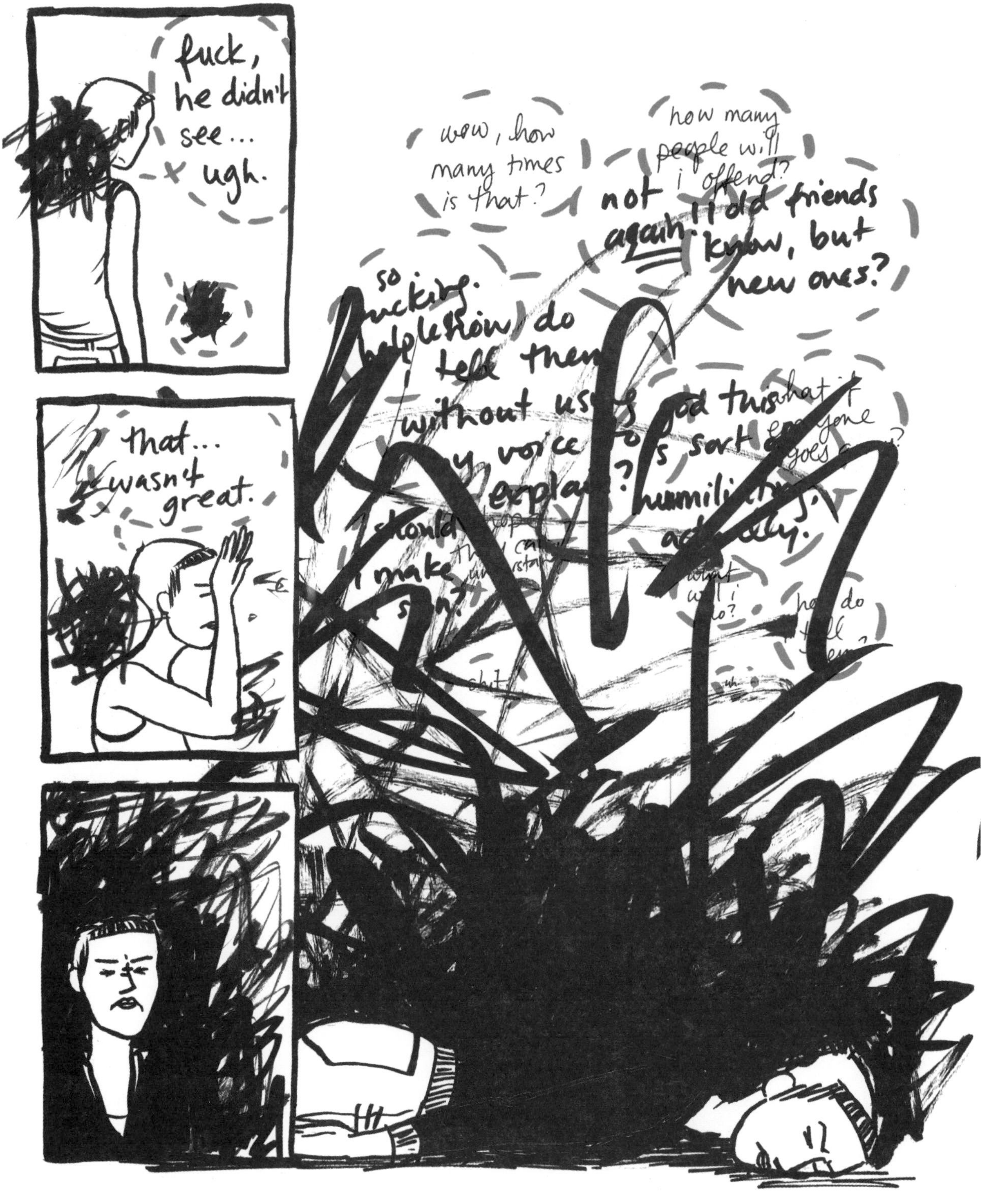
fuck, he didn't see... ugh.
wow, how many times is that?
how many people will i offend?
not again.
old friends know, but new ones?
that... wasn't great.

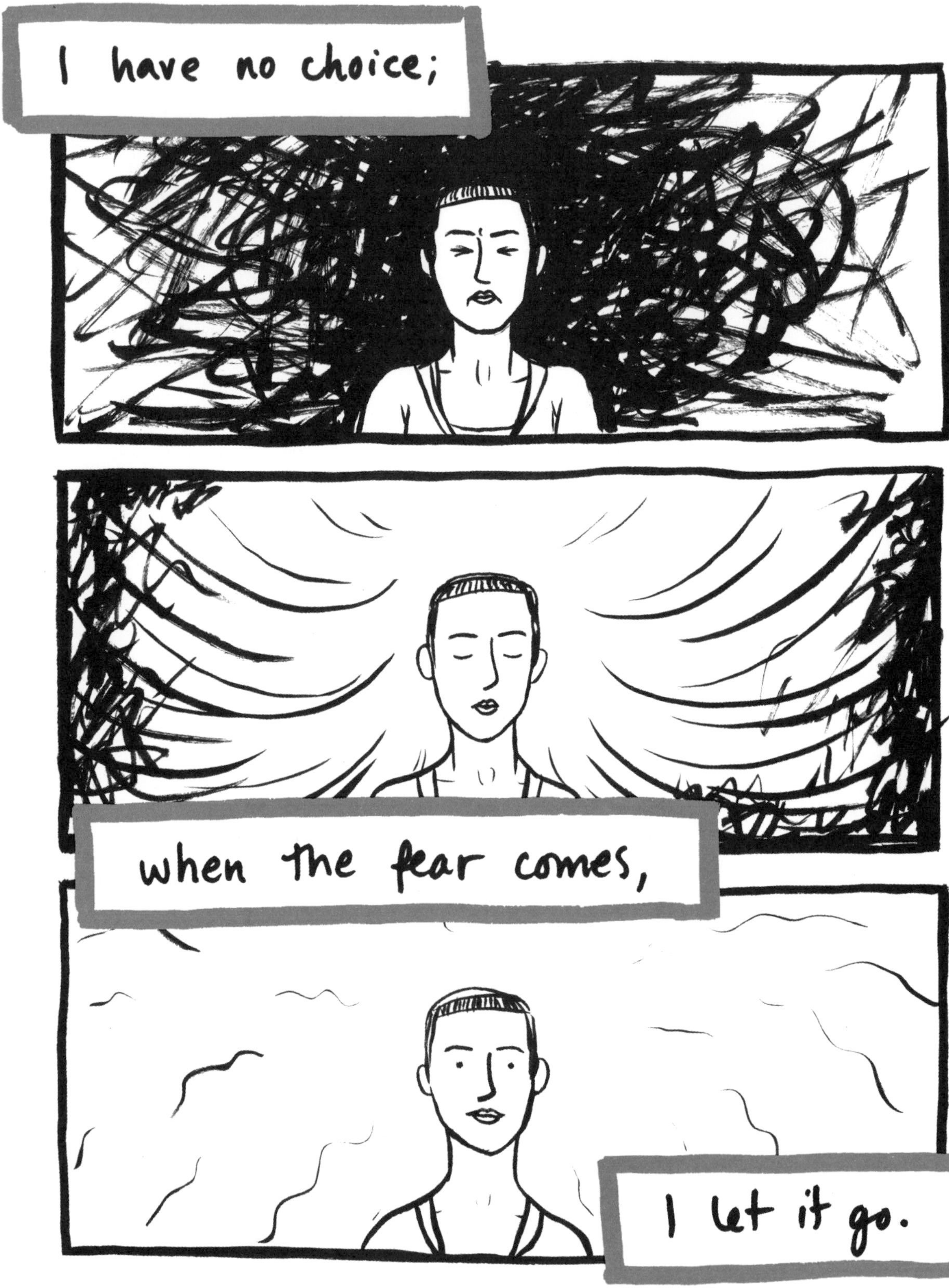
I have no choice;
when the fear comes,
I let it go.

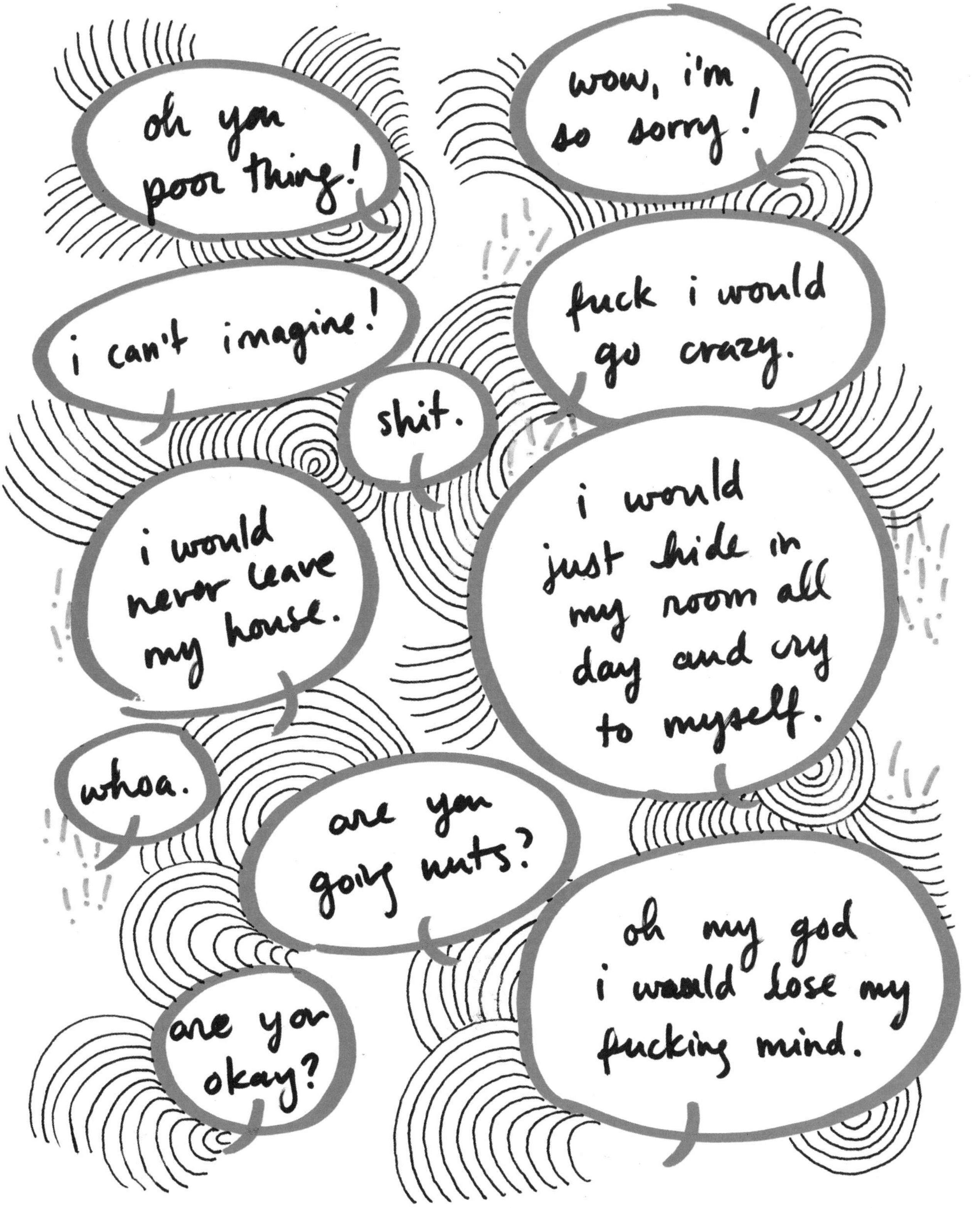
oh you poor thing!
wow, i'm so sorry!
i can't imagine!
fuck i would go crazy.
shit.
i would never leave my house.
i would just hide in my room all day and cry to myself.
whoa.
are you going nuts?
are you okay?
oh my god i would lose my fucking mind.

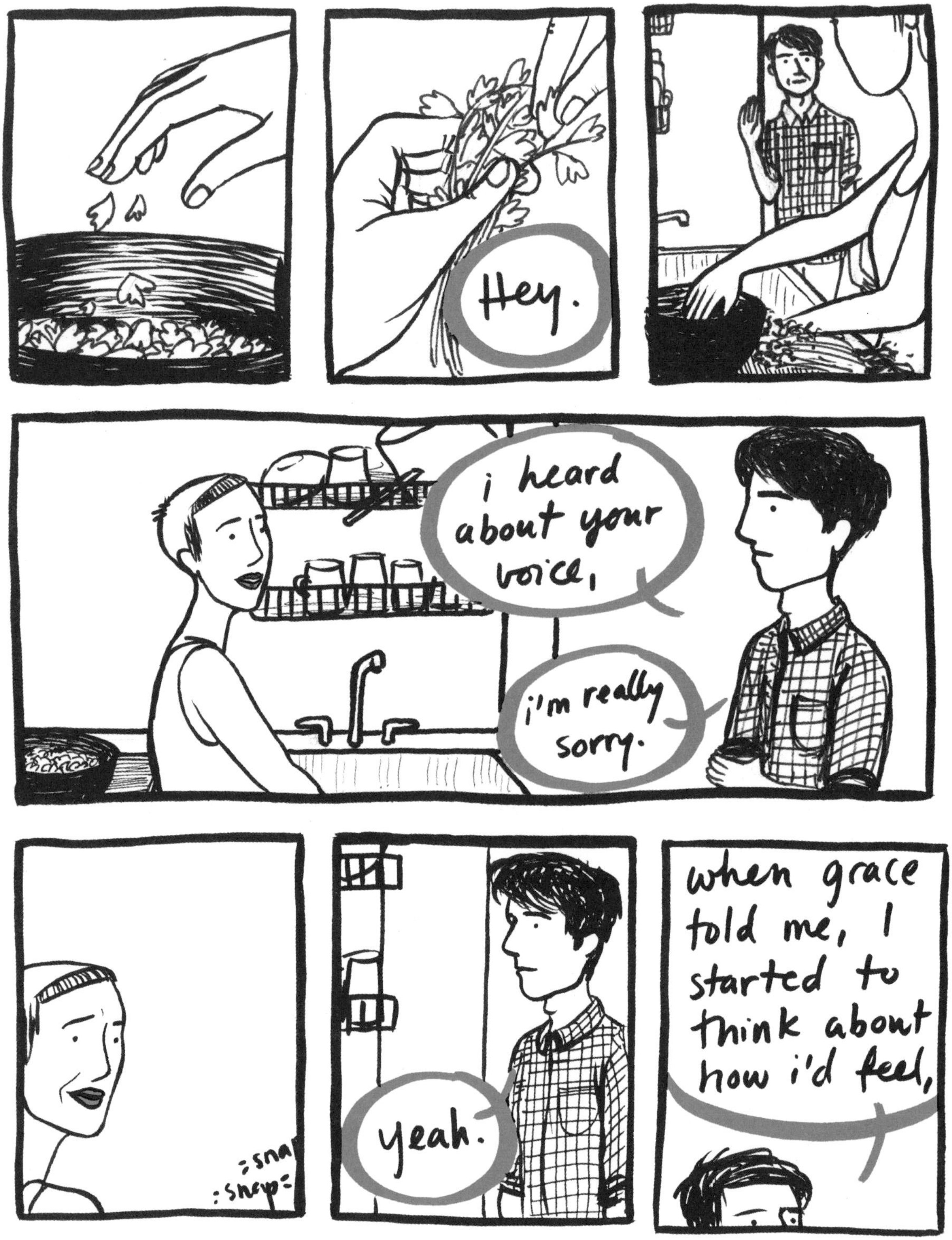
Hey.
i heard about your voice,
i'm really sorry.
:snap
:snap:
yeah.
when grace told me, I started to think about how i'd feel,

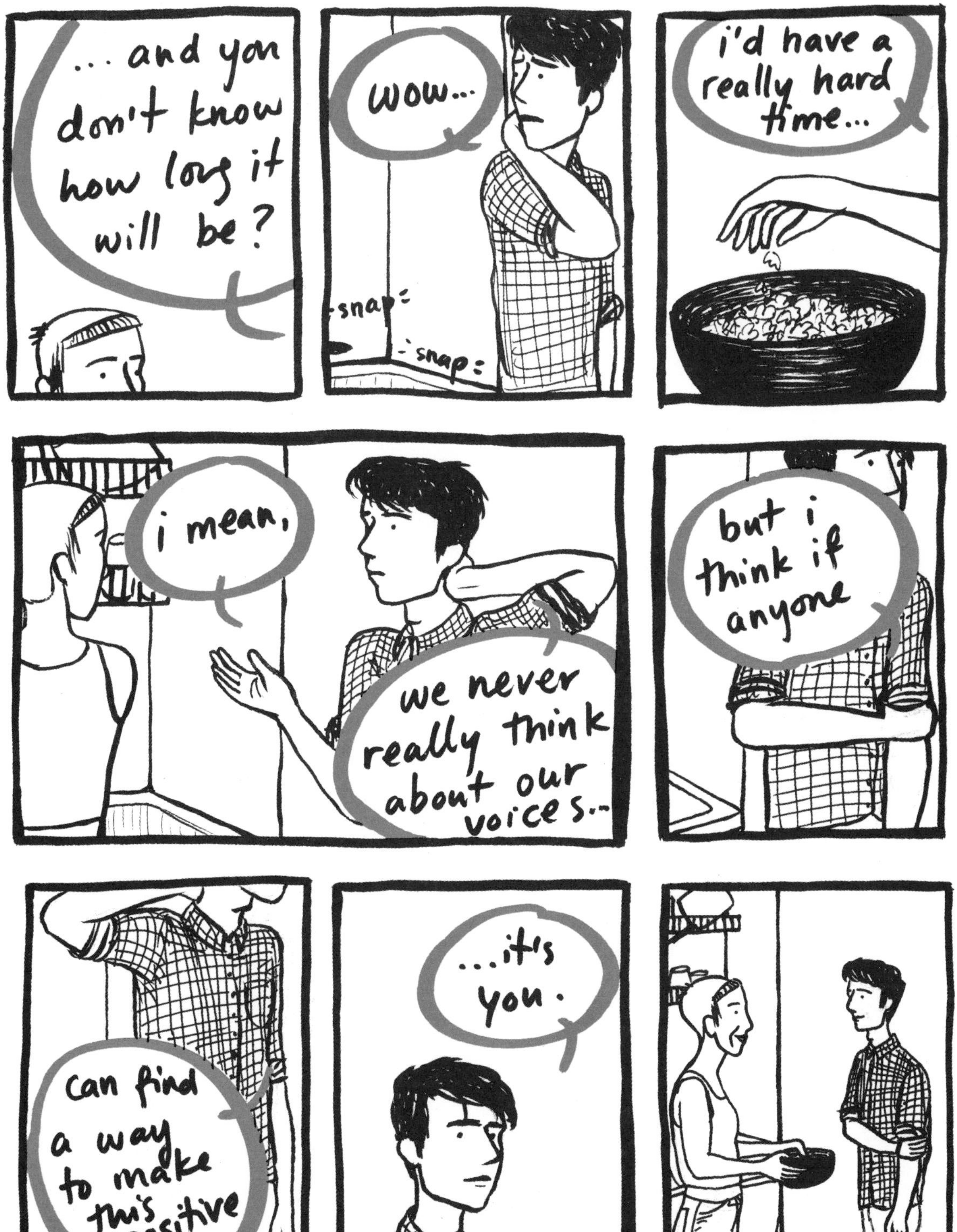
... and you don't know how long it will be?
wow...
snap
snap
i'd have a really hard time...
i mean,
we never really think about our voices...
but i think if anyone
can find a way to make this positive
...it's you.

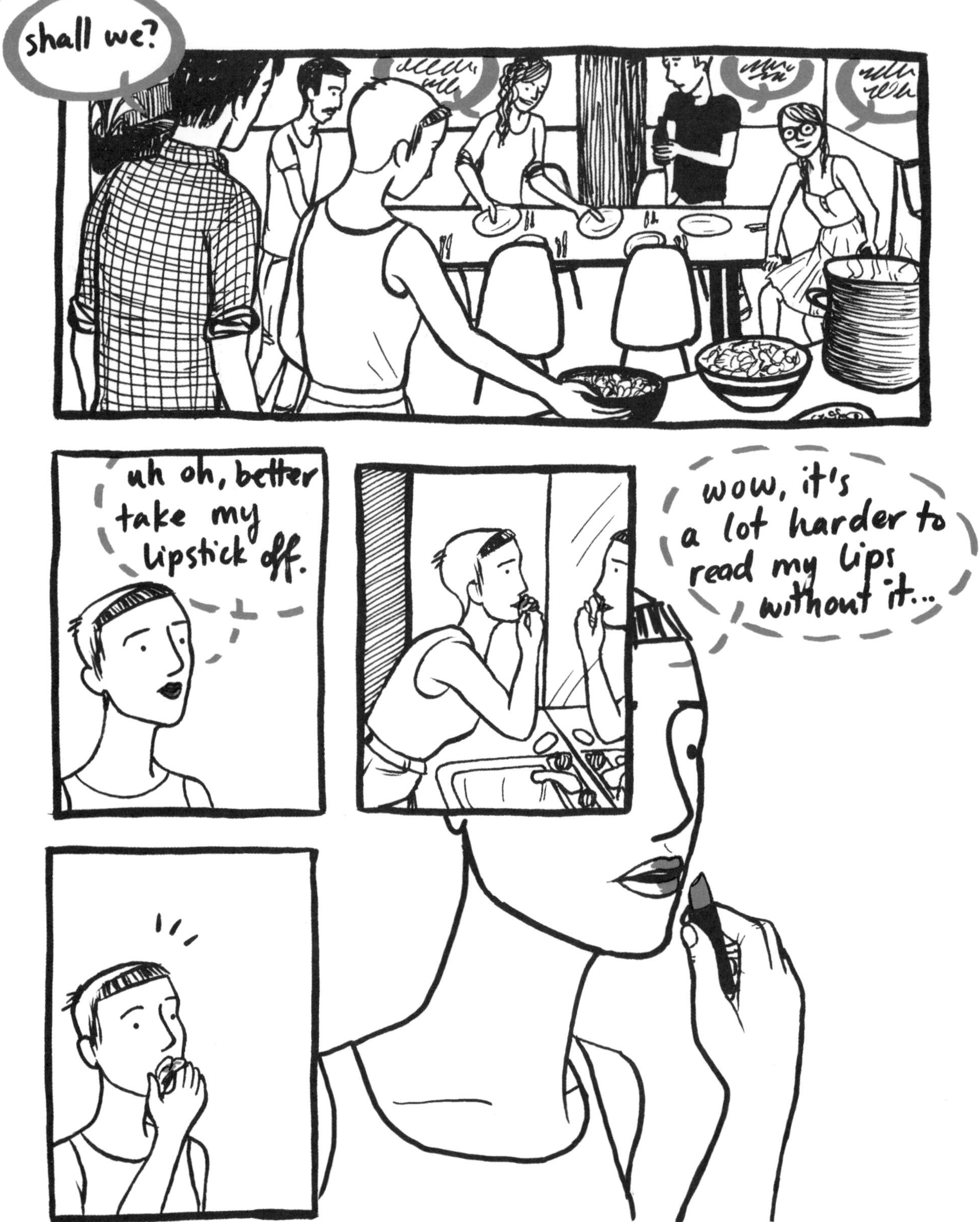
shall we?
uh oh, better take my lipstick off.
wow, it's a lot harder to read my lips without it...

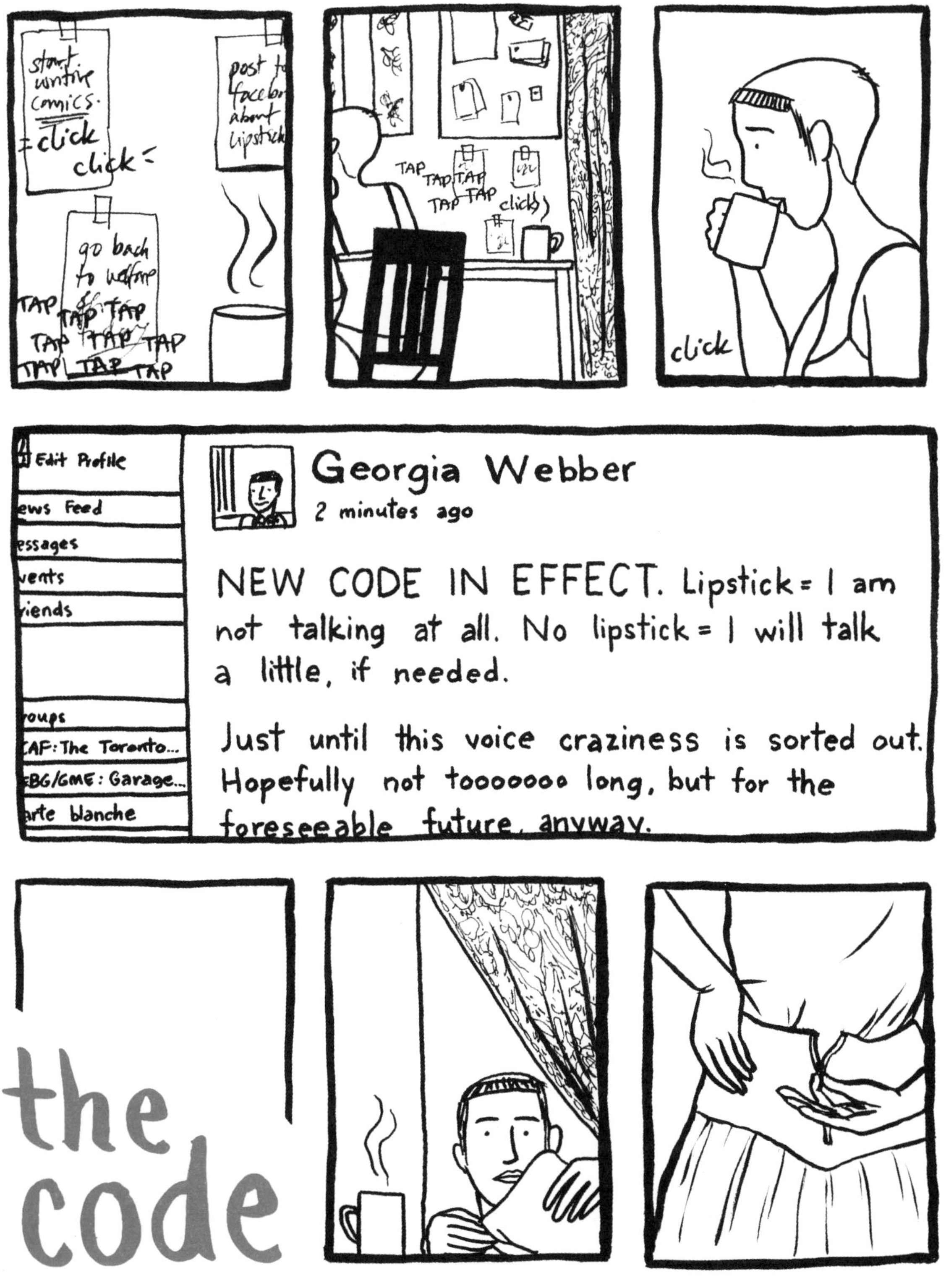
start writing comics.
click click
TAP TAP TAP TAP TAP TAP TAP TAP
TAP TAP TAP TAP TAP click
click
Edit Profile
Georgia Webber
2 minutes ago
NEW CODE IN EFFECT. Lipstick = I am not talking at all. No lipstick = I will talk a little, if needed.
Just until this voice craziness is sorted out. Hopefully not tooooooo long, but for the foreseeable future, anyway.
the code

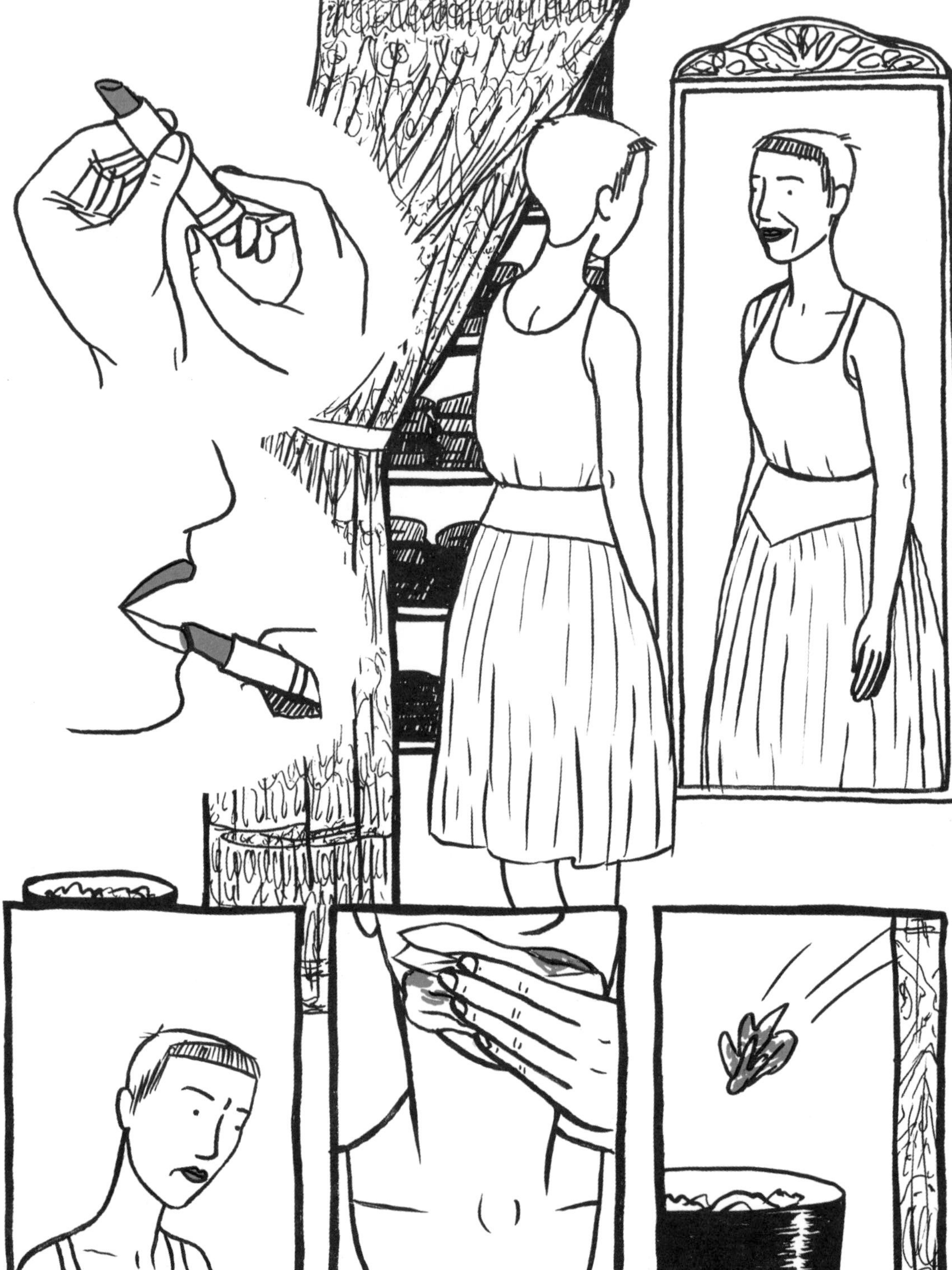

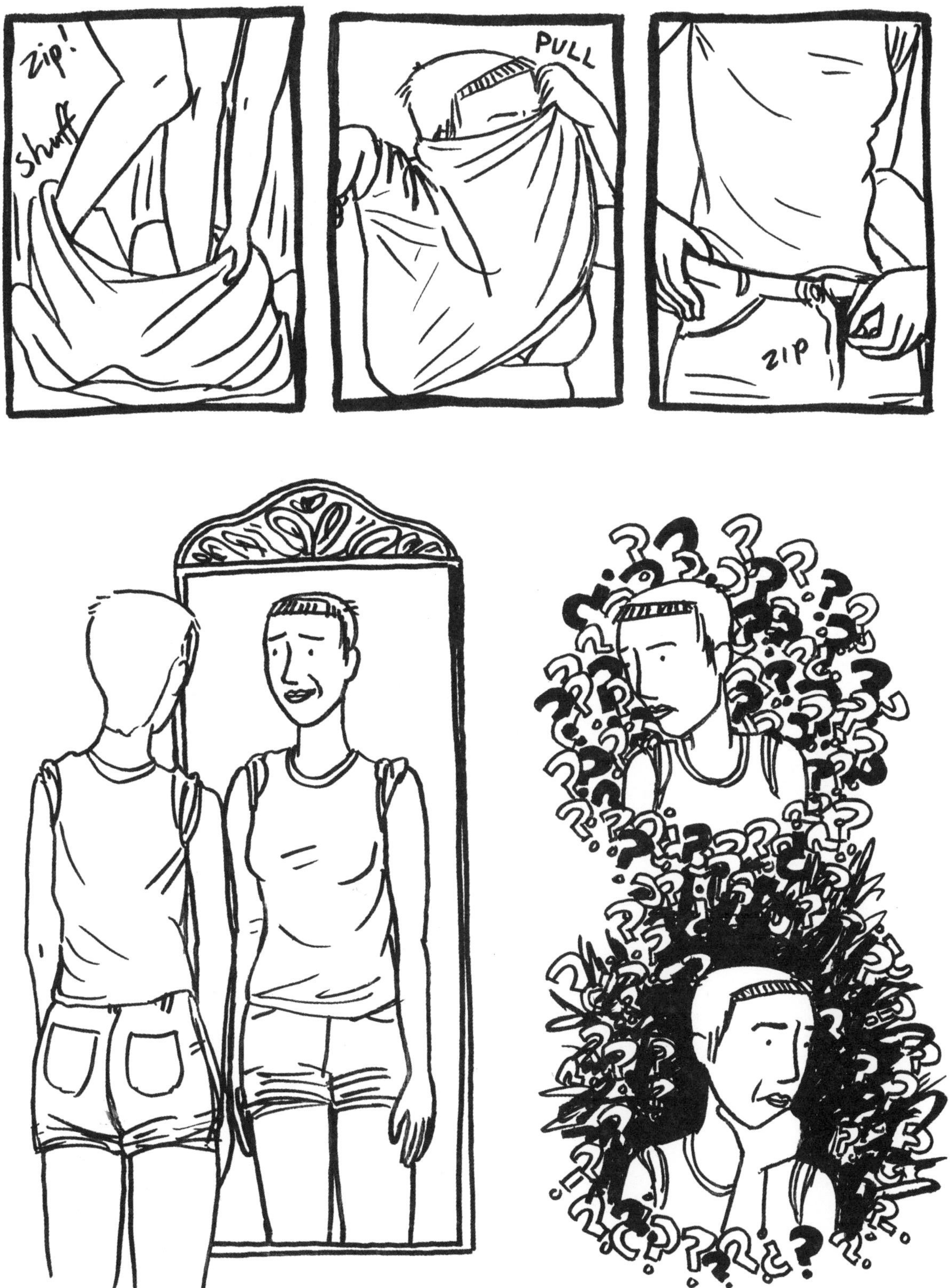
zip!
shuff
PULL
zip

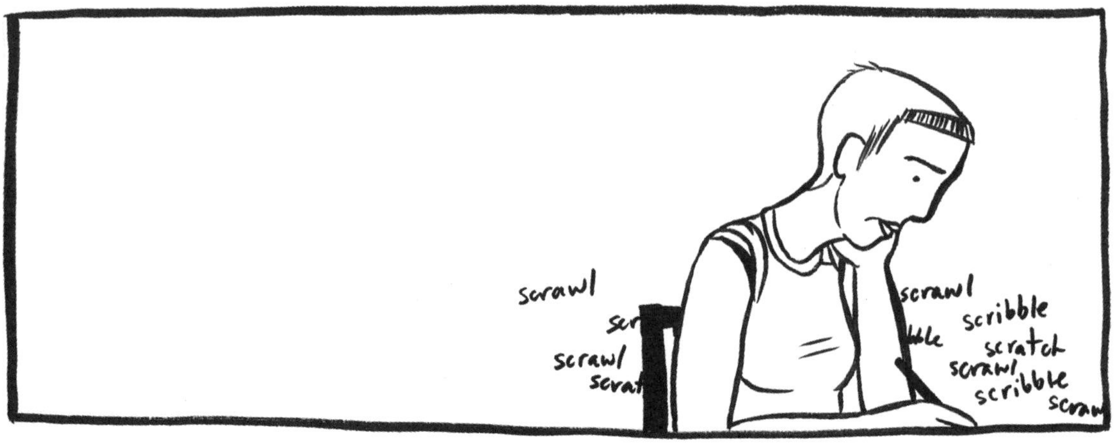
scrawl
scr
scrawl
scrat
scrawl
scribble
bble
scratch
scrawl
scribble
scraw

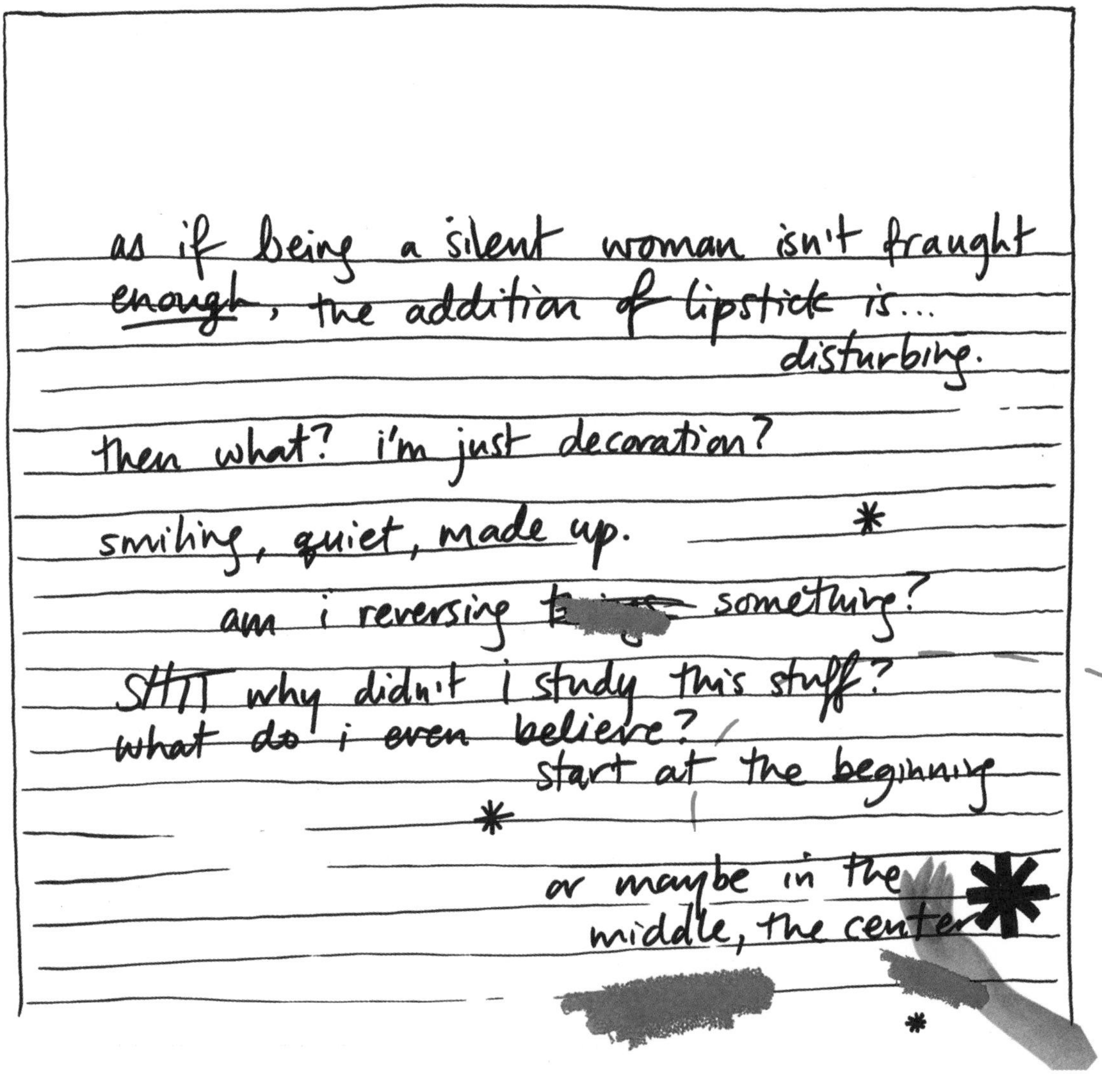
as if being a silent woman isn't fraught enough, the addition of lipstick is...
disturbing.
then what? i'm just decoration?
smiling, quiet, made up.
*
am i reversing something?
SHIT why didn't i study this stuff?
what do i even believe?
start at the beginning
*
or maybe in the middle, the center
*
*

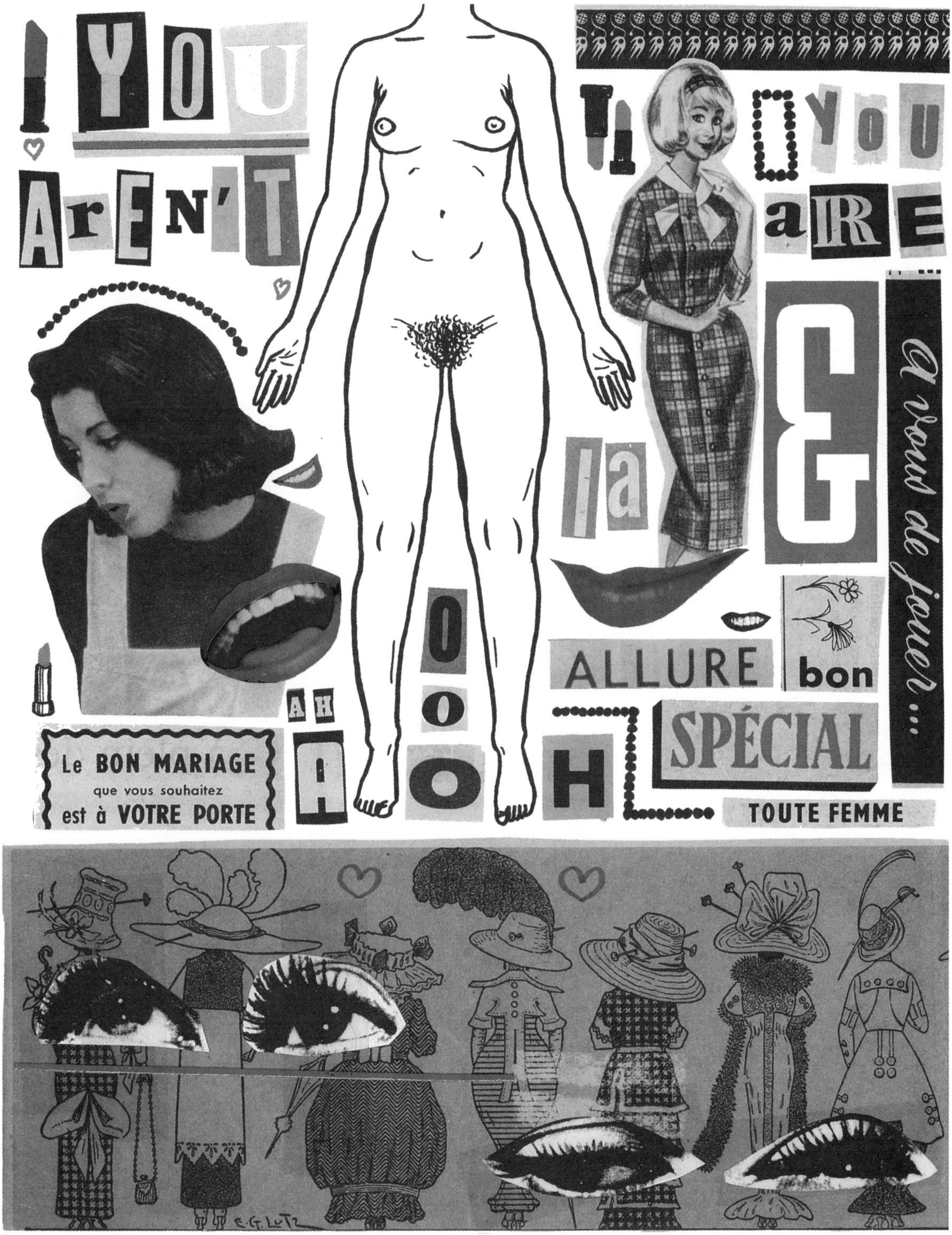
I YOU
YOU AREN'T
I YOU ARE
la
A vous de jouer…
ALLURE
bon
SPÉCIAL
TOUTE FEMME
Le BON MARIAGE
que vous souhaitez
est à VOTRE PORTE
AH
A O H
E.G. LUTZ

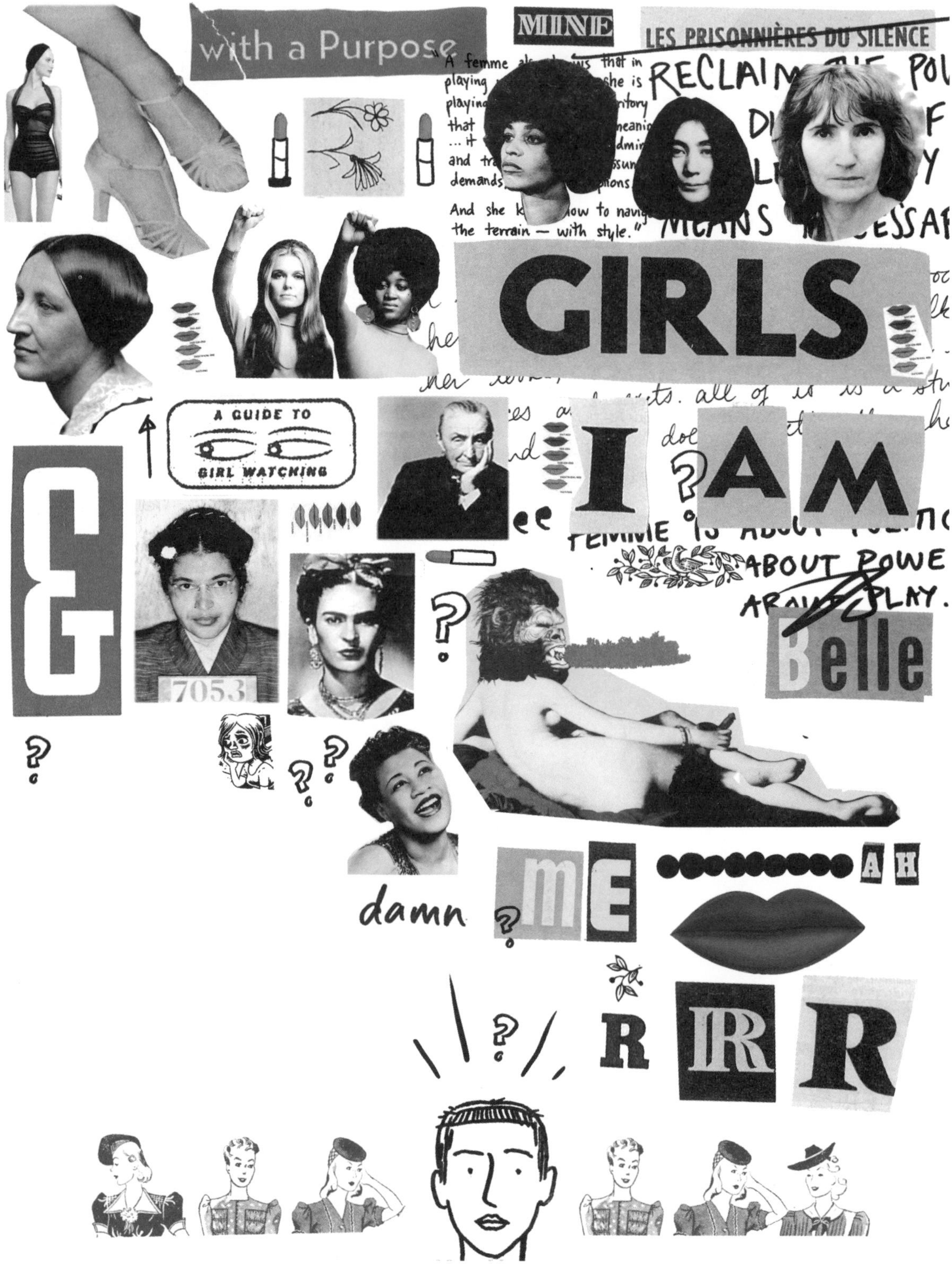
with a Purpose
MINE
LES PRISONNIÈRES DU SILENCE
And she k
the terrain — with style."
GIRLS
A GUIDE TO
GIRL WATCHING
I AM
ABOUT POWE
Belle
7053
damn
me
A H
R R R

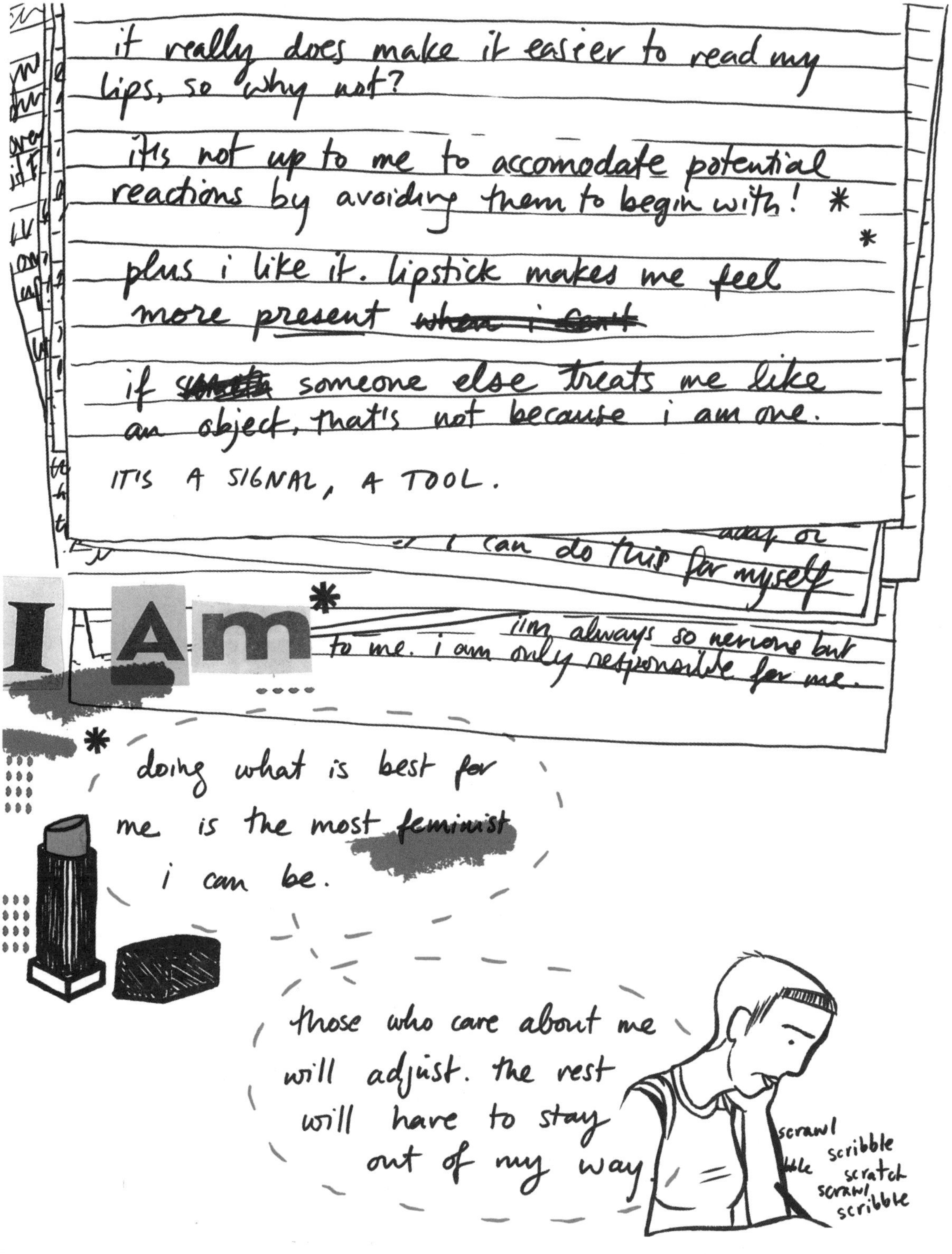

it really does make it easier to read my lips, so why not?
it's not up to me to accomodate potential reactions by avoiding them to begin with! *
*
plus i like it. lipstick makes me feel more present ~~when i can't~~
if someone else treats me like an object, that's not because i am one.
IT'S A SIGNAL, A TOOL.
i can do this for myself
I Am*
i'm always so nervous but
to me. i am only responsible for me.
* doing what is best for me is the most feminist i can be.
those who care about me will adjust. the rest will have to stay out of my way.
scrawl
scribble
scratch
scrawl
scribble

...but it's still a negotiation every day.

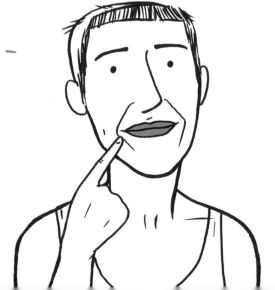

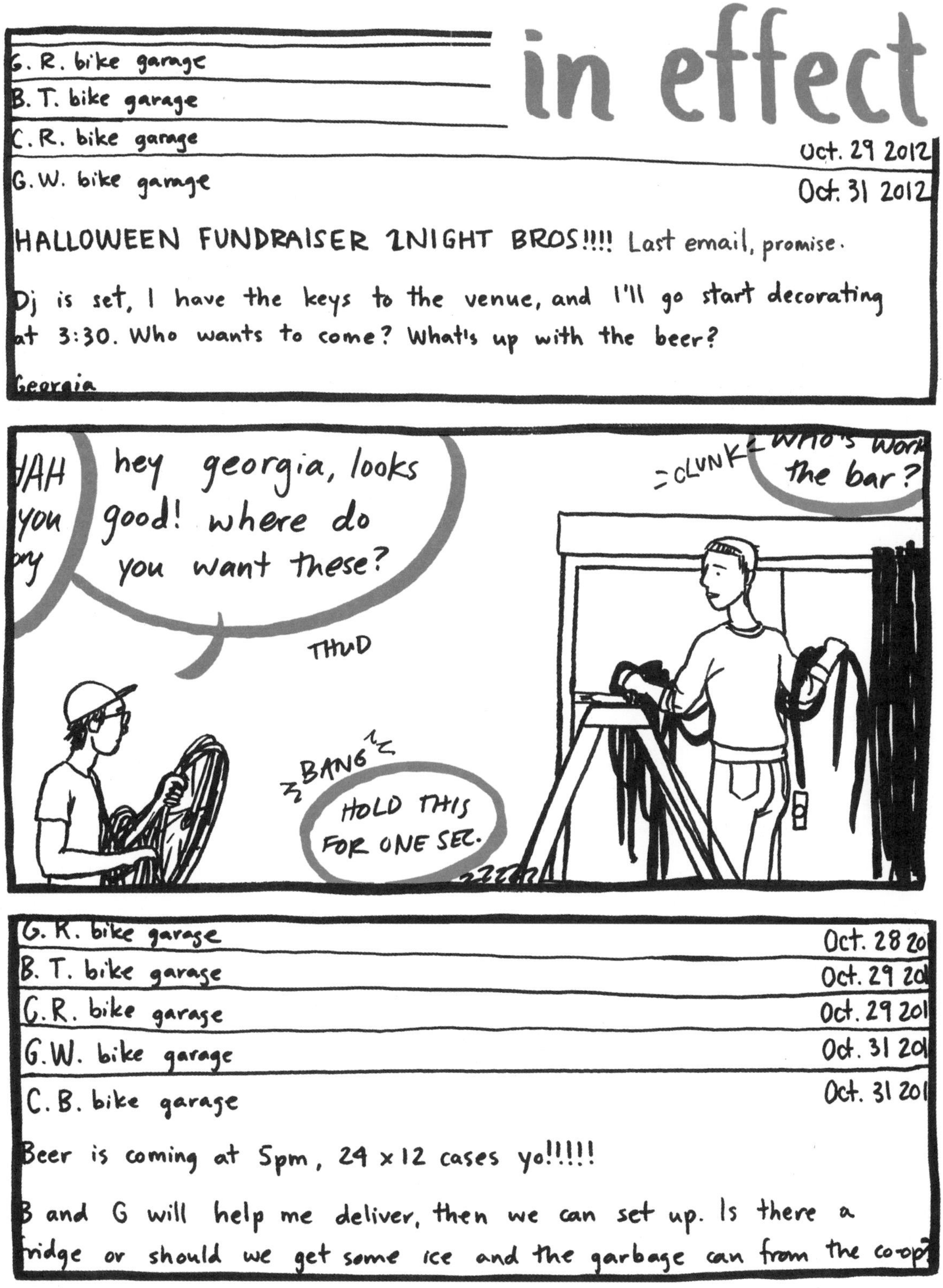

G.R. bike garage	
B.T. bike garage	
C.R. bike garage	Oct. 29 2012
G.W. bike garage	Oct. 31 2012

HALLOWEEN FUNDRAISER 2NIGHT BROS!!!! Last email, promise.

Dj is set, I have the keys to the venue, and I'll go start decorating at 3:30. Who wants to come? What's up with the beer?

Georgia

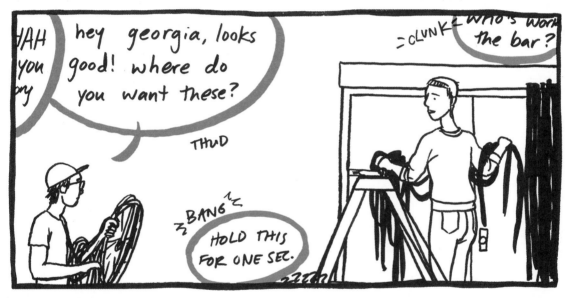

G.R. bike garage	Oct. 28 20
B.T. bike garage	Oct. 29 20
C.R. bike garage	Oct. 29 20
G.W. bike garage	Oct. 31 20
C.B. bike garage	Oct. 31 20

Beer is coming at 5pm, 24 x12 cases yo!!!!!

B and G will help me deliver, then we can set up. Is there a fridge or should we get some ice and the garbage can from the co-op?

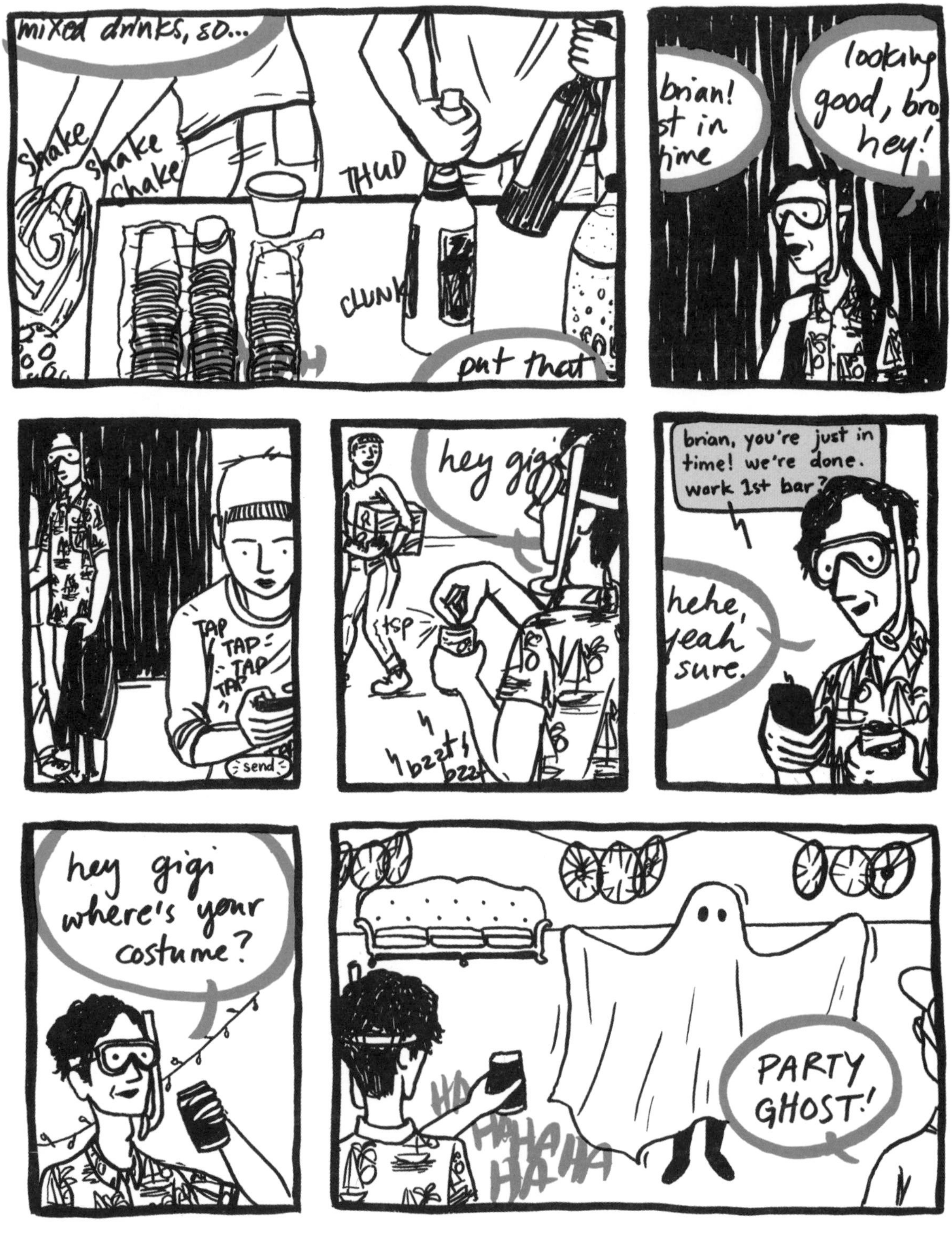
mixed drinks, so...
shake shake shake
THUD
CLUNK
put that
brian!
looking good, bro hey!
TAP TAP TAP TAP
send
hey gigi
tsp
bzzt bzz
brian, you're just in time! we're done. work 1st bar?
hehe, yeah sure.
hey gigi where's your costume?
PARTY GHOST!
HA HA HA HA HA HA

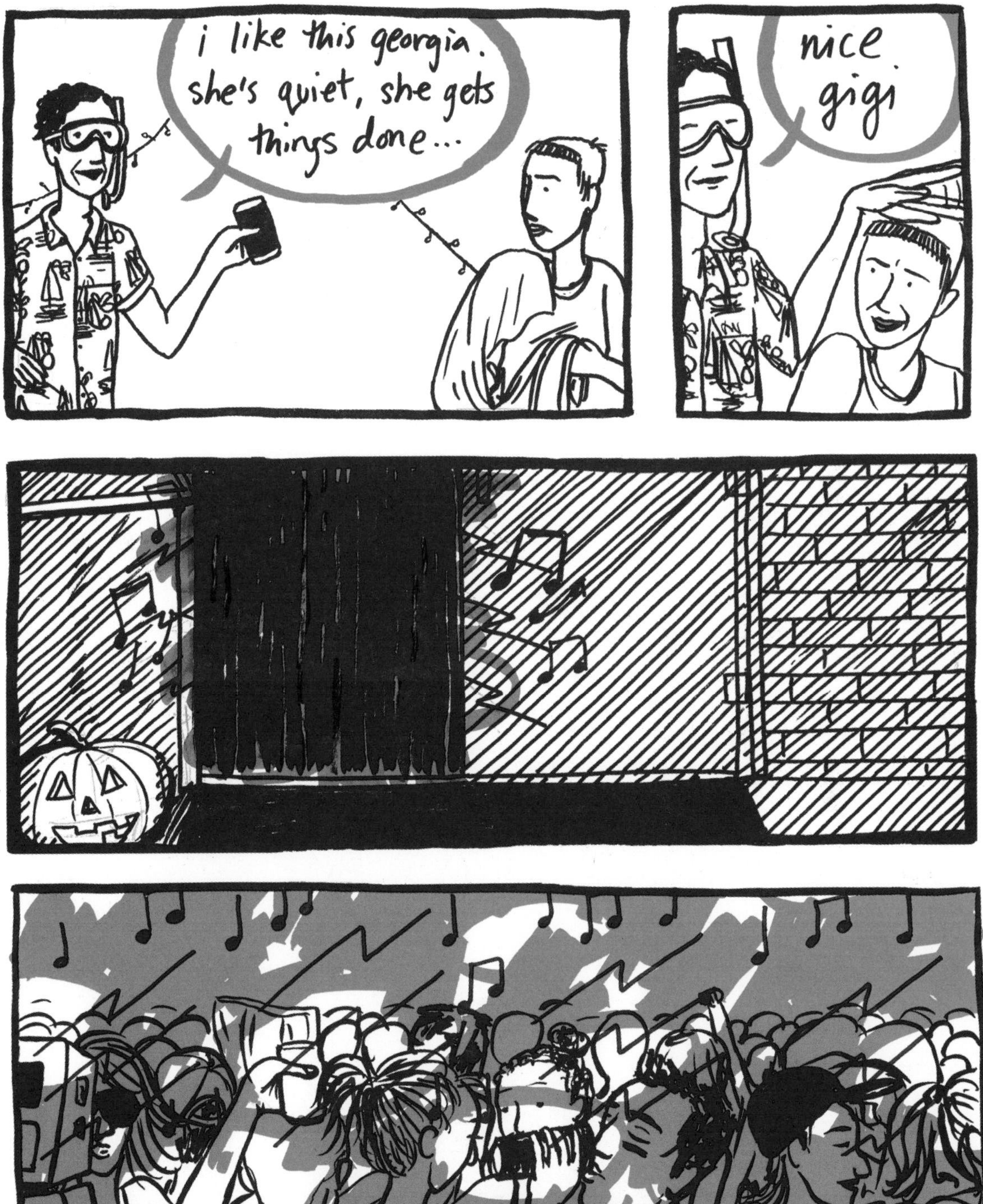
i like this georgia. she's quiet, she gets things done...
nice gigi

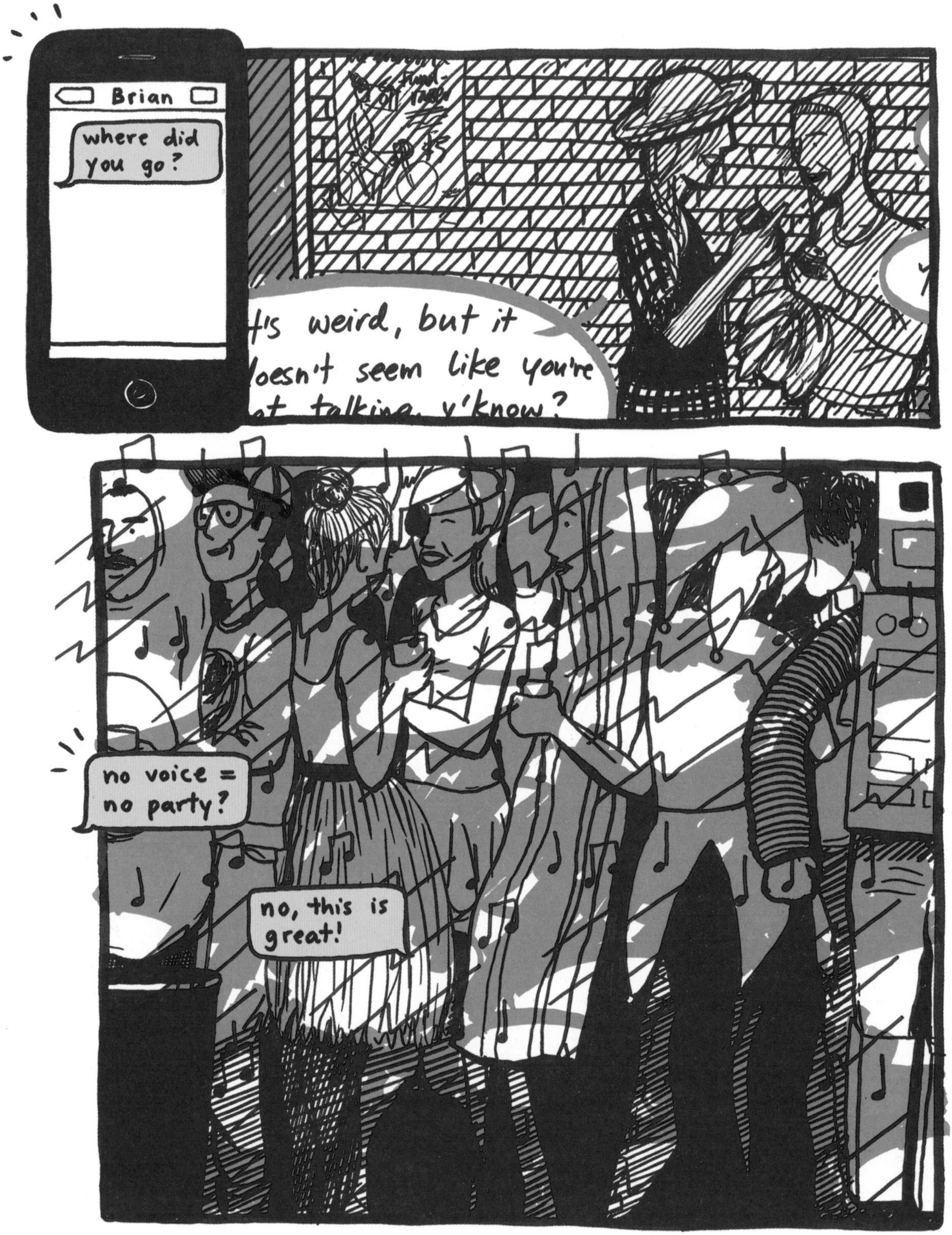
Brian
where did you go?
t's weird, but it
oesn't seem like you're
t talking, y'know?
no voice = no party?
no, this is great!

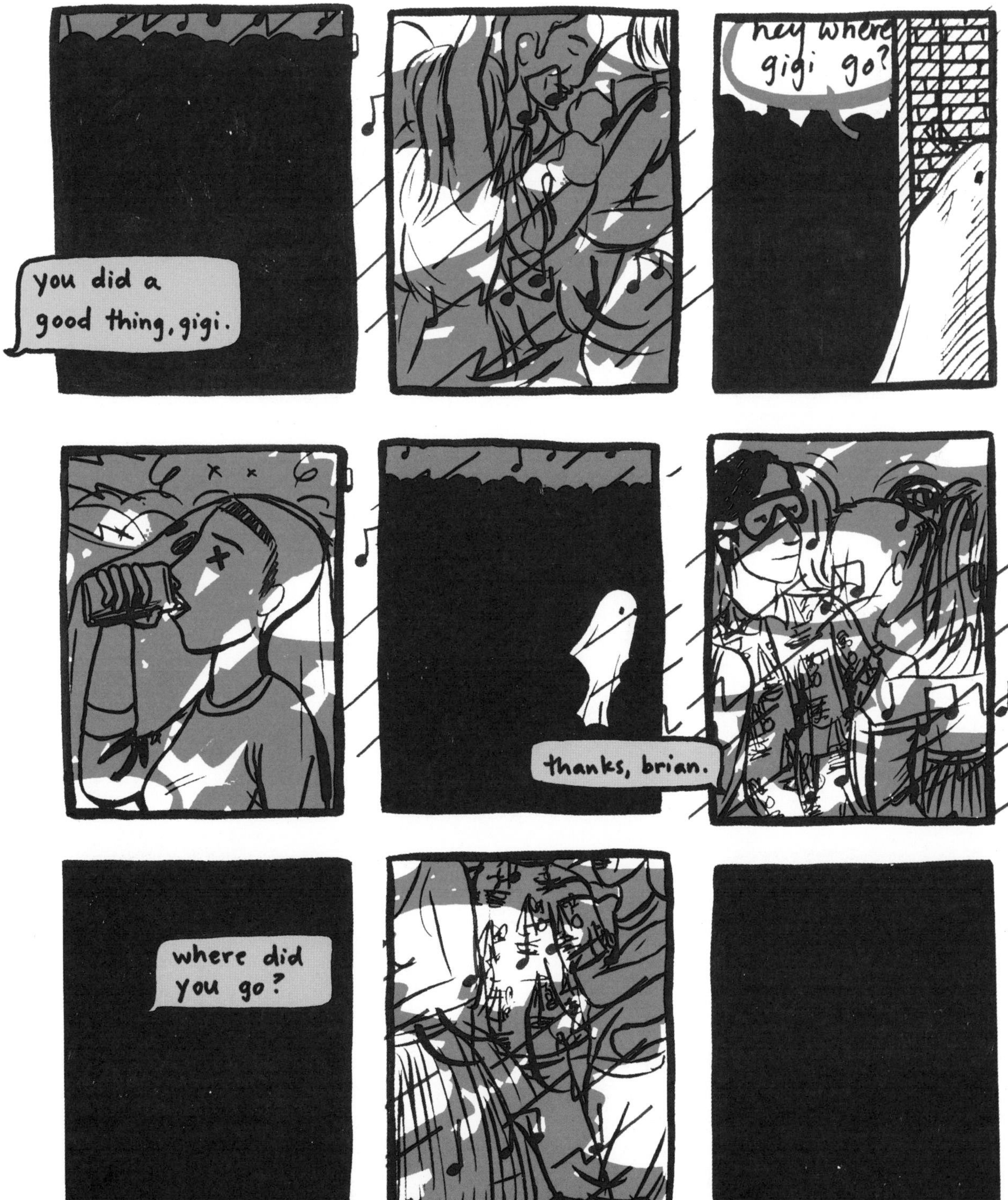
you did a good thing, gigi.
hey where gigi go?
thanks, brian.
where did you go?

gh
shit
no talk
stupid
roll
ffuckk
was brian really hitting on me??
after saying he liked me better silent?
asking for me all...
uugghh gross
liked him—

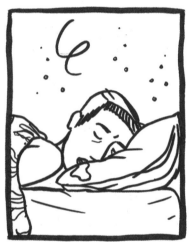

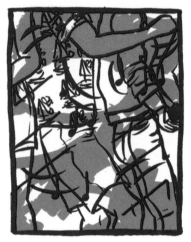

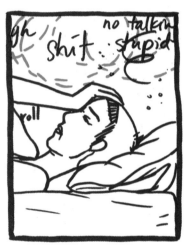

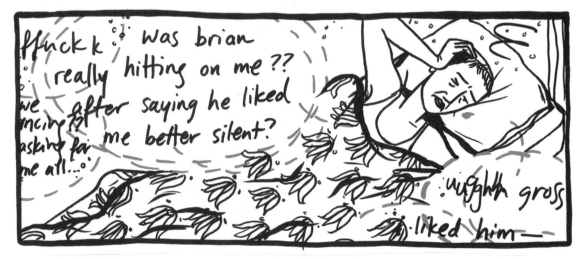

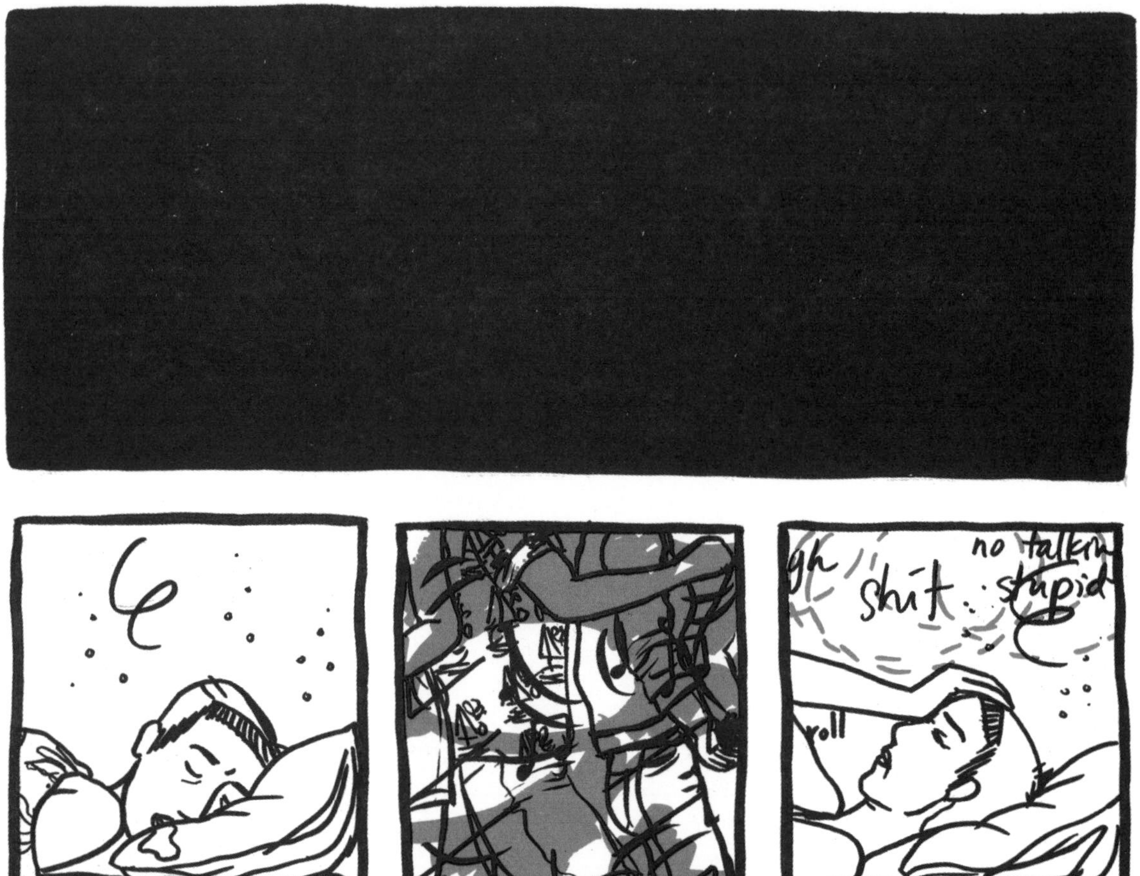

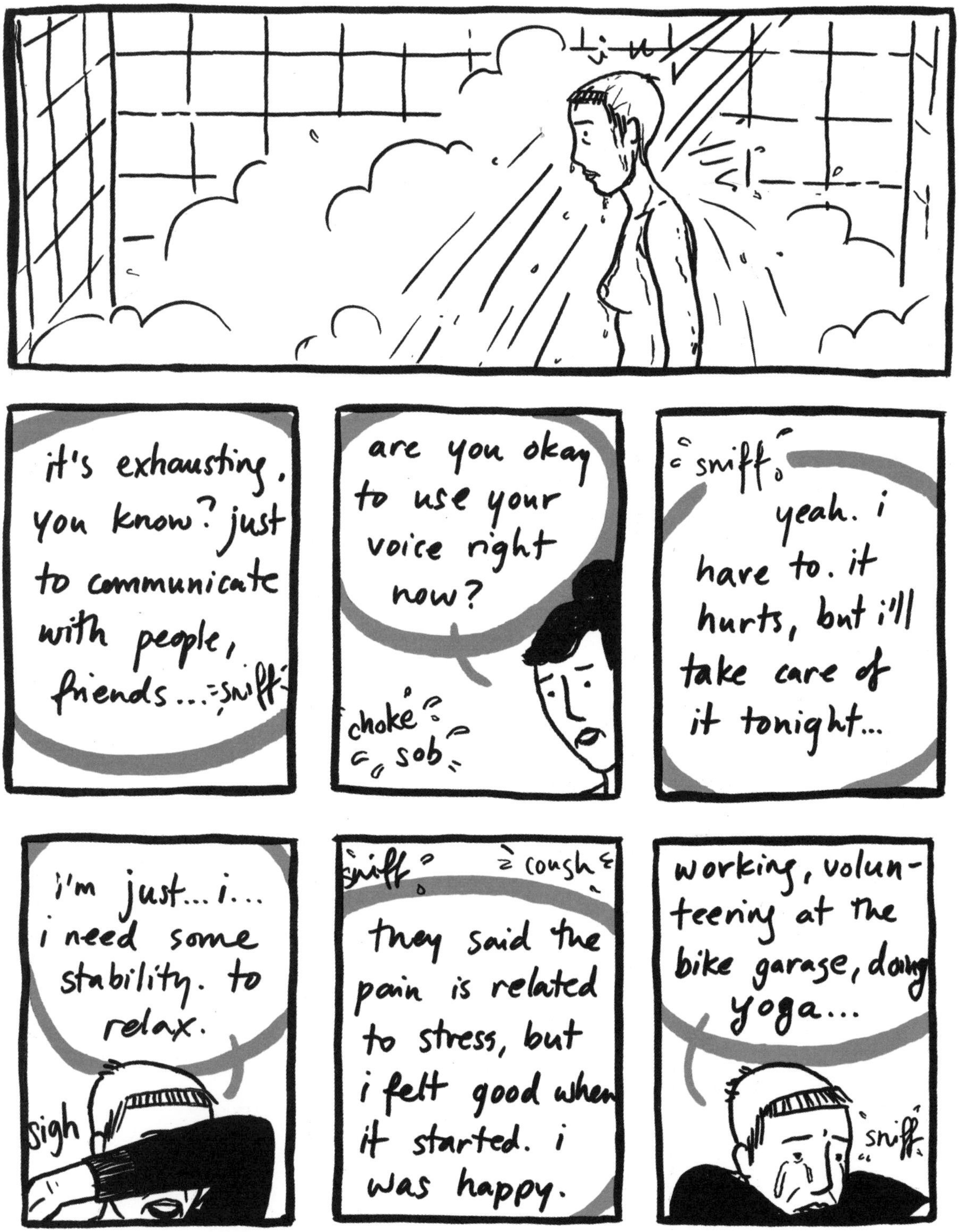
it's exhausting, you know? just to communicate with people, friends... sniff
are you okay to use your voice right now?
choke sob
sniff
yeah. i have to. it hurts, but i'll take care of it tonight...
i'm just... i... i need some stability. to relax.
sigh
sniff cough
they said the pain is related to stress, but i felt good when it started. i was happy.
working, volunteering at the bike garage, doing yoga...
sniff

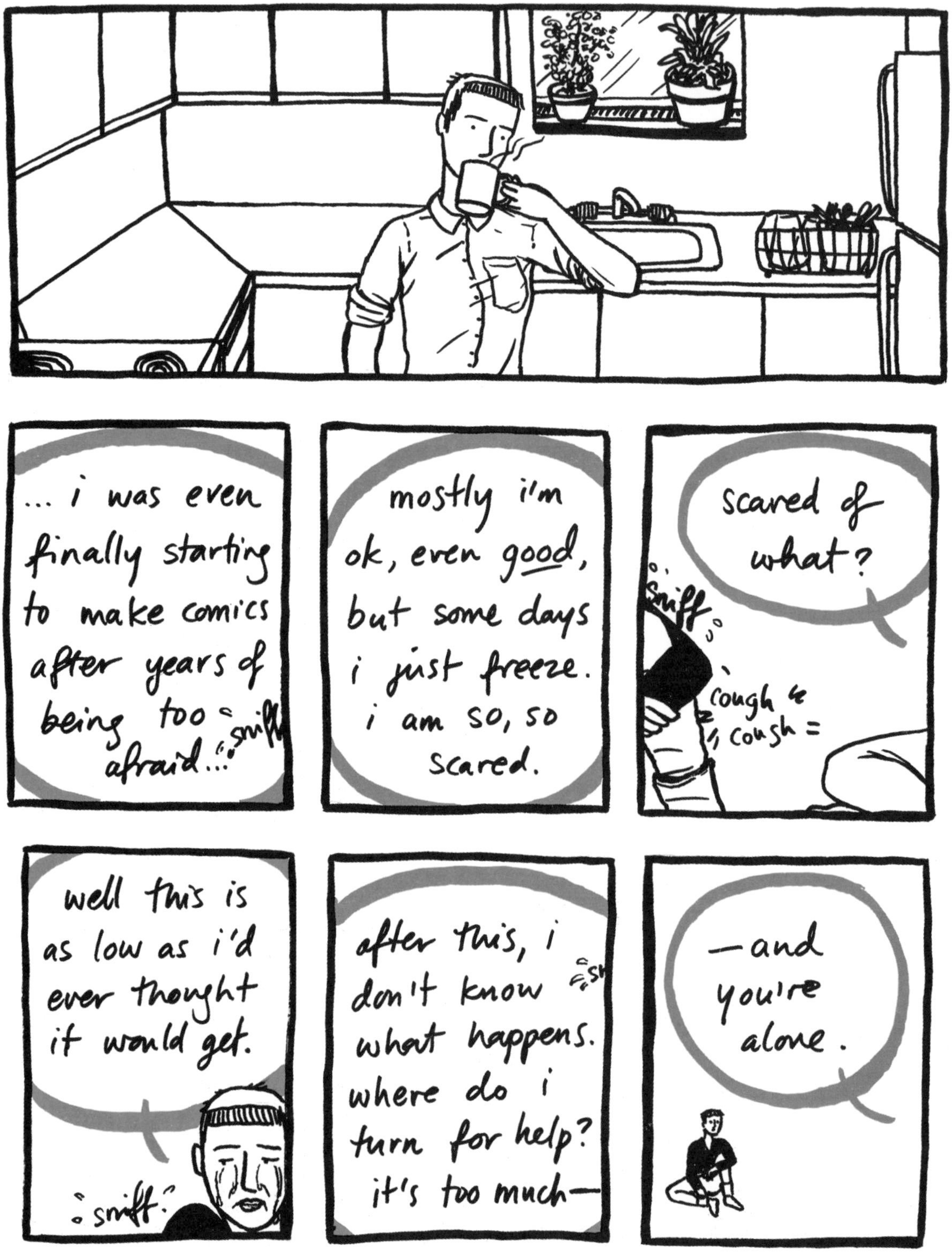
... i was even finally starting to make comics after years of being too afraid...
sniff
mostly i'm ok, even good, but some days i just freeze. i am so, so scared.
scared of what?
sniff
cough
cough
well this is as low as i'd ever thought it would get.
sniff
after this, i don't know what happens. where do i turn for help? it's too much—
—and you're alone.

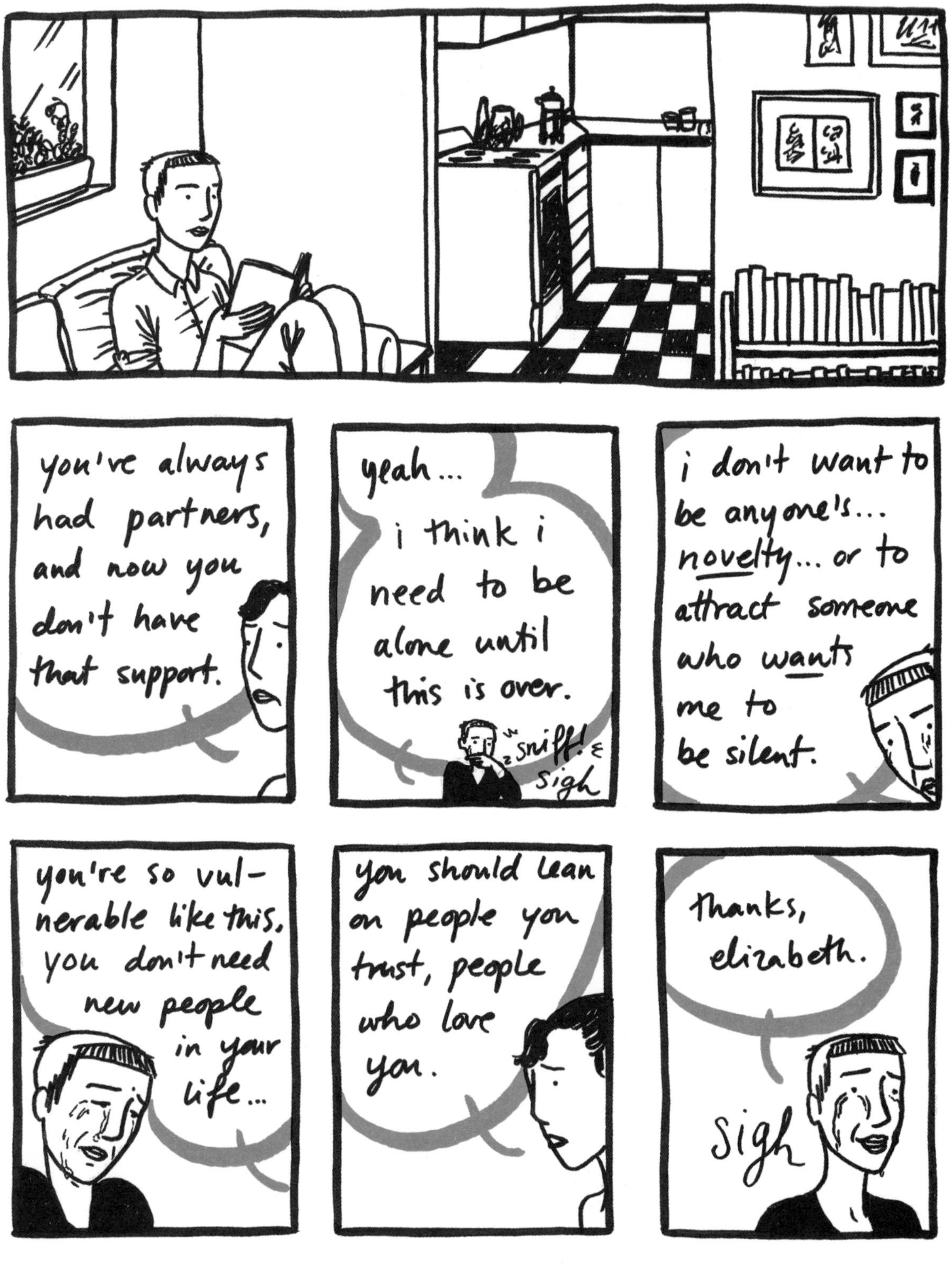
you've always had partners, and now you don't have that support.
yeah...
i think i need to be alone until this is over.
sniff! & sigh
i don't want to be anyone's... novelty... or to attract someone who wants me to be silent.
you're so vul-nerable like this. you don't need new people in your life...
you should lean on people you trust, people who love you.
thanks, elizabeth.
sigh

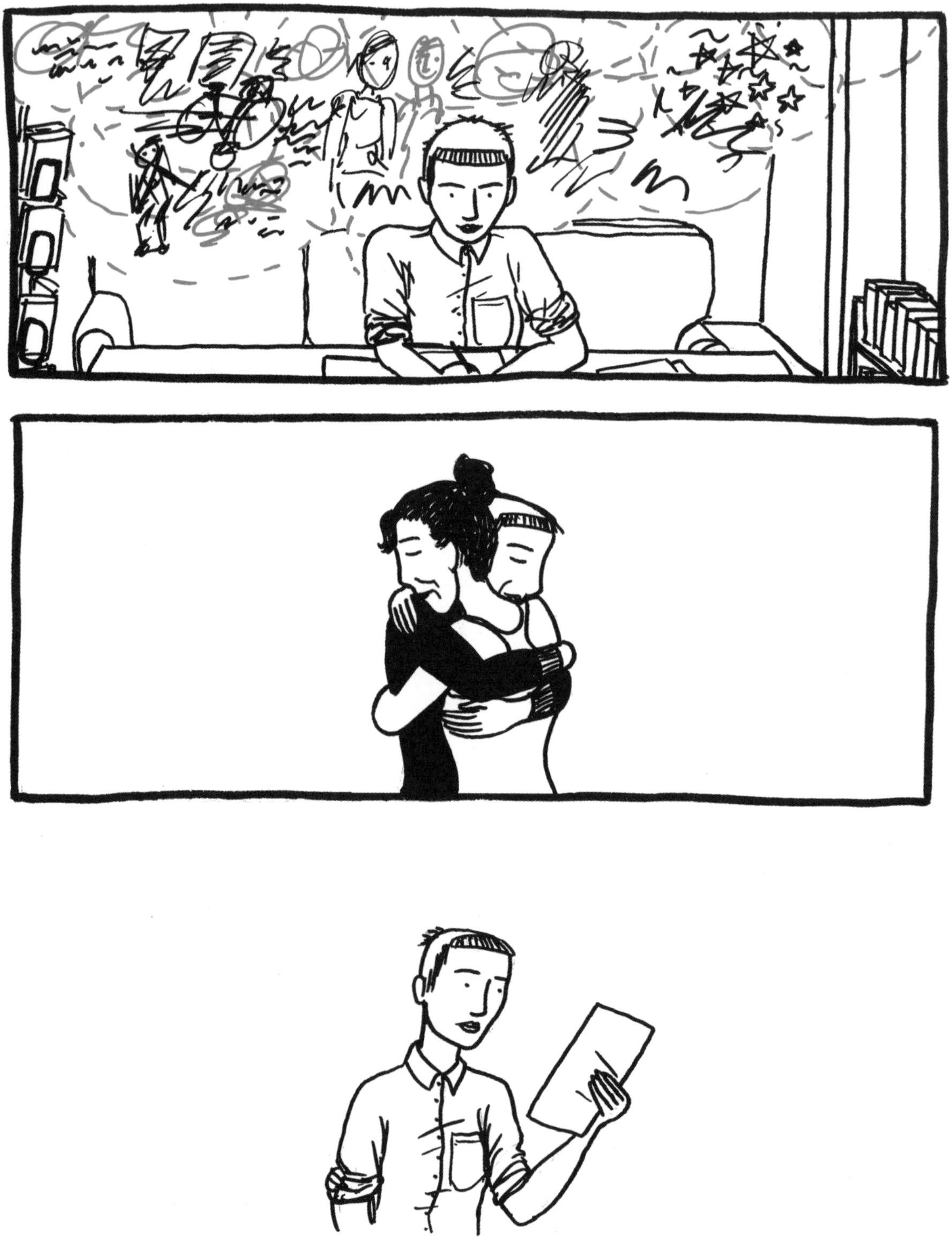

paperwork

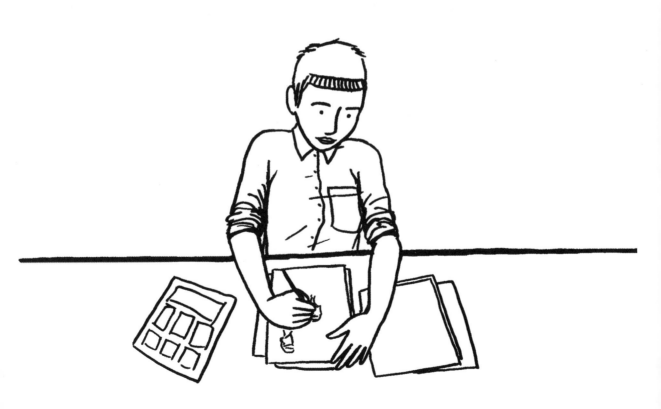

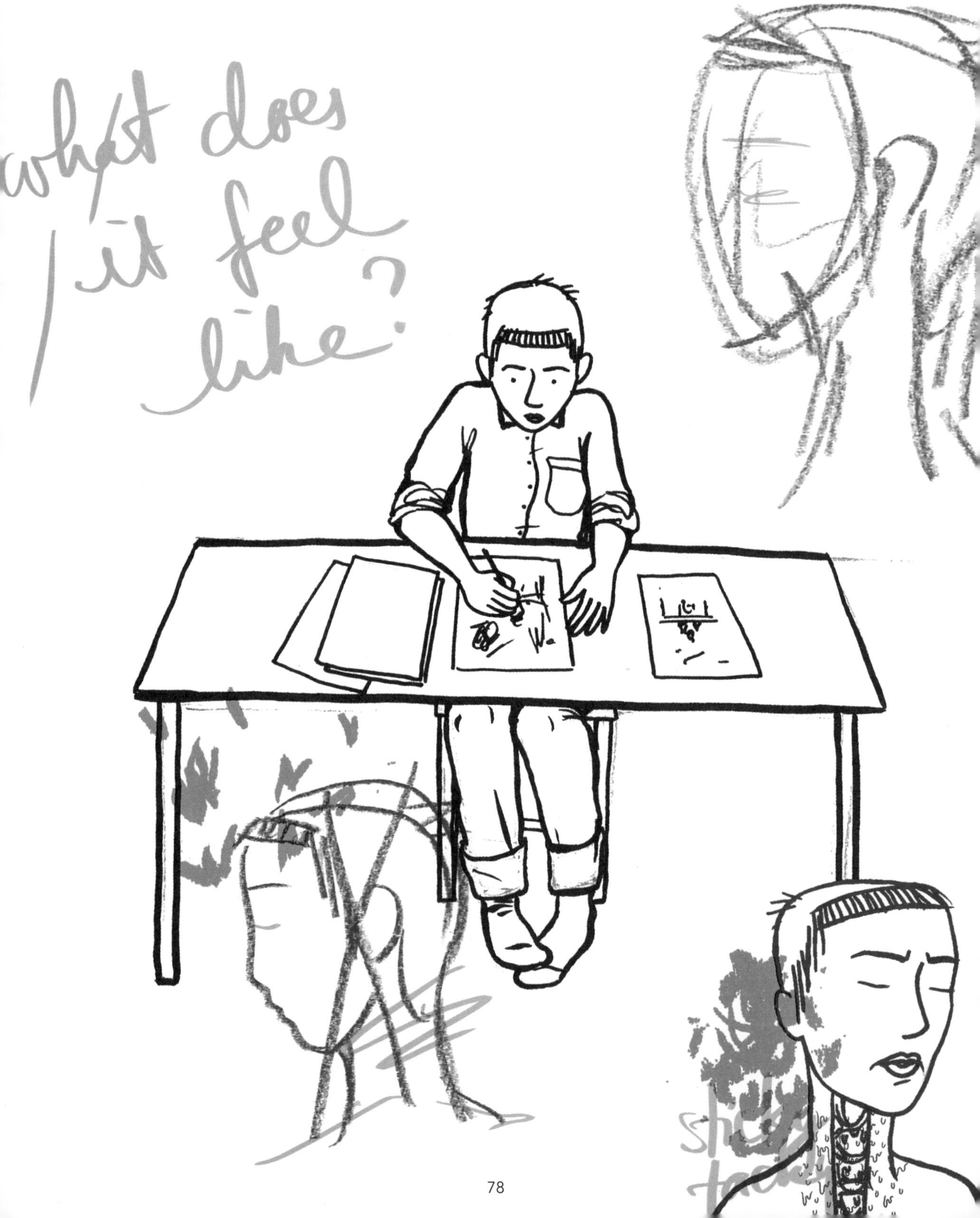
what does it feel like?

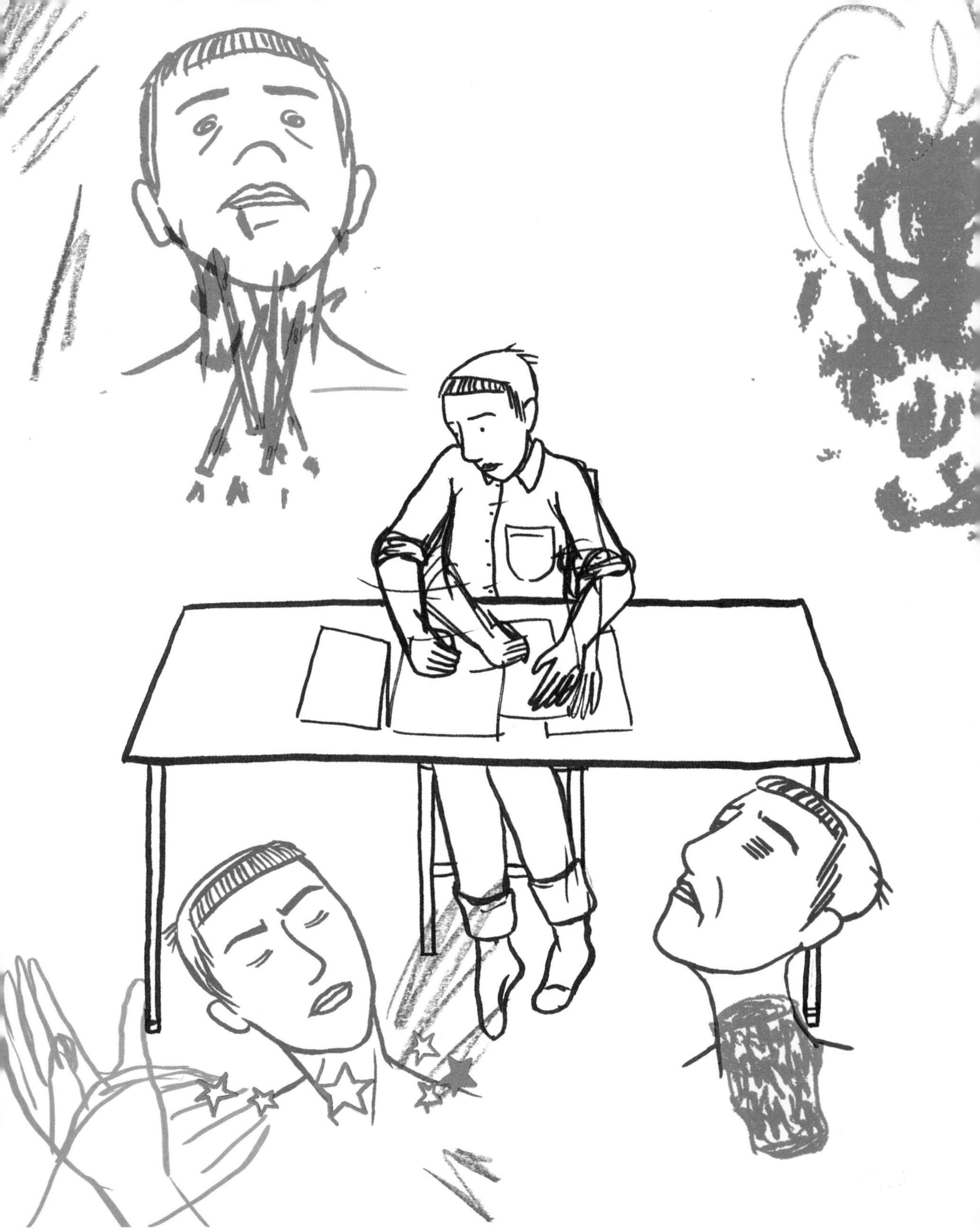

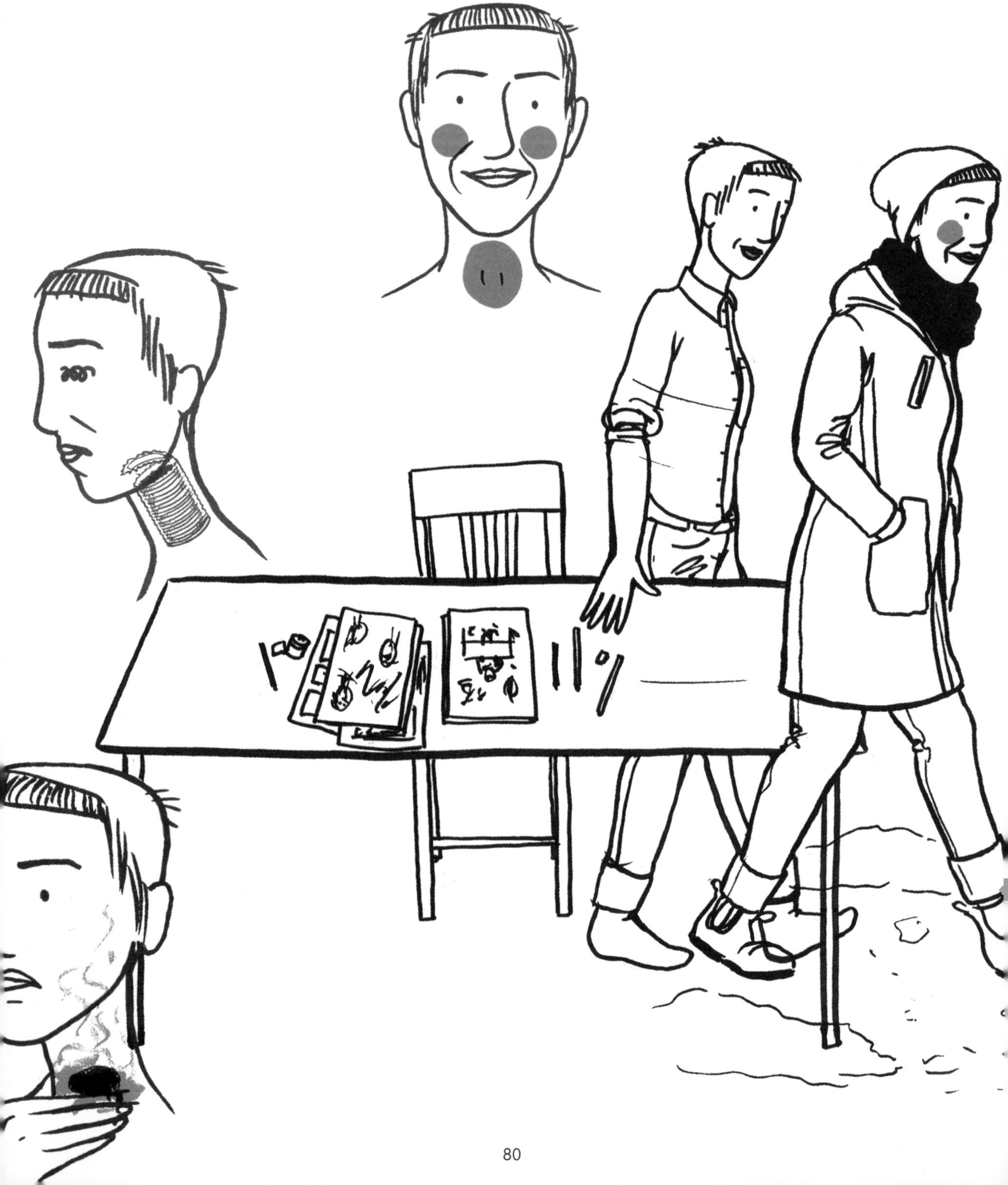

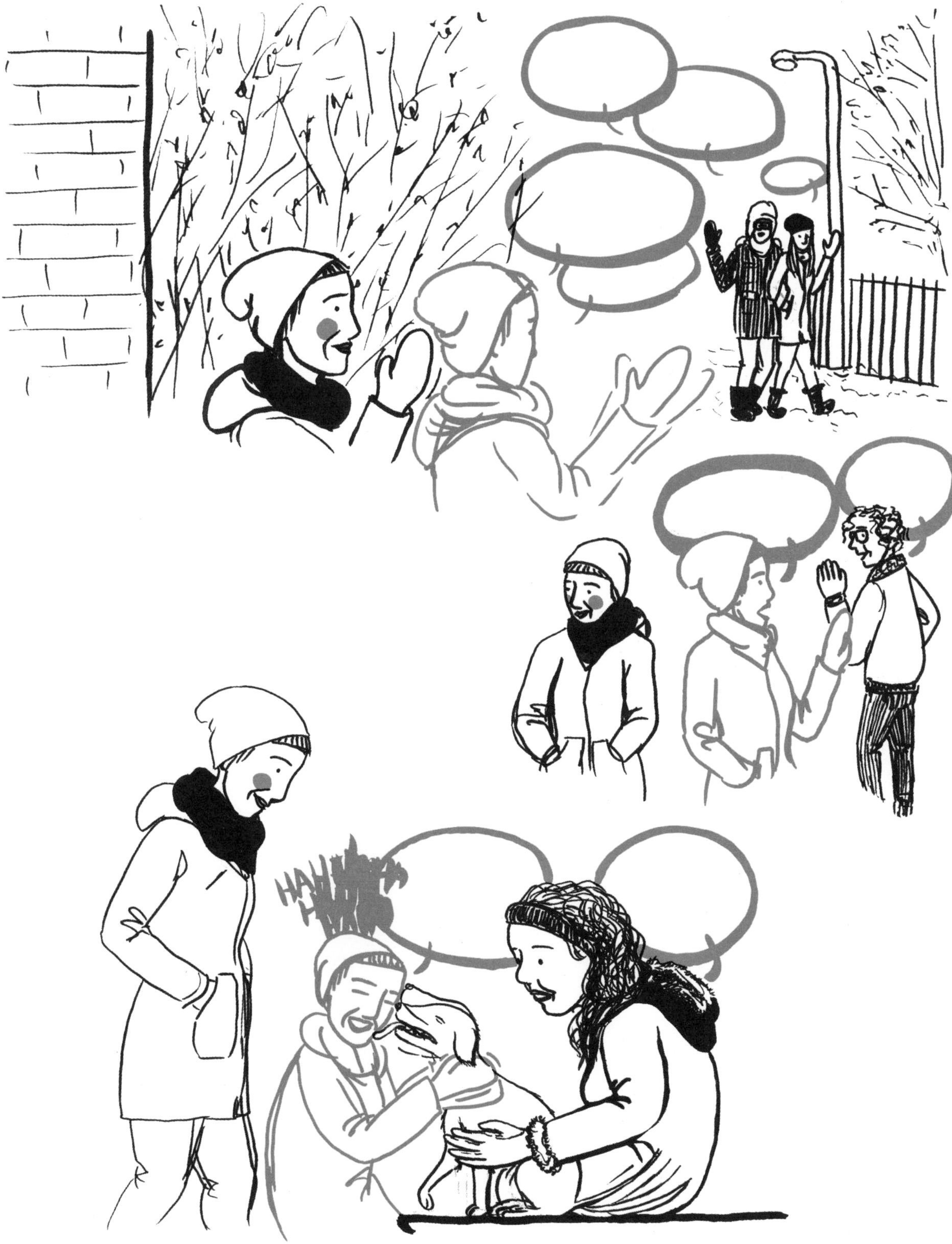
HAH

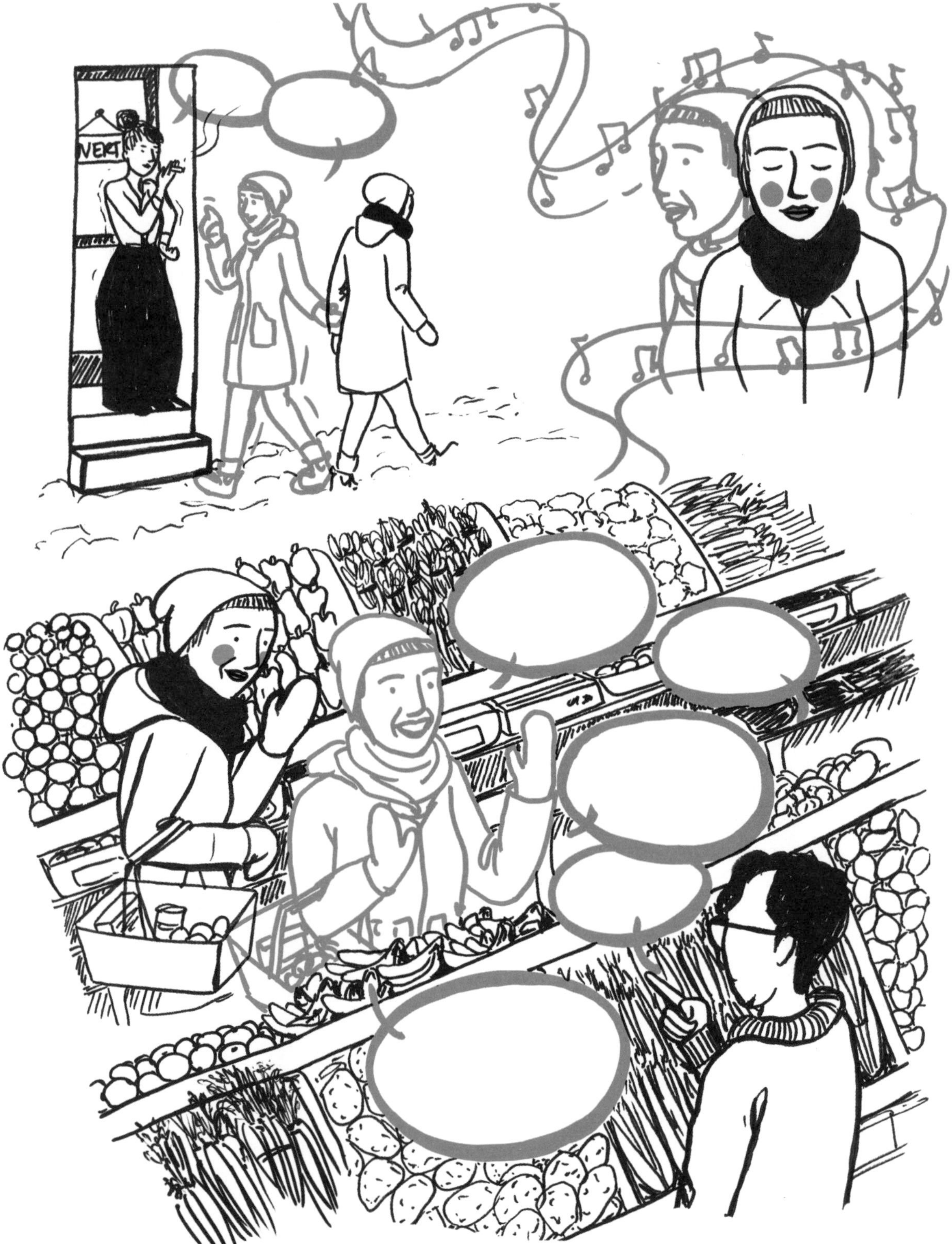
VERT

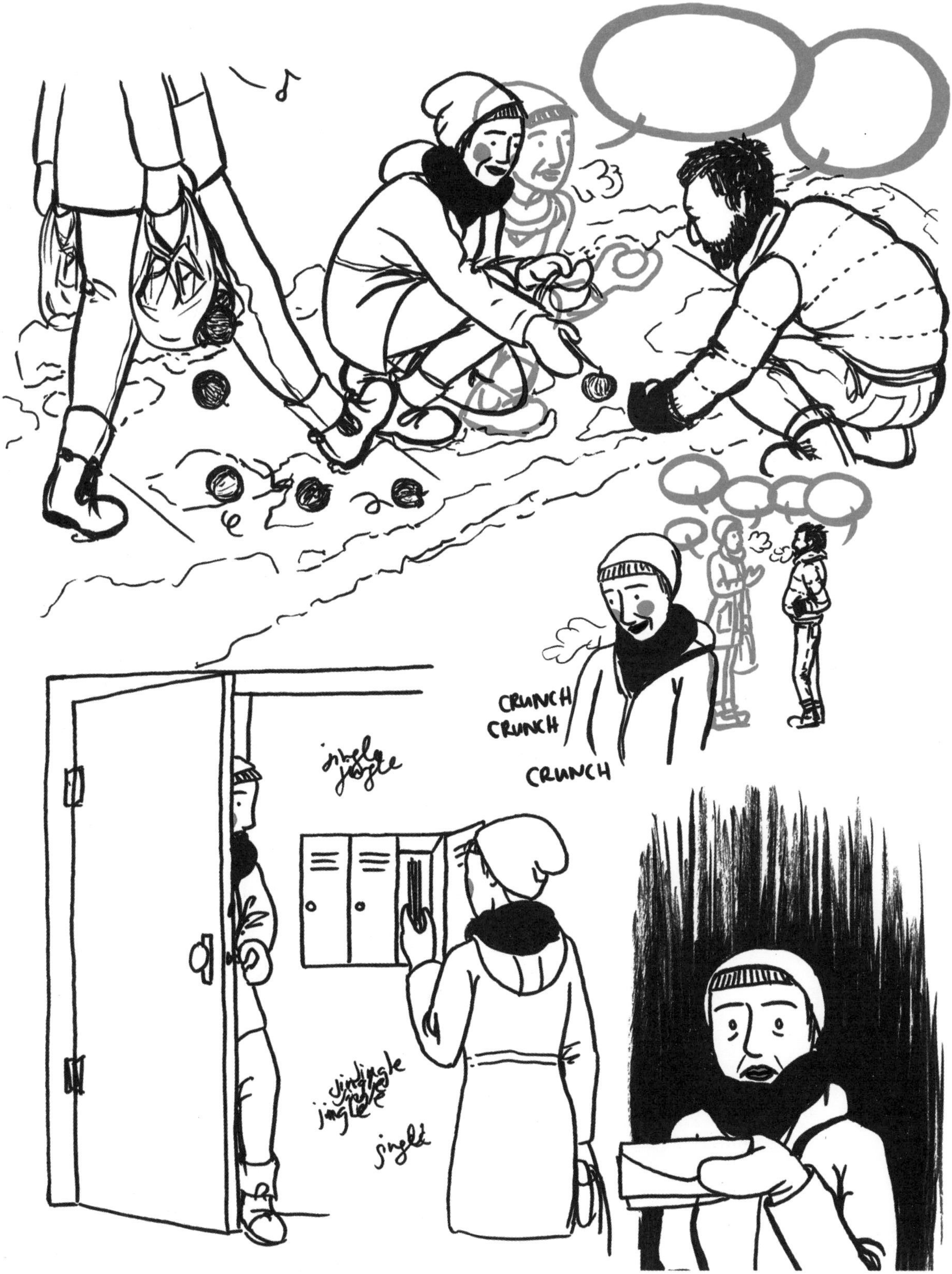
CRUNCH
CRUNCH
CRUNCH
jingle jingle
jingle jingle
jingle
jingle

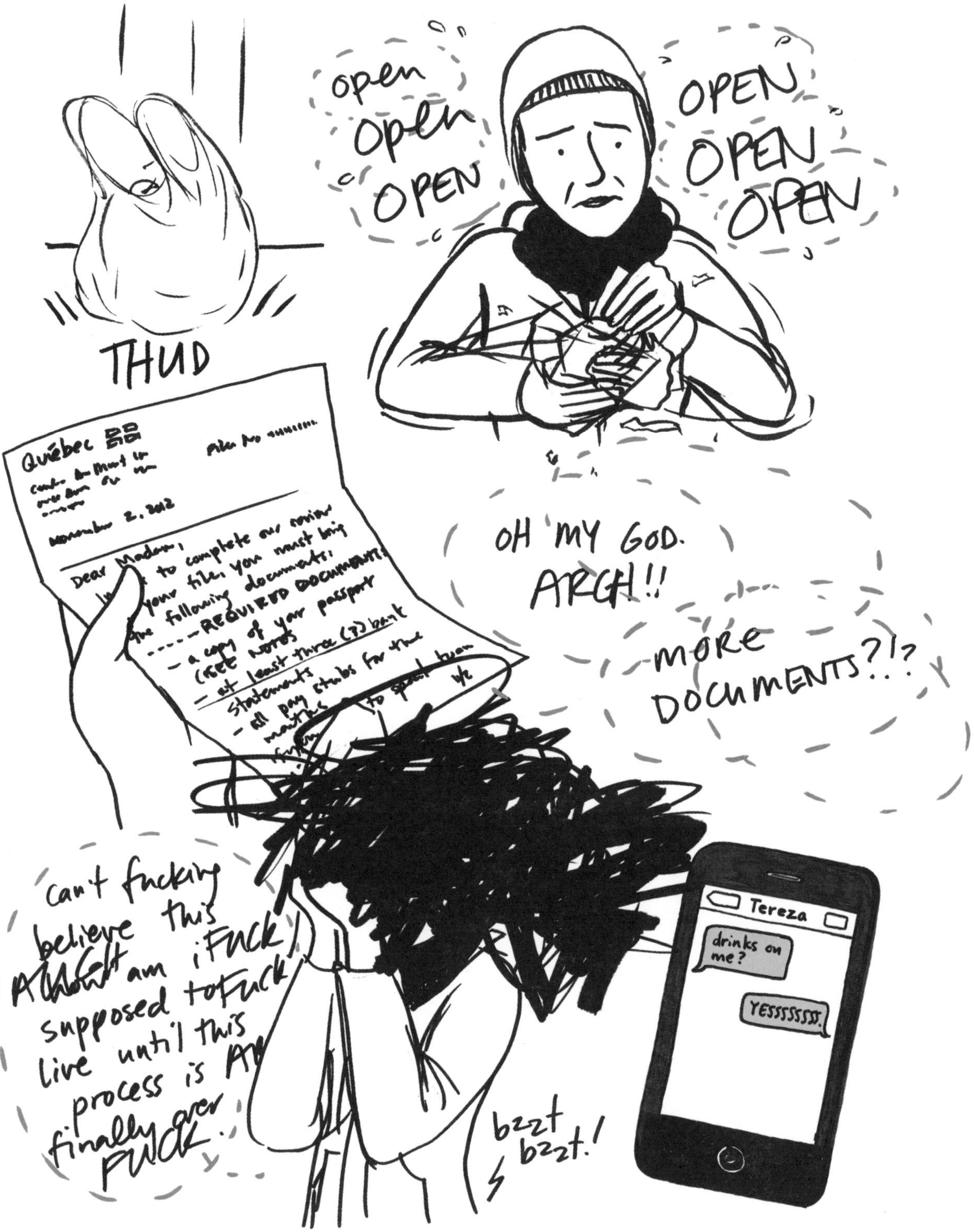
THUD
open
Open
OPEN
OPEN
OPEN
OPEN
Québec
November 2, 2012
Dear Madam,
to complete our review
your file, you must bring
following documents:
REQUIRED DOCUMENTS:
a copy of your passport
(SEE NOTES)
at least three (3) bank
statements
all pay stubs for the
OH MY GOD.
ARGH!!
MORE
DOCUMENTS?!?
can't fucking believe this AAUGH how am i FUCK supposed to FUCK live until this process is AA finally over FUCK
Tereza
drinks on me?
YESSSSSSSS.
bzzt
bzzt!

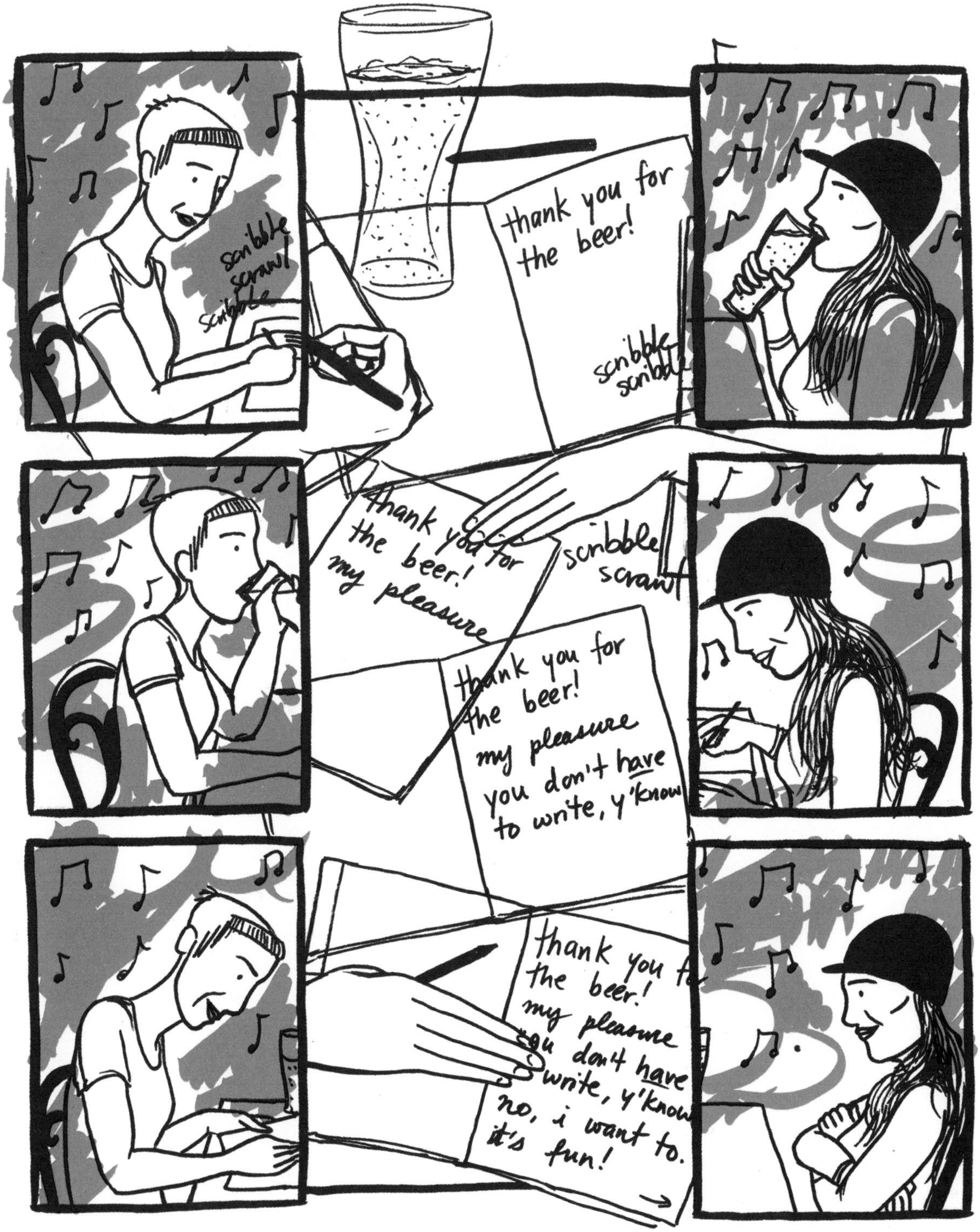

scribble
scrawl
scribble
thank you for the beer!
scribble
scribble
thank you for the beer!
my pleasure
scribble
scrawl
thank you for the beer!
my pleasure
you don't have to write, y'know
thank you fo[r]
the beer!
my pleasure
you don't have
write, y'know
no, i want to.
it's fun!

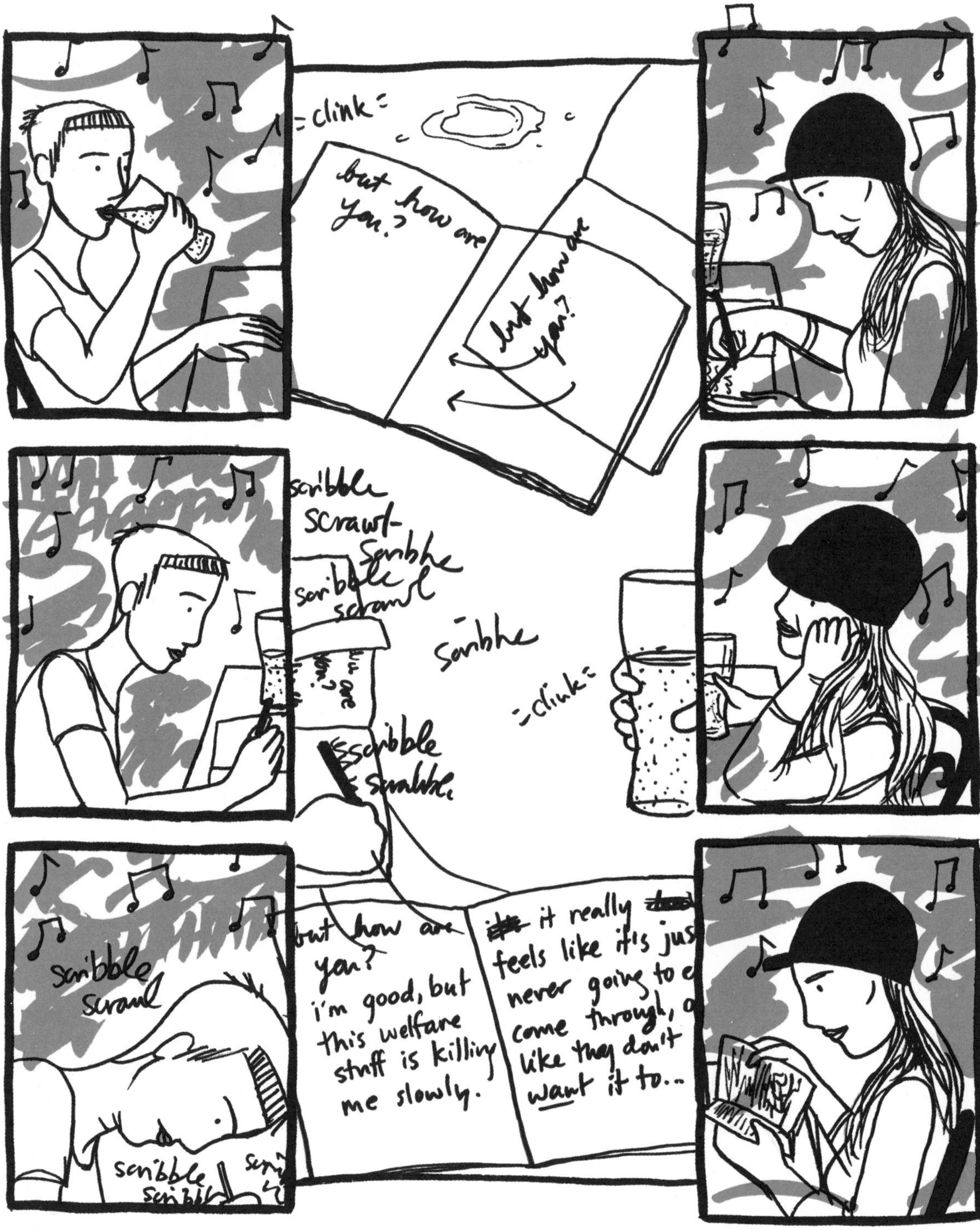
=clink=
but how are you?
but how are you?
scribble
scrawl
scribble
scribble
scrawl
scribble
=clink=
scribble
scrawl
scribble
scrawl
scribble
but how are you?
i'm good, but this welfare stuff is killing me slowly.
it really feels like it's jus never going to e come through, a like they don't want it to...

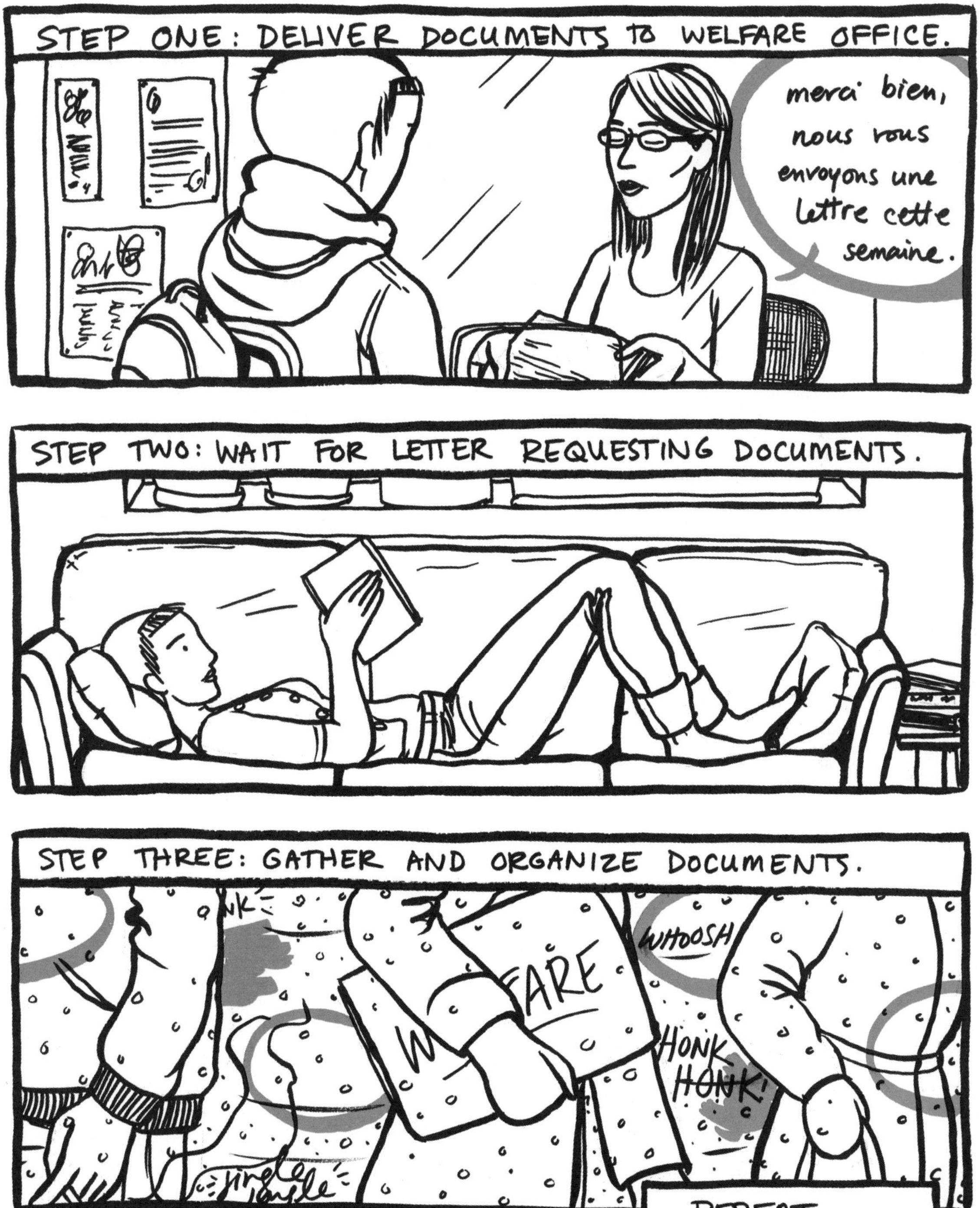
STEP ONE: DELIVER DOCUMENTS TO WELFARE OFFICE.
merci bien, nous vous envoyons une lettre cette semaine.
STEP TWO: WAIT FOR LETTER REQUESTING DOCUMENTS.
STEP THREE: GATHER AND ORGANIZE DOCUMENTS.
WHOOSH
HONK HONK!
jingle jingle
REPEAT.

STEP ONE
bzzt pip bzzt pip bzzt pip bzzt
A21
ES GÉNÉRAL
ICES D'EMPLOI B
S VOLONTAIRES C
NEXT
→A06
bonjour madame. ça va bien?
Québec
November 7, 2012
Dear Madam,
To enable us to complete our study of your file, you must send us:
------REQUIRED DOCUMENTS:
- all the pay slips for the months of SEPT + OCTOBER
- your record of employment
- proof of application
- see notes
celles-ci sont les documents pour votre dossier
merci bien, nous vous envoyons une lettre cette semaine.
STEP TWO
keep breathing

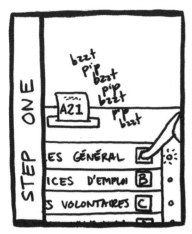

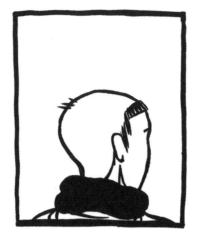

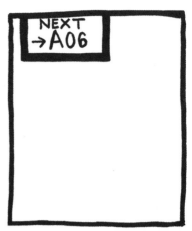

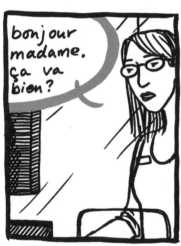

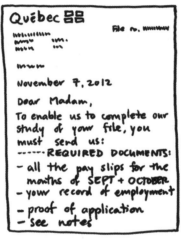

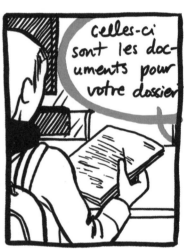

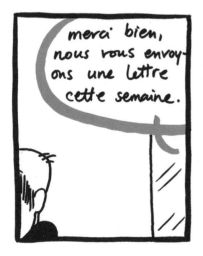

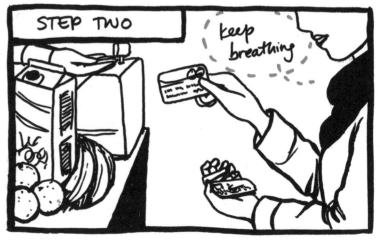

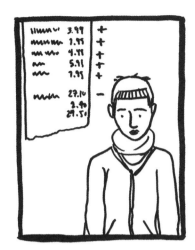

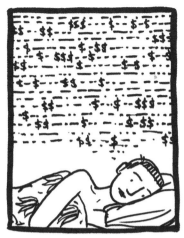

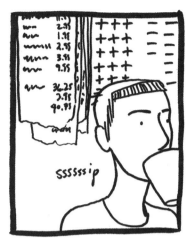

ssssssip
STEP THREE
Québec
GEORGIA WEBBER
Québec
page 1 of 3
File no.
November 12, 2012
Dear Madam,
To enable us to complete our study of your file, you must send us:
REQUIRED DOCUMENTS:
- all the pay stubs for the months of JULY - AUG
- account booklets or statements, including capital stock booklet. (See notes: 2 accounts.)
clink
scribble
scribble
clink
CRUNCH
CRUNCH
WELFARE

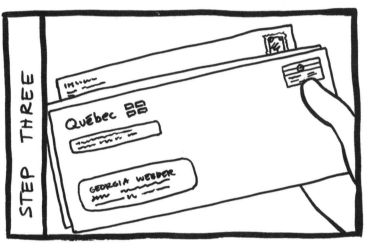

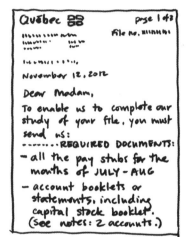

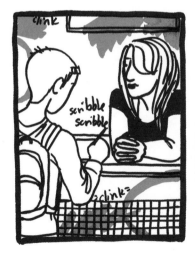

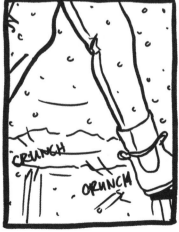

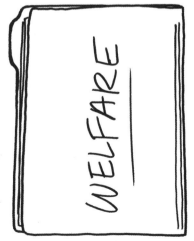

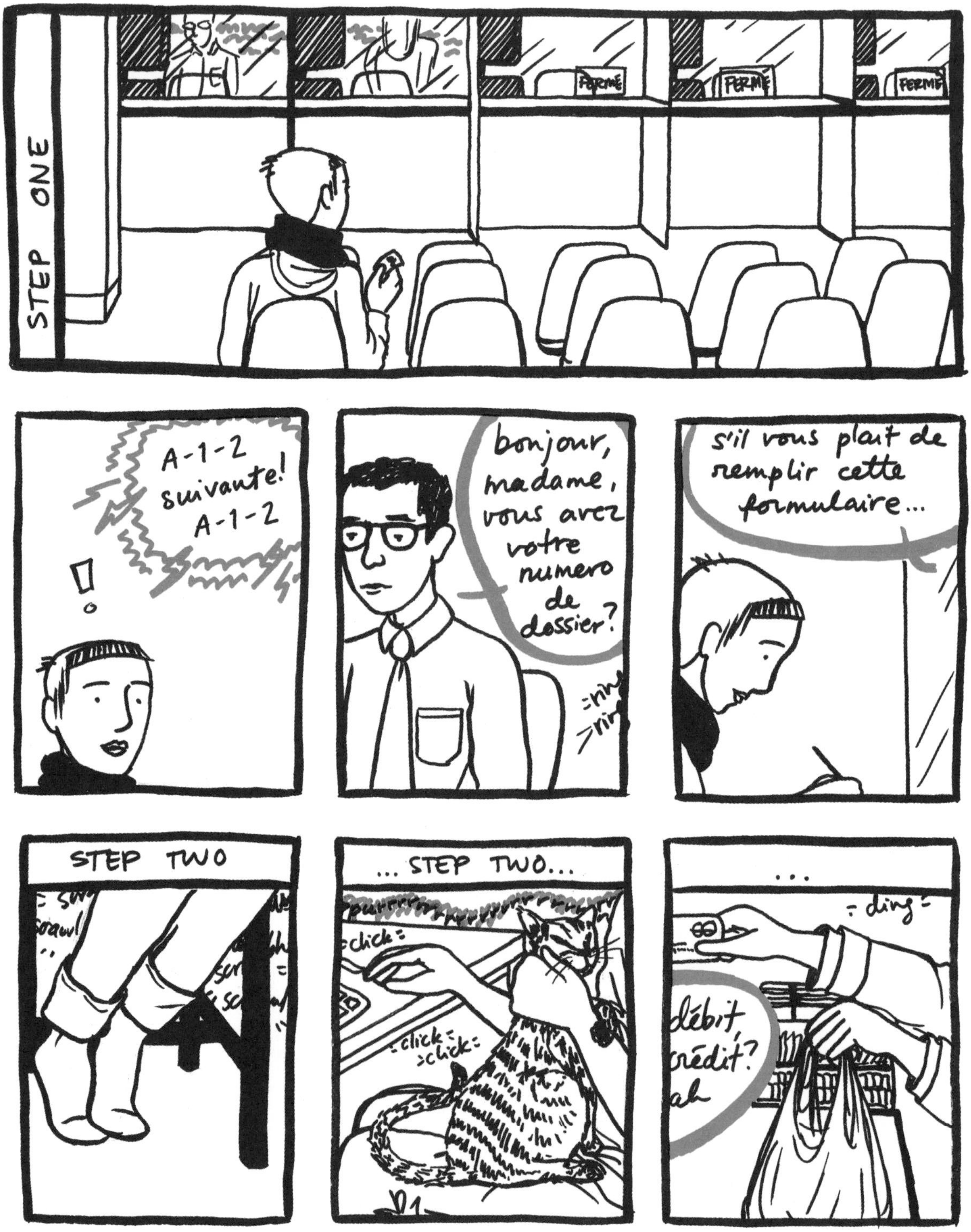
STEP ONE
FERMÉ
FERMÉ
FERMÉ
A-1-2 suivante! A-1-2
!
bonjour, madame, vous avez votre numero de dossier?
s'il vous plait de remplir cette formulaire...
STEP TWO
... STEP TWO...
click
click click
...
ding
débit,

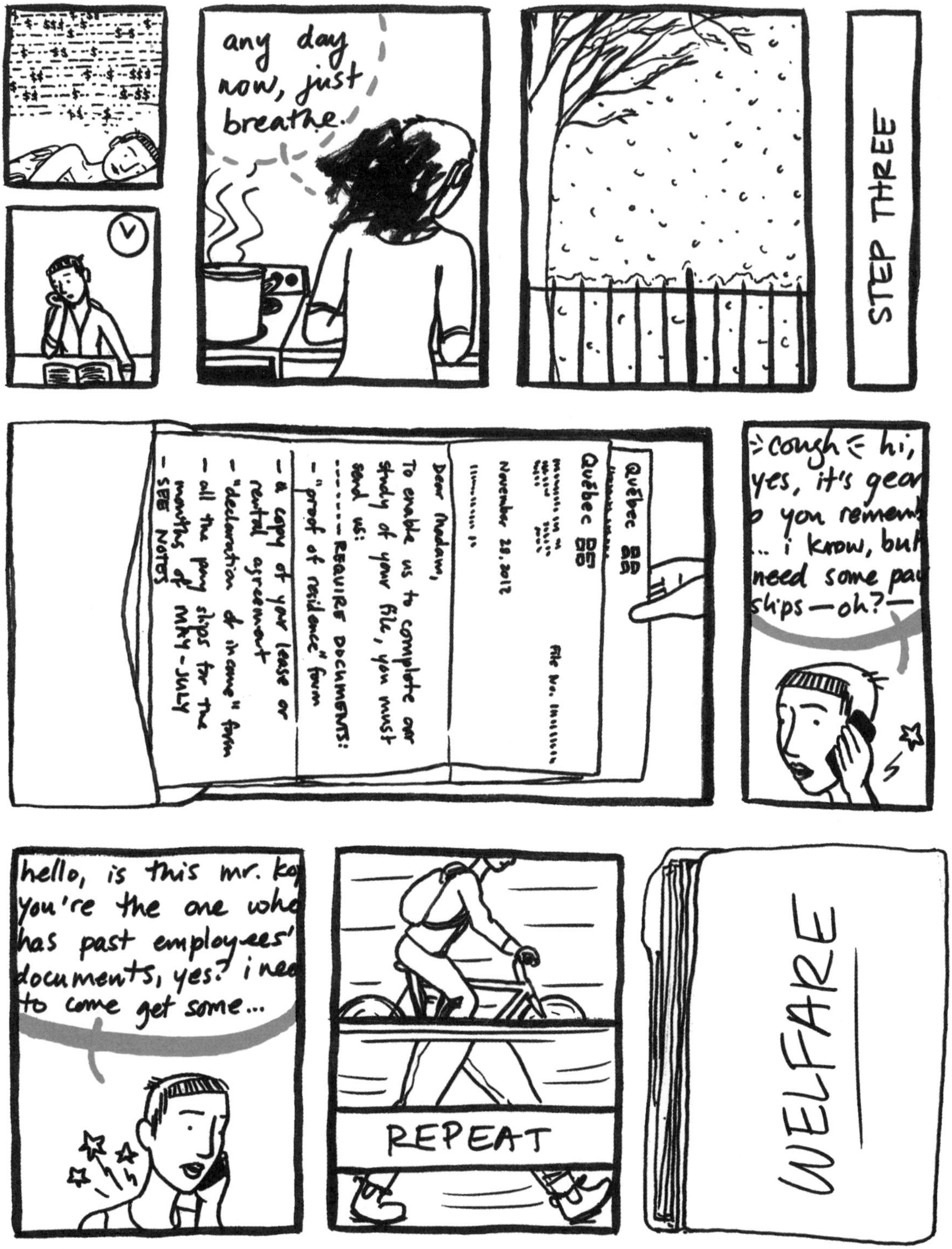
any day now, just breathe.
STEP THREE
Québec
November 28, 2012
File No.
Dear Madam,
To enable us to complete our study of your file, you must send us:
REQUIRED DOCUMENTS:
- "proof of residence" form
- a copy of your lease or rental agreement
- "declaration of income" form
- all the pay slips for the months of MAY-JULY
- SEE NOTES
cough hi, yes, it's geor
o you remem
... i know, but
need some pa
slips—oh?—
hello, is this mr. ko
you're the one who
has past employees'
documents, yes? i nee
to come get some...
REPEAT
WELFARE

STEP ONE
bzzt pip bzzt pip bzzt pip bzzt
A21
NEXT →A06
bonjour madam, ça va bien?
Québec
November 9, 2012
Dear Madam,
To enable us to complete our study of your file, you must send us:
REQUIRED DOCUMENTS:
- all the pay slips for the months of SEPT + OCTOBER
celles-ci sont les documents pour votre dossier
STEP ONE
hein?
Sébastien
c'est la femme qui ne parle pas.
how long will it take?
STEP TWO
DECEMBER
STEP TWO
pace
pace
STEP TWO
STEP THREE
A-1-2
Québec
Québec
Québec
Québec
PAY STUBS
PAY STUBS EM CAFÉ

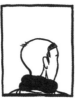

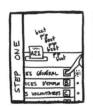

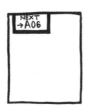

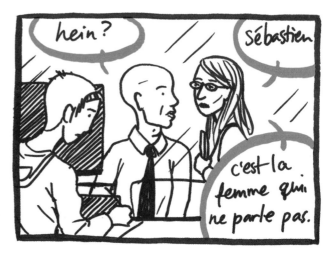

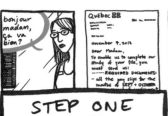

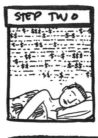

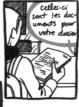

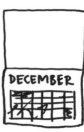

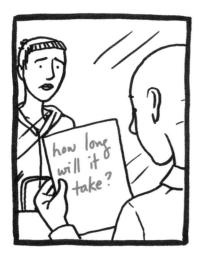

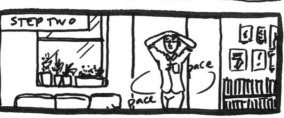

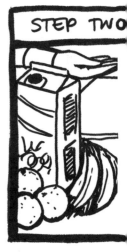

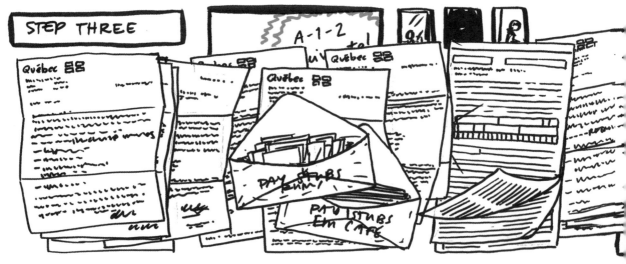

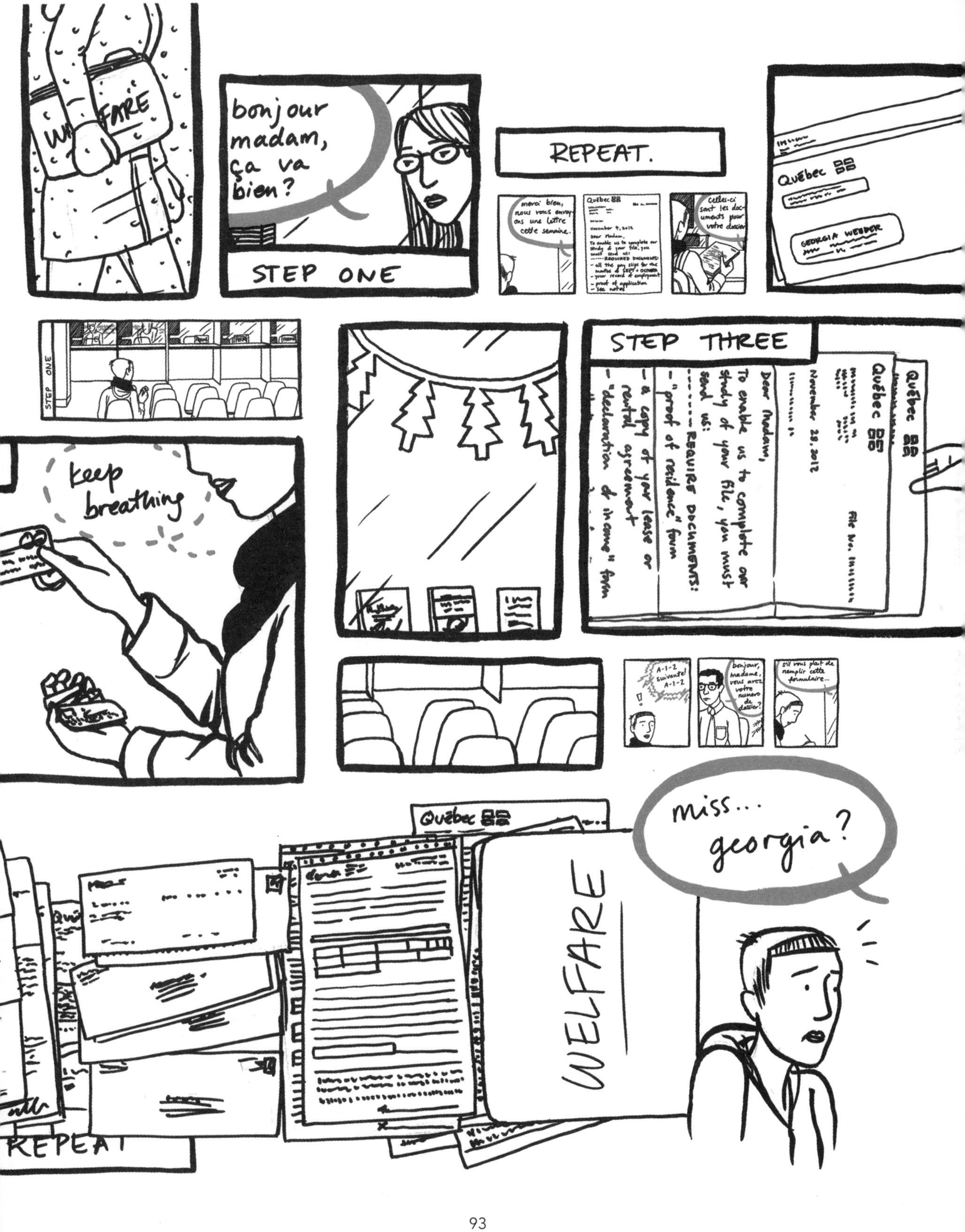
WELFARE
bonjour madam, ça va bien?
STEP ONE
REPEAT.
merci bien, nous vous envoyons une lettre cette semaine.
celles-ci sont les documents pour votre dossier
Québec
GEORGIA WEBBER
STEP ONE
keep breathing
STEP THREE
Québec
November 28, 2012
Dear Madam,
To enable us to complete our study of your file, you must send us:
------- REQUIRED DOCUMENTS:
- "proof of residence" form
- a copy of your lease or rental agreement
- "declaration of income" form
A-1-2 suivante! A-1-2
bonjour, madame, vous avez votre numero de dossier?
s'il vous plaît de remplir cette formulaire...
Québec
WELFARE
miss... georgia?
REPEAT

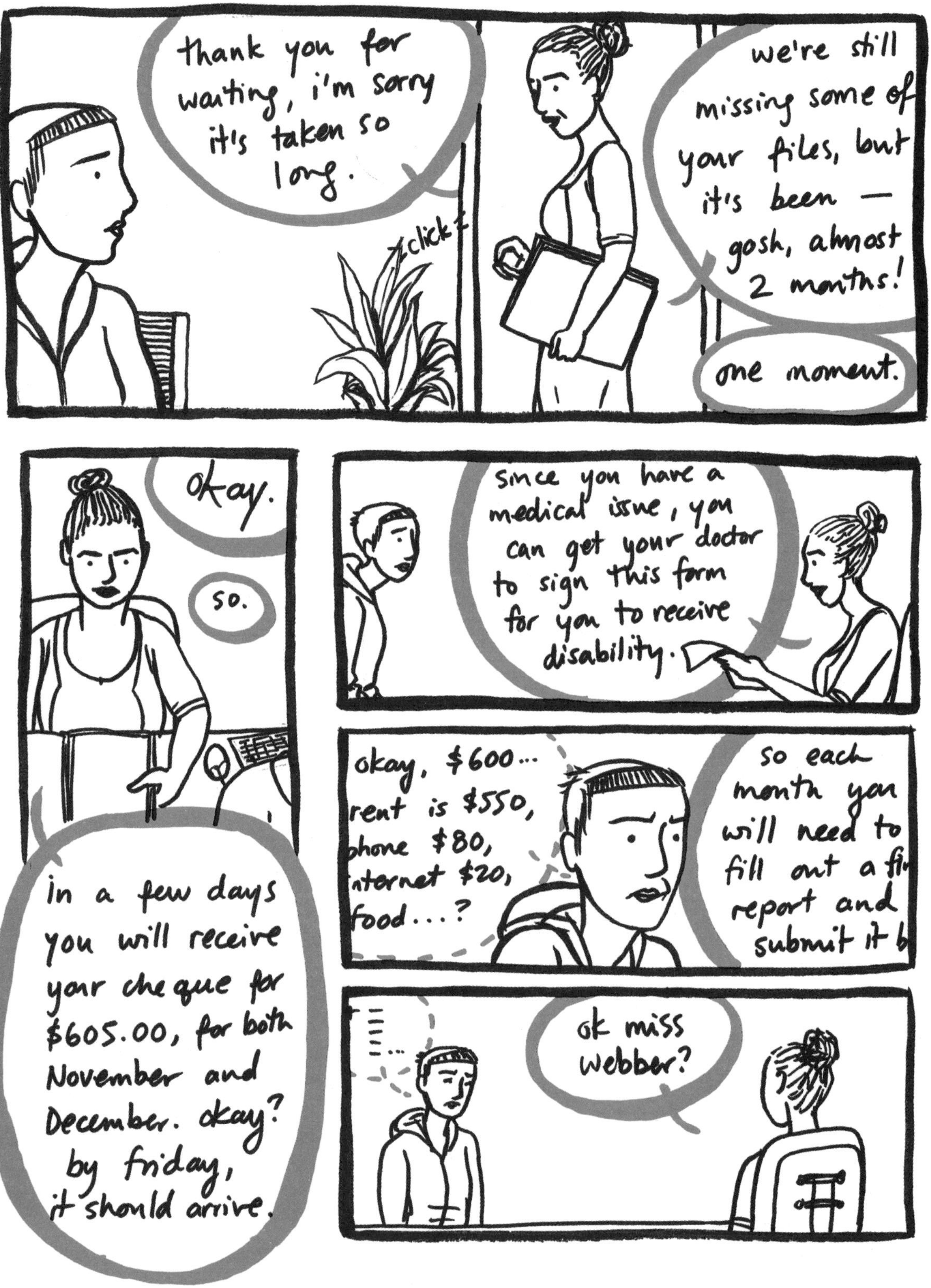
thank you for waiting, i'm sorry it's taken so long.
click
we're still missing some of your files, but it's been — gosh, almost 2 months!
one moment.
okay.
so.
in a few days you will receive your cheque for $605.00, for both November and December. okay? by friday, it should arrive.
since you have a medical issue, you can get your doctor to sign this form for you to receive disability.
okay, $600... rent is $550, phone $80, internet $20, food...?
so each month you will need to fill out a
report and submit it
ok miss webber?

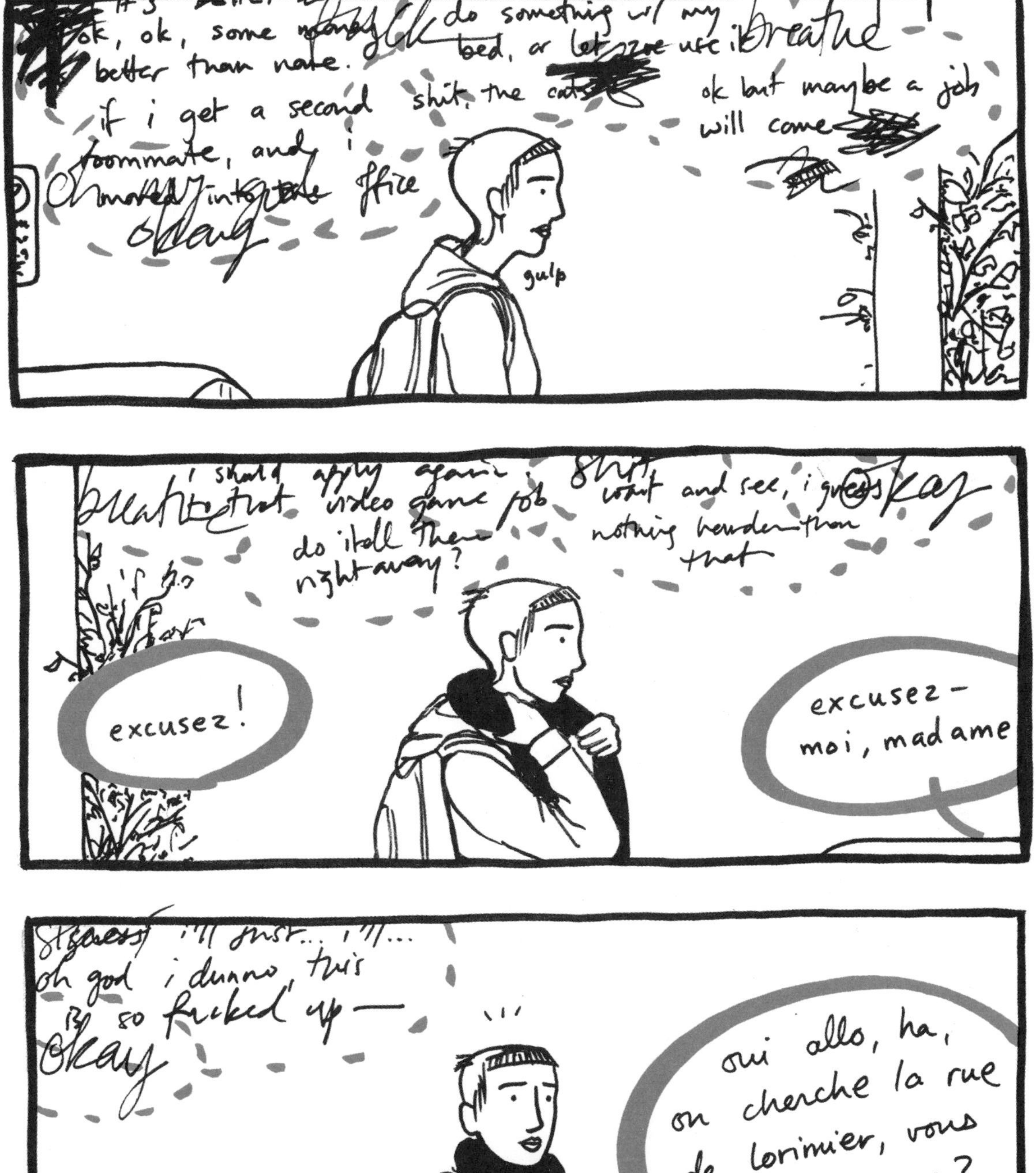
ok, ok, some
better than none.
do something w/ my
bed, or
breathe
if i get a second
roommate, and i
okay
shit, the cats
ok but maybe a job
will come
gulp
i should apply again
video game job
breathe
shit
wait and see, i guess
okay
do it all there
right away?
nothing harder than
that
excusez!
excusez-moi, madame
i'll just... i'll...
oh god i dunno this
is so fucked up —
okay
oui allo, ha, on cherche la rue de lorimier, vous la connaissez?

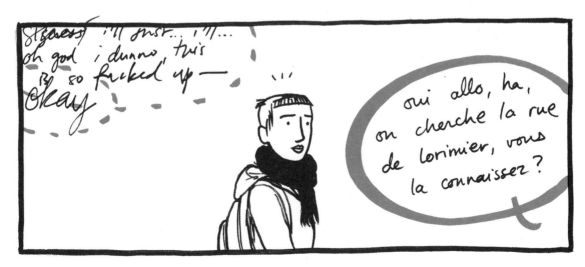

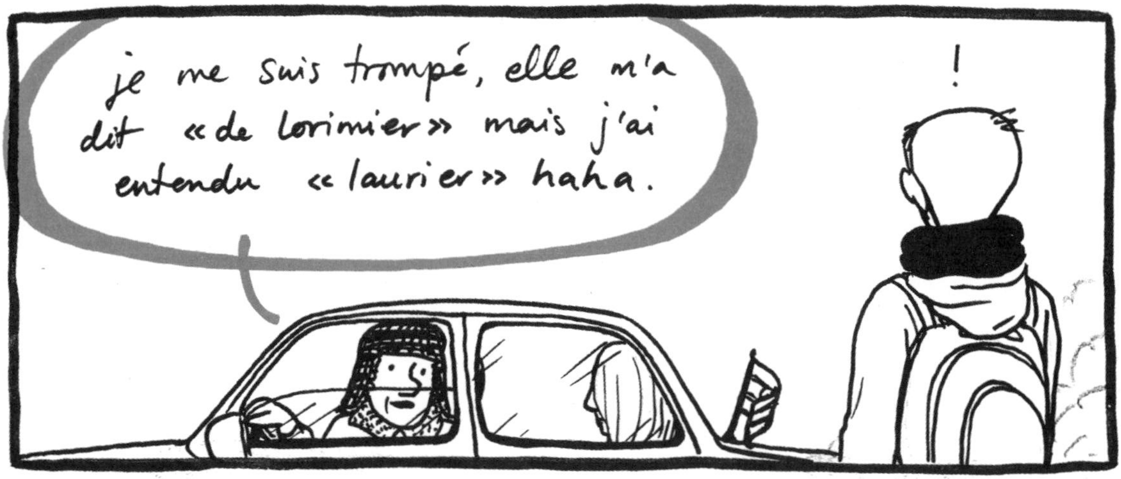
je me suis trompé, elle m'a dit «de lorimier» mais j'ai entendu «laurier» haha.
!

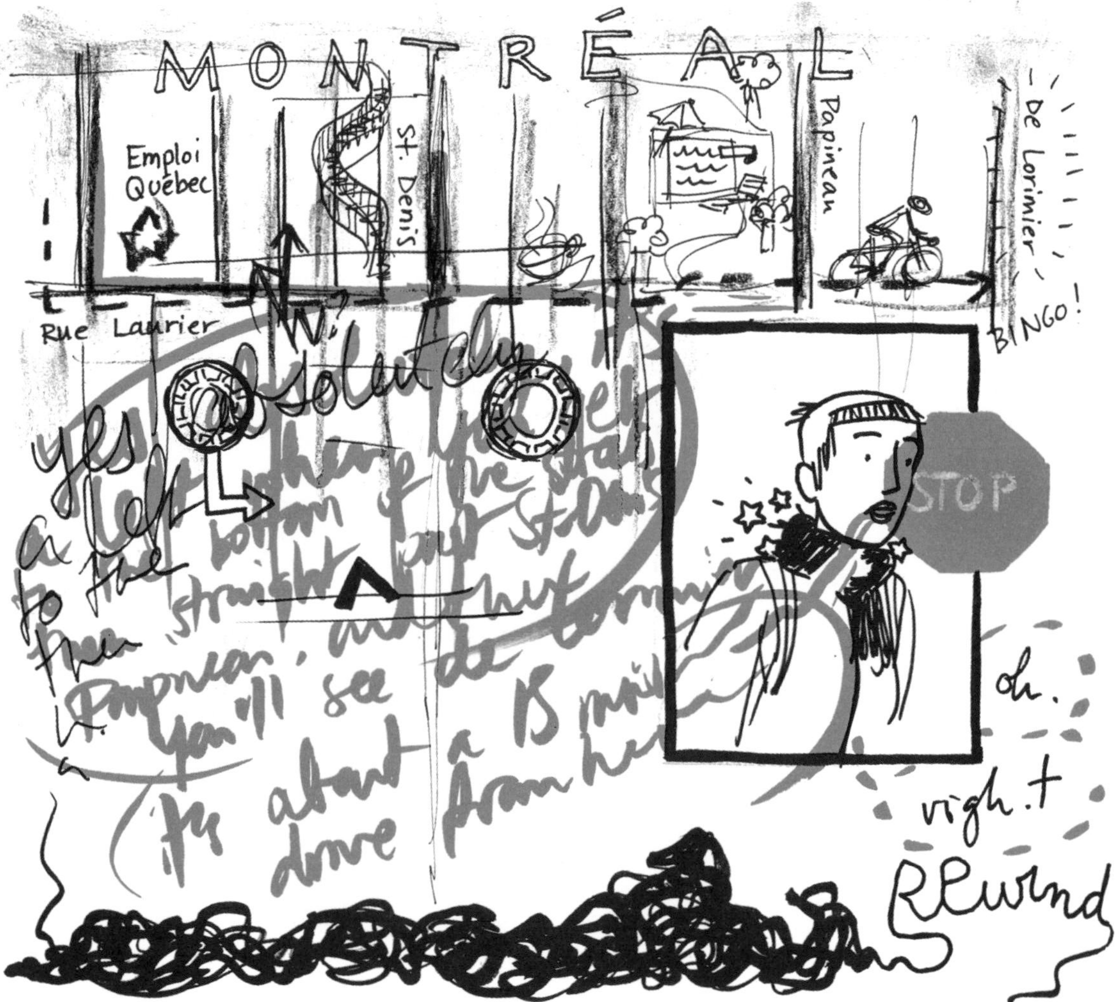
MONTRÉAL
Emploi Québec
St. Denis
Papineau
De Lorimier
Rue Laurier
BINGO!
STOP
oh.
right
REWIND

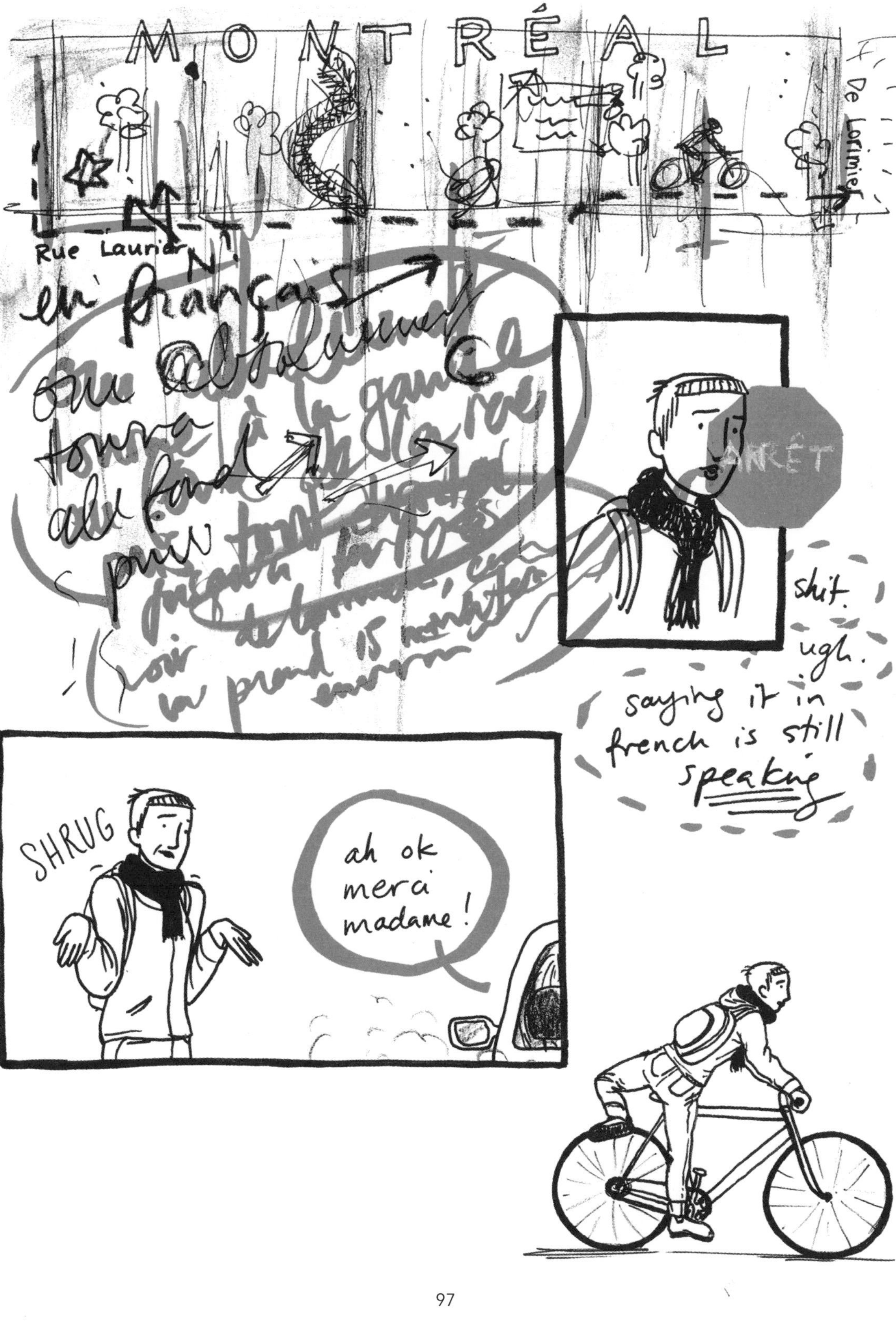
MONTRÉAL
Rue Laurier
N
De Lorimier
en français
ARRÊT
shit.
ugh.
saying it in french is still speaking
SHRUG
ah ok merci madame!

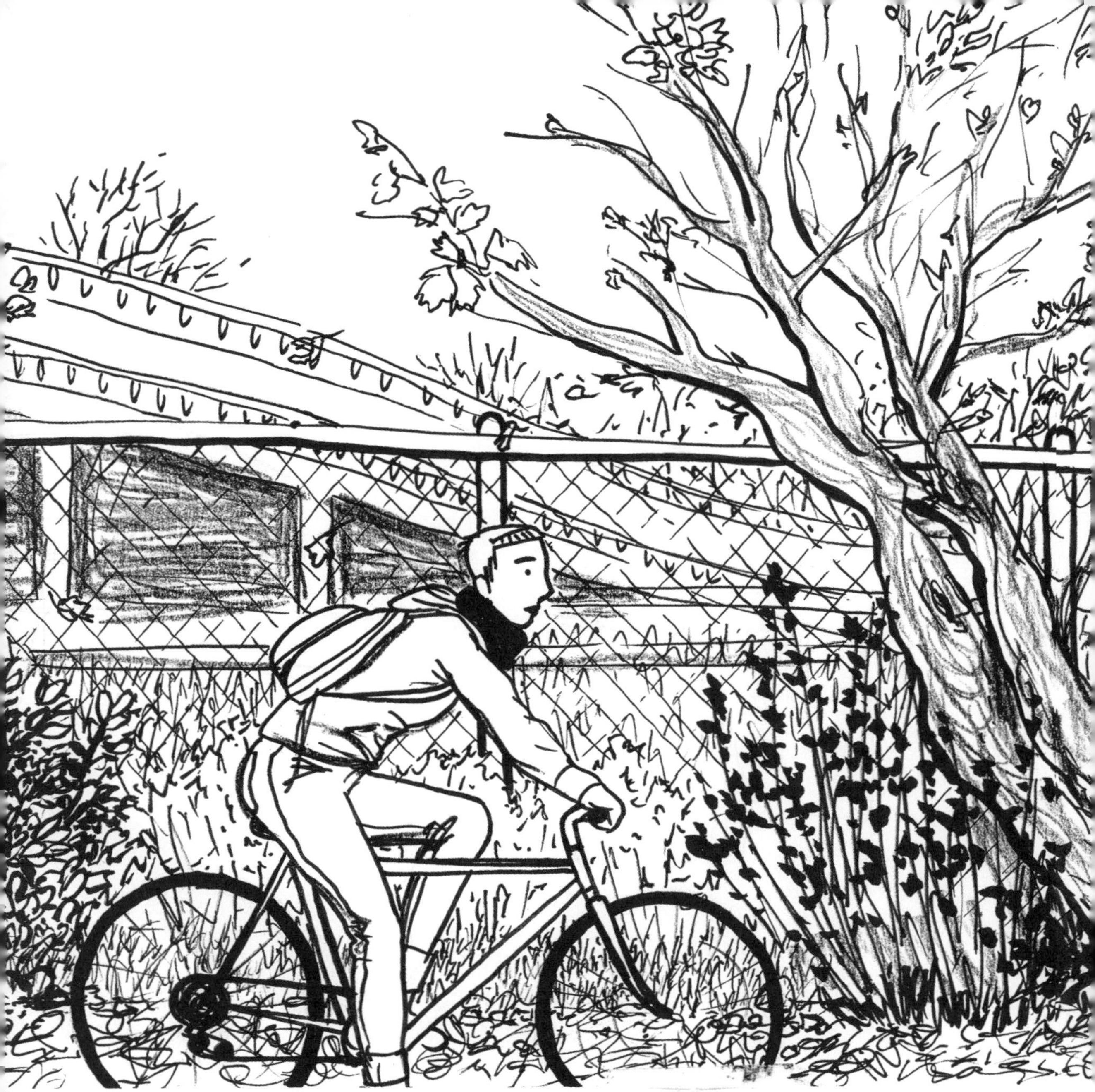

montréal, my home, is a city of languages.

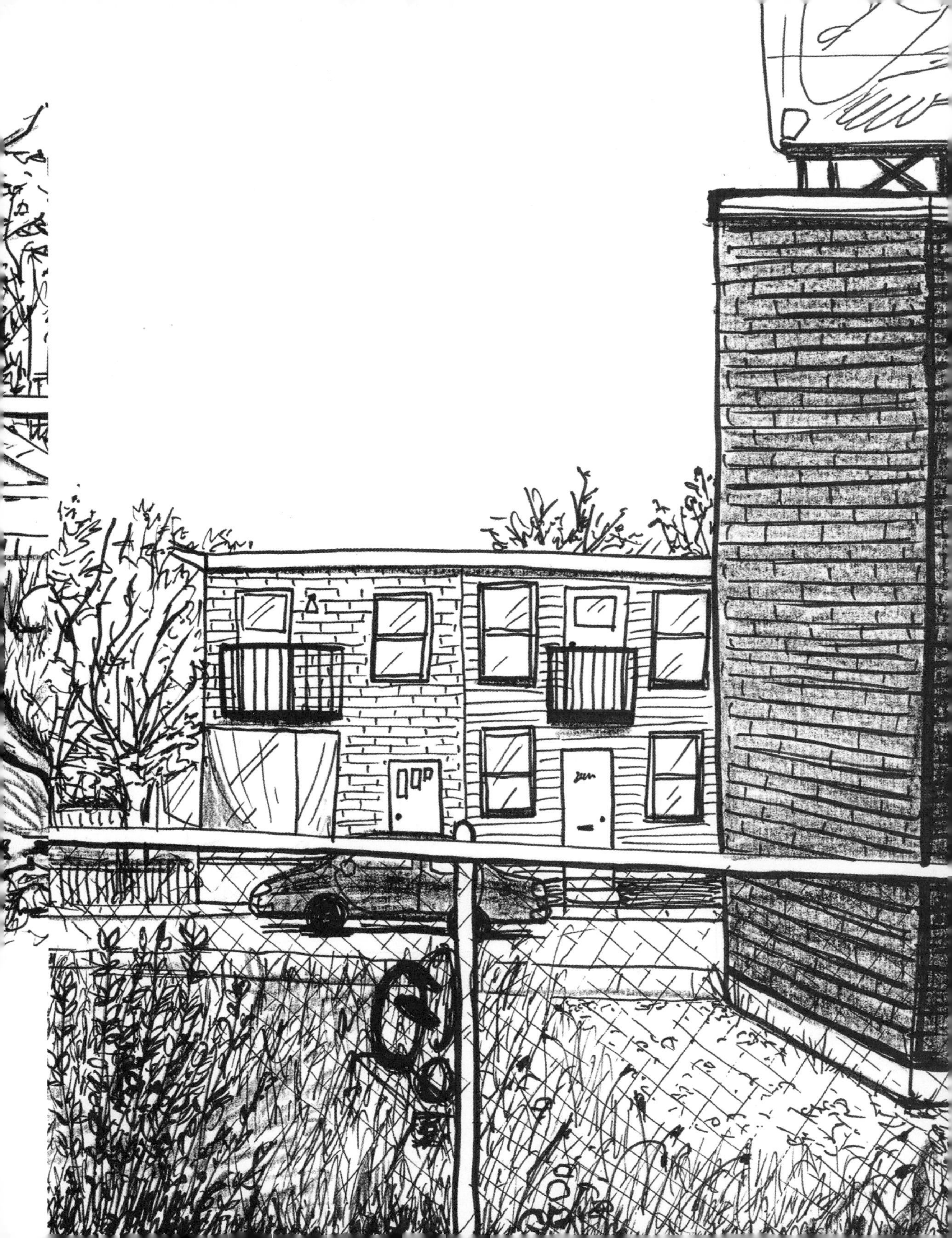

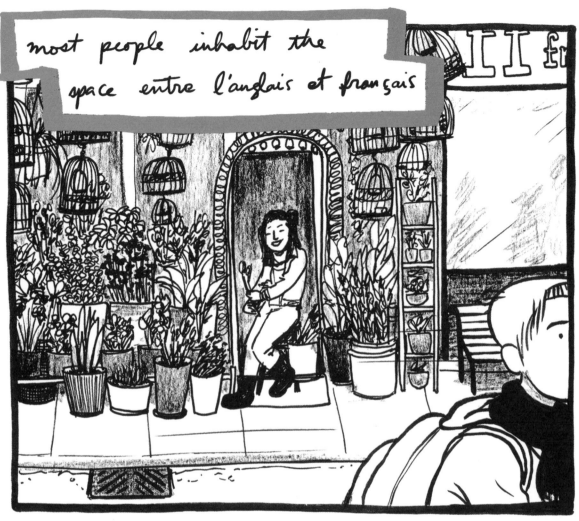

most people inhabit the
space entre l'anglais et français

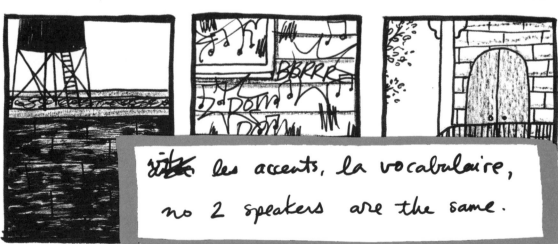

les accents, la vocabulaire,
no 2 speakers are the same.

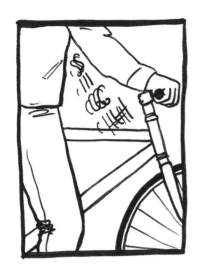
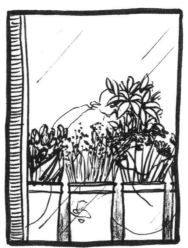
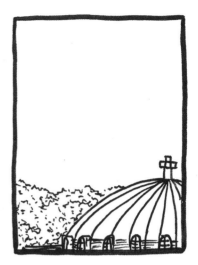

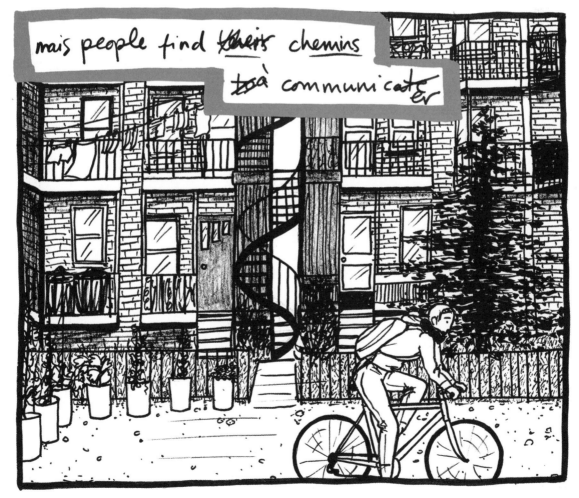
mais people find ~~their~~ chemins ~~to~~ à communicat~~e~~er

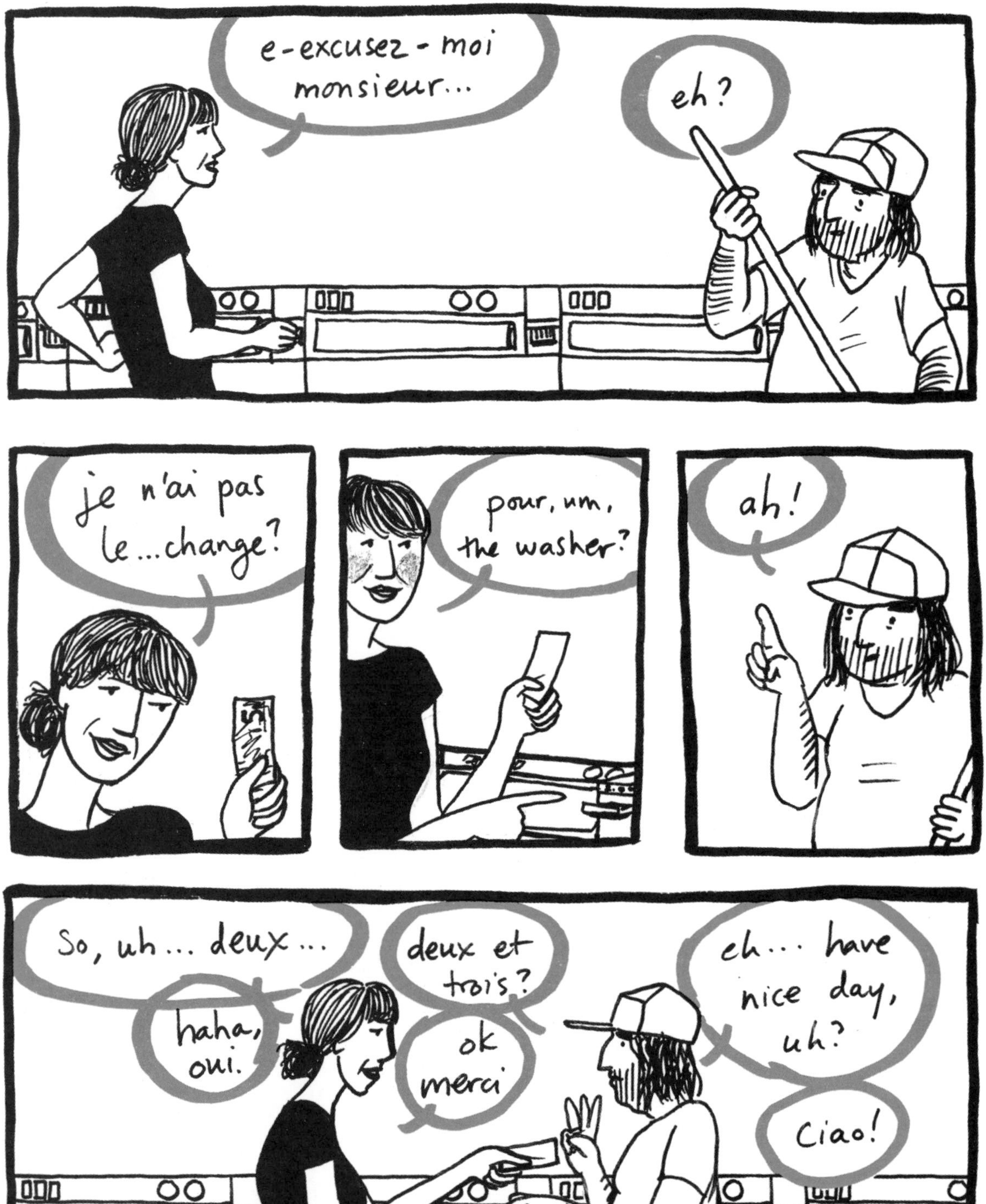
e-excusez-moi monsieur...
eh?
je n'ai pas le...change?
pour, um, the washer?
ah!
So, uh... deux...
haha, oui.
deux et trois?
ok merci
eh... have nice day, uh?
Ciao!

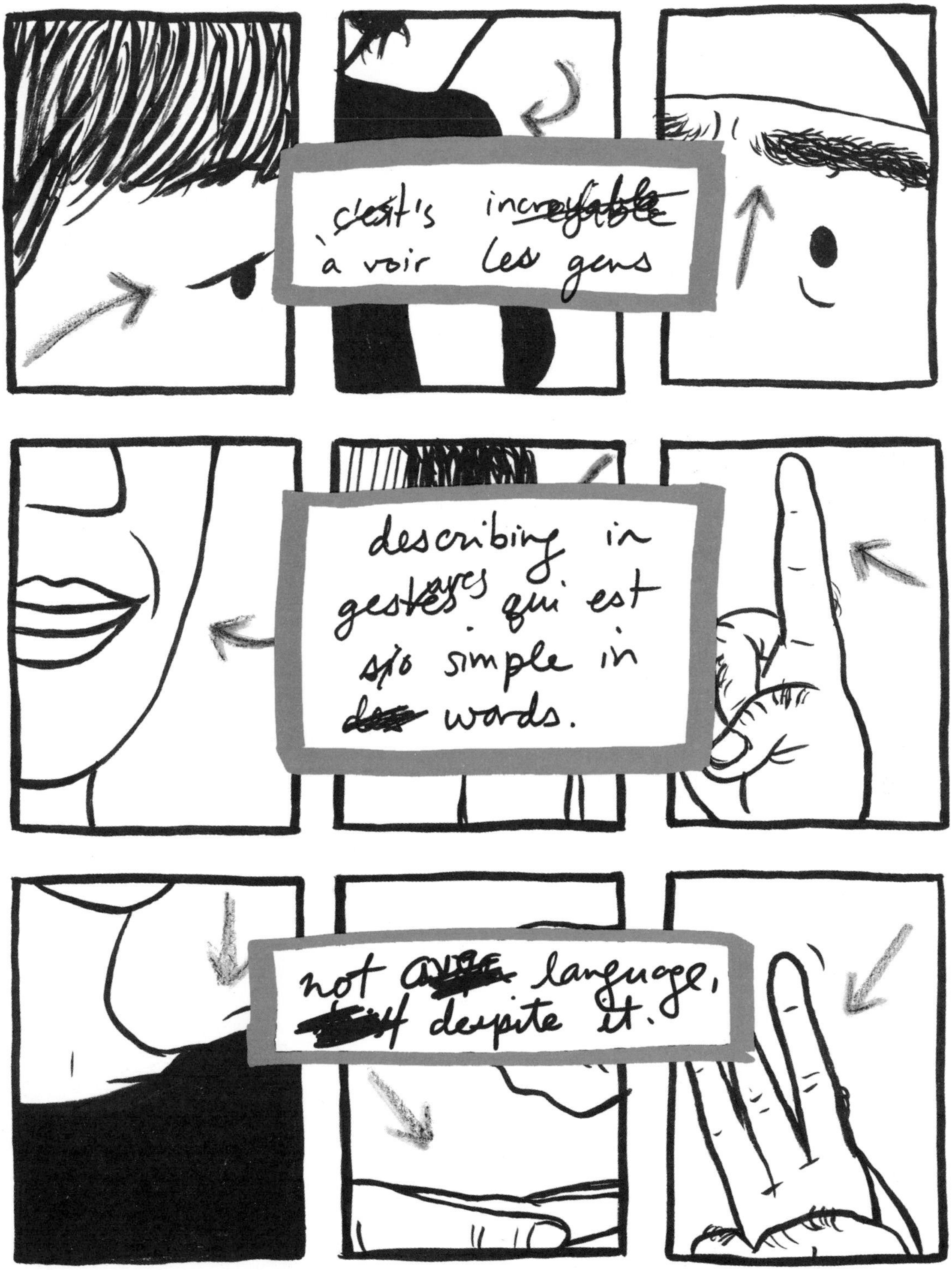

it's incredible à voir les gens
describing in gestures qui est so simple in words.
not language, despite it.

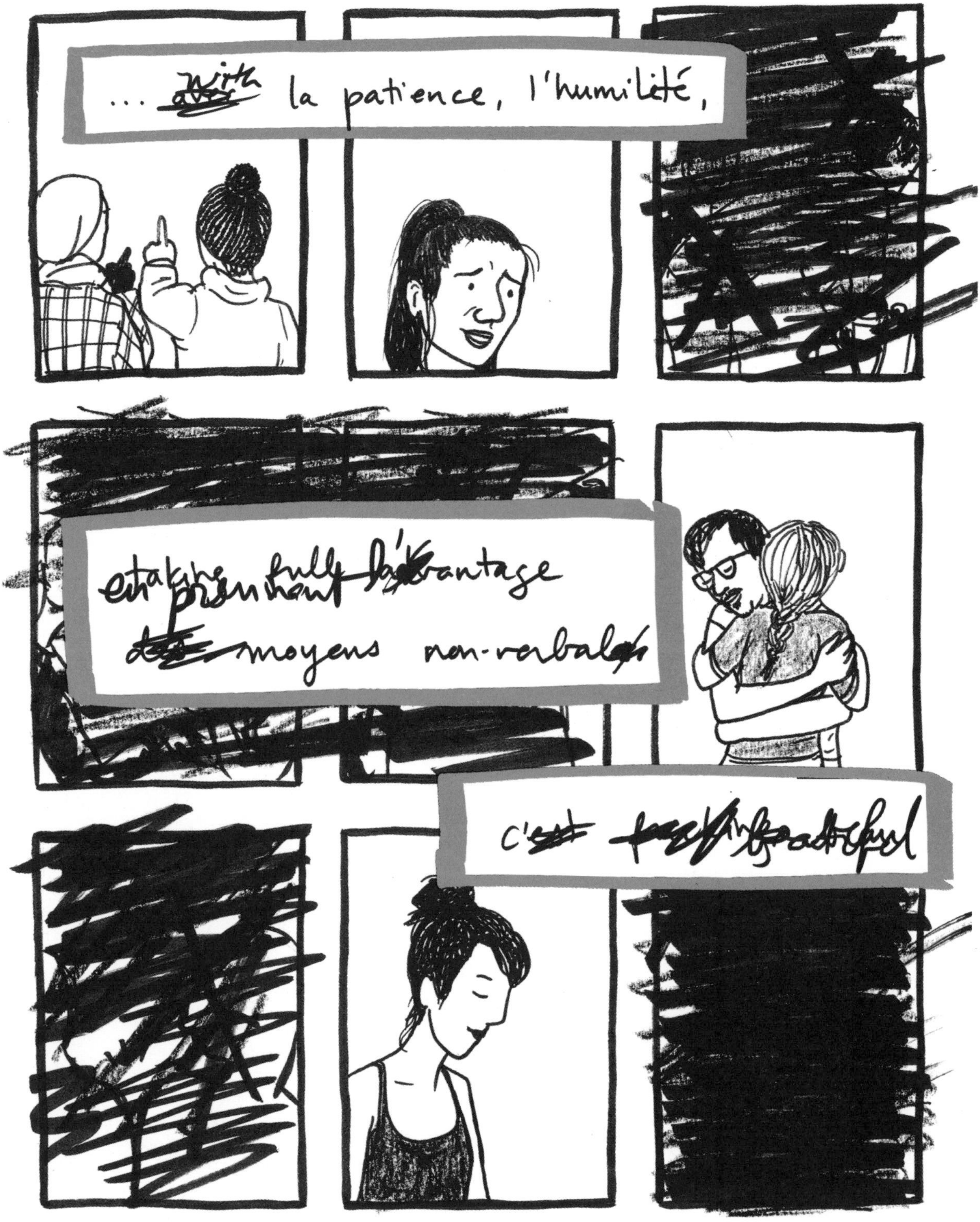
... with la patience, l'humilité,
taking full
en prenant l'avantage
moyens non-verbal
c'

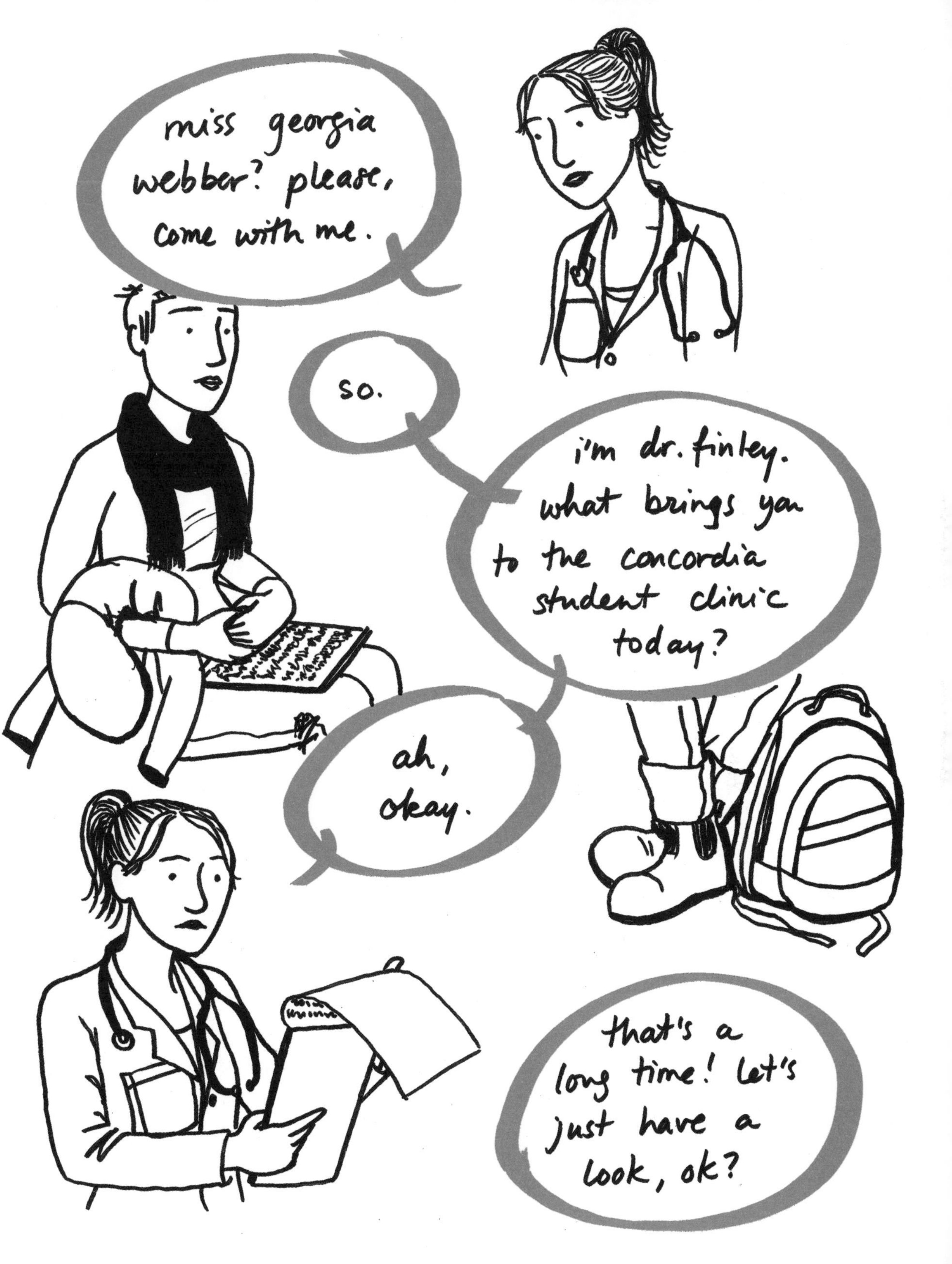
miss georgia webber? please, come with me.
so.
i'm dr. finley. what brings you to the concordia student clinic today?
ah, okay.
that's a long time! let's just have a look, ok?

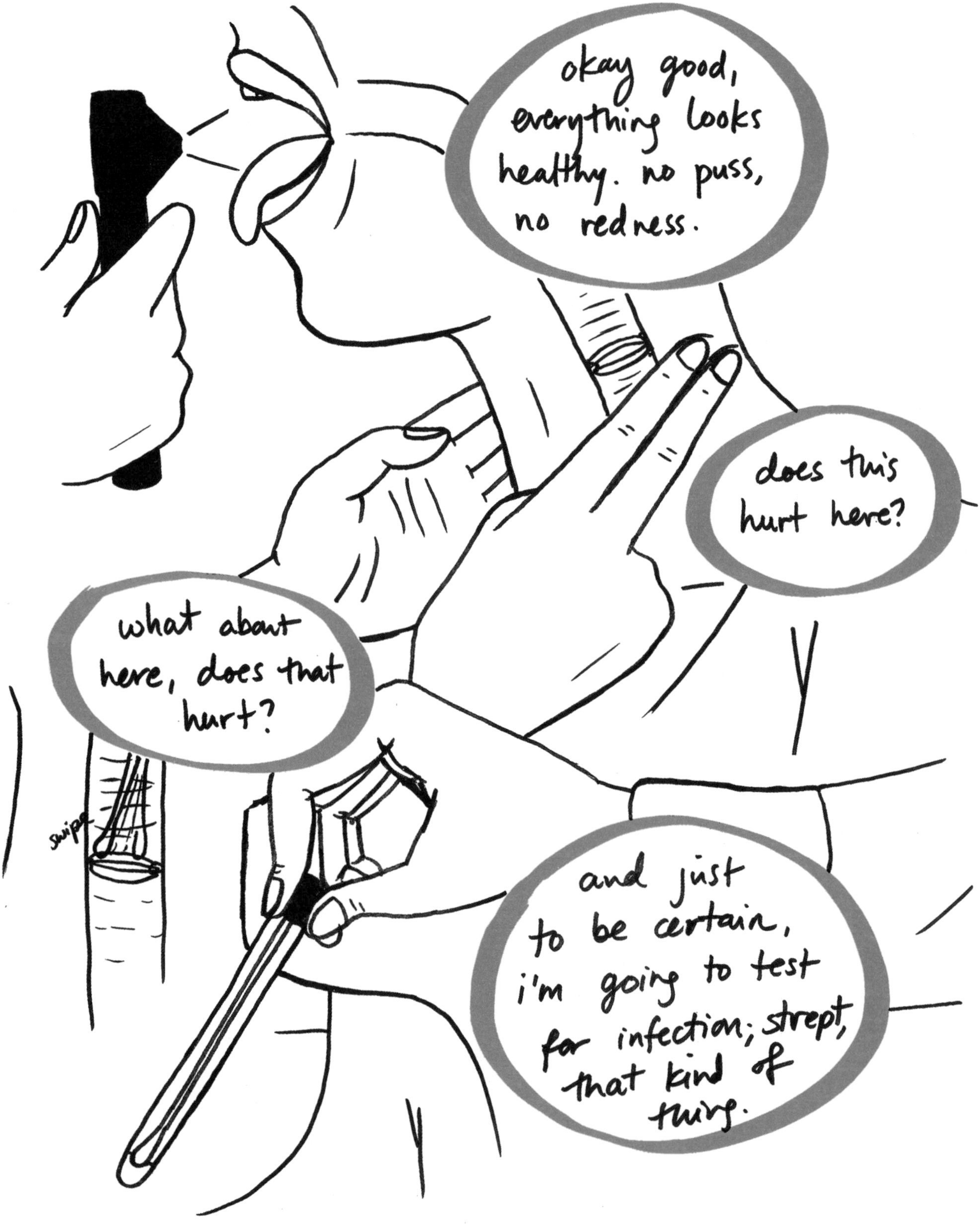
okay good, everything looks healthy. no puss, no redness.
does this hurt here?
what about here, does that hurt?
swipe
and just to be certain, i'm going to test for infection; strept, that kind of thing.

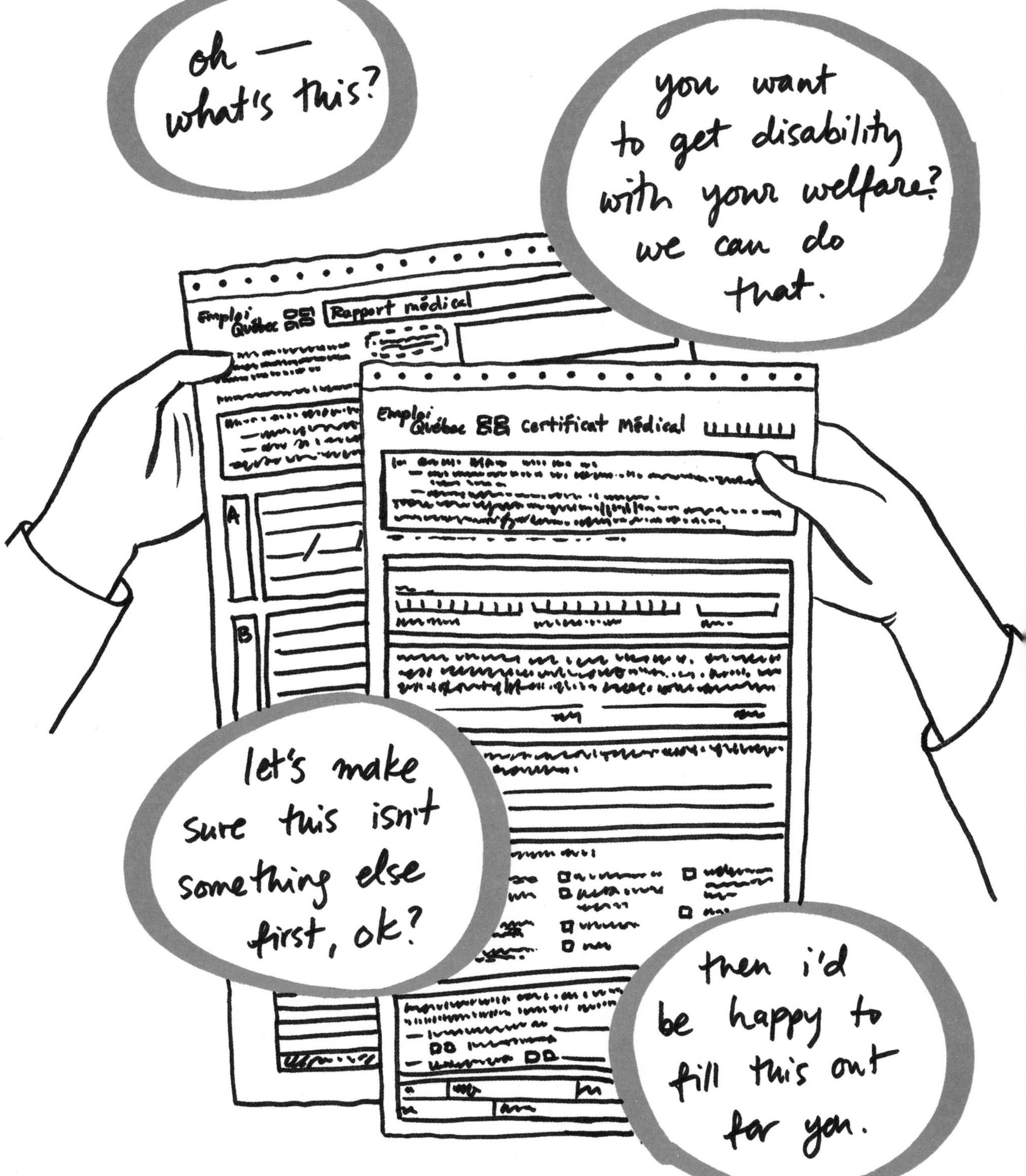
oh — what's this?
you want to get disability with your welfare? we can do that.
Emploi Québec Rapport médical
Emploi Québec certificat médical
A
B
let's make sure this isn't something else first, ok?
then i'd be happy to fill this out for you.

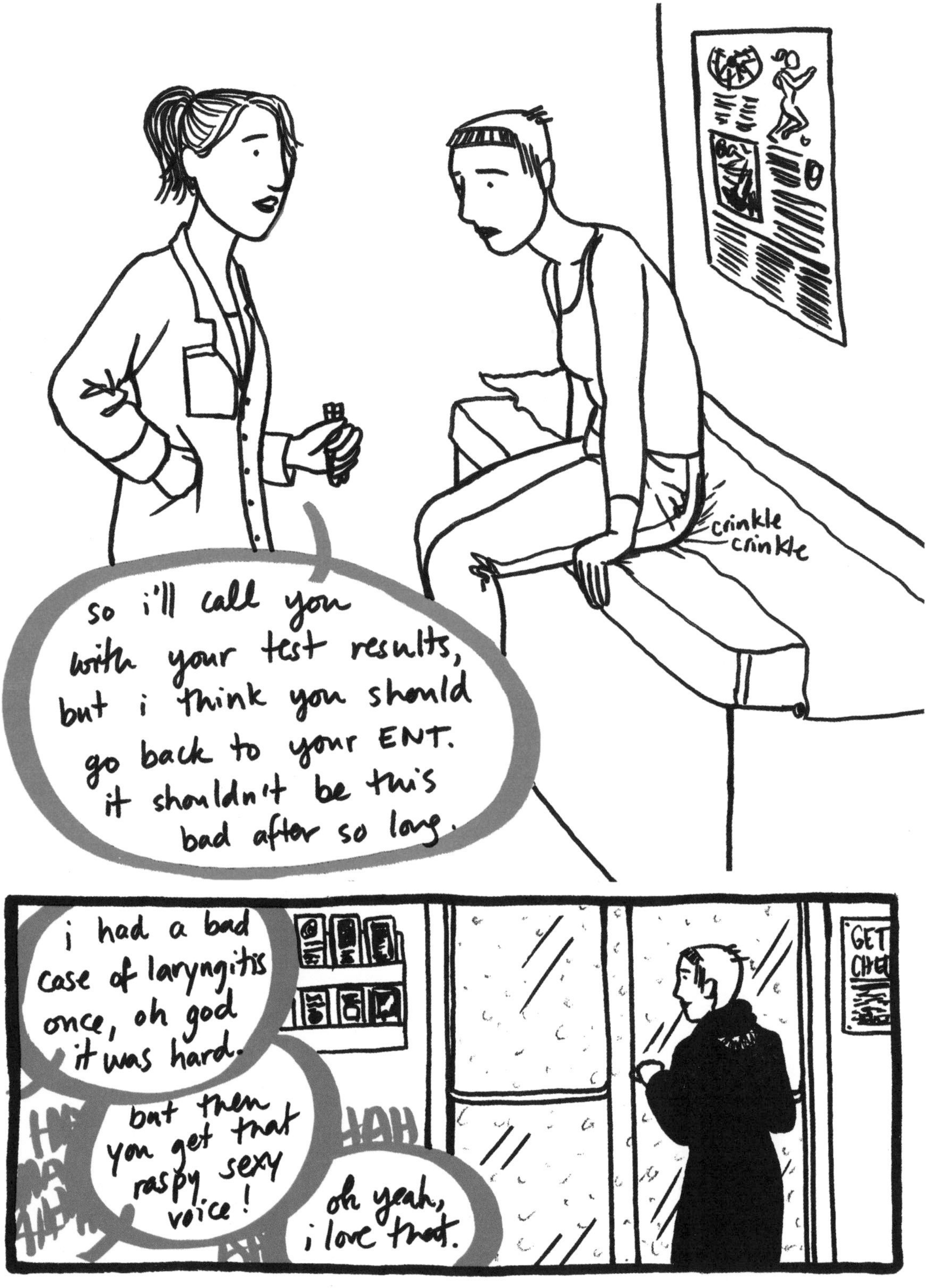
crinkle crinkle
so i'll call you with your test results, but i think you should go back to your ENT. it shouldn't be this bad after so long.
i had a bad case of laryngitis once, oh god it was hard.
but then you get that raspy sexy voice!
oh yeah, i love that.

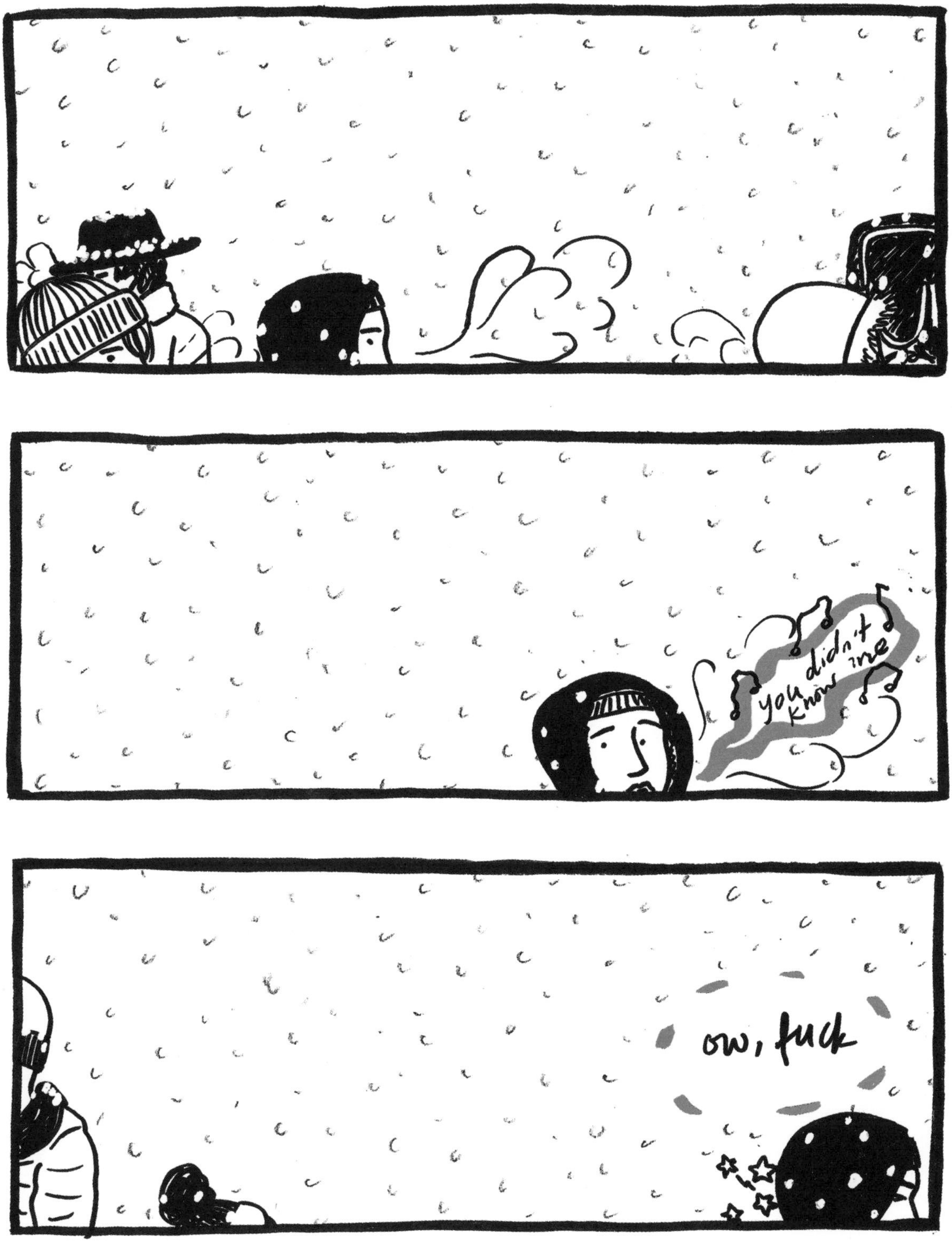
you didn't know me
ow, fuck

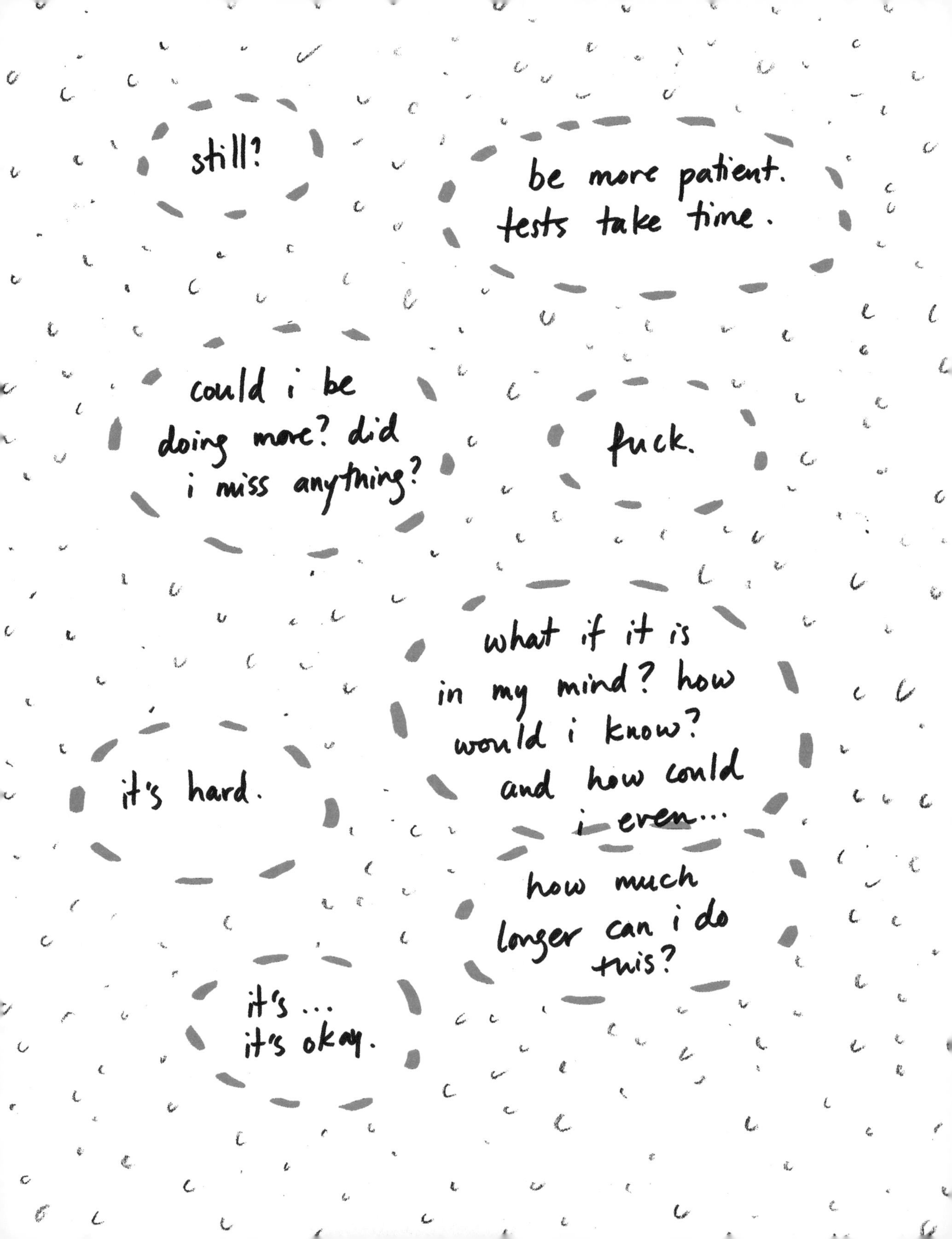
still?
be more patient. tests take time.
could i be doing more? did i miss anything?
fuck.
what if it is in my mind? how would i know? and how could i even...
it's hard.
how much longer can i do this?
it's... it's okay.

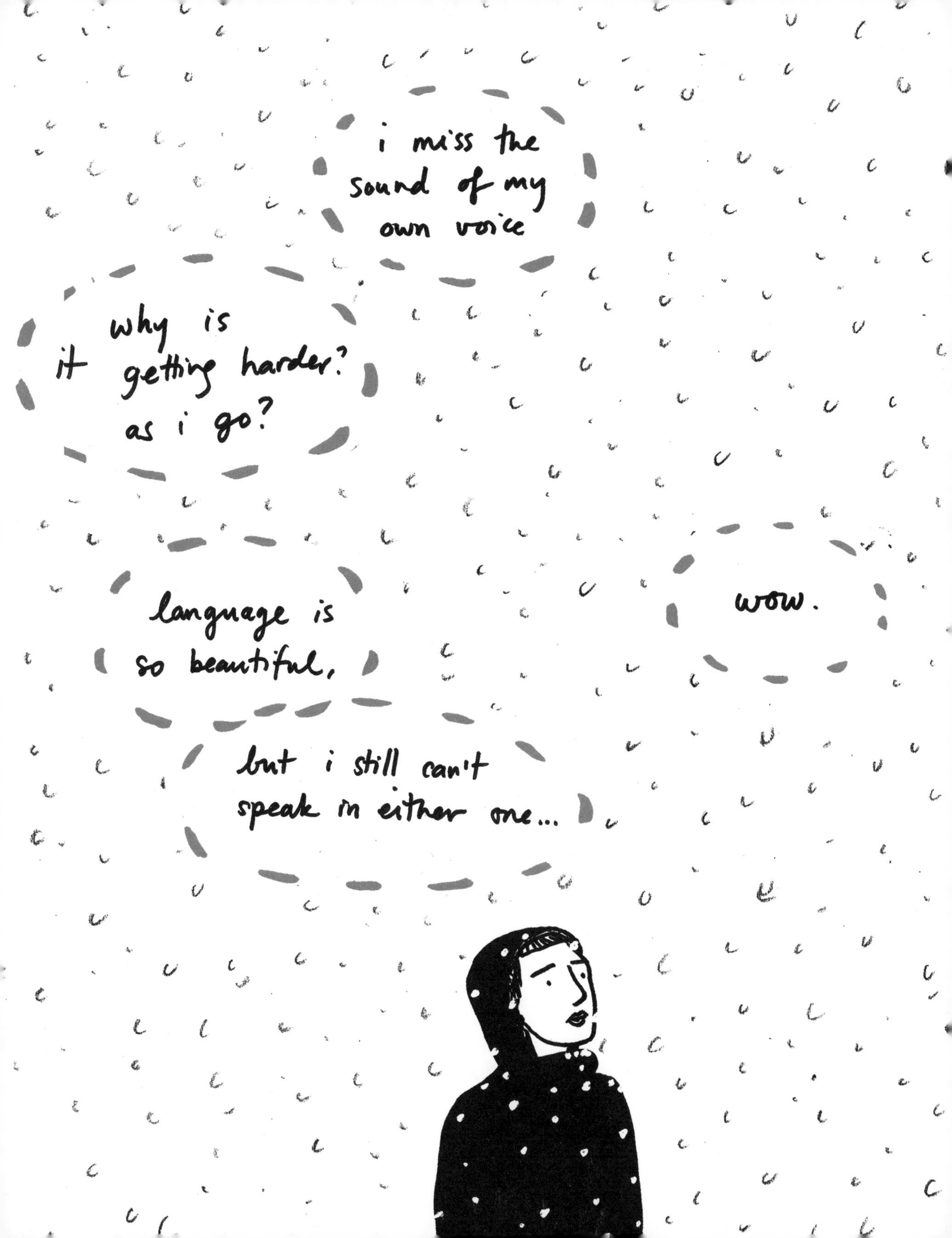
i miss the sound of my own voice
why is it getting harder? as i go?
language is so beautiful,
wow.
but i still can't speak in either one...

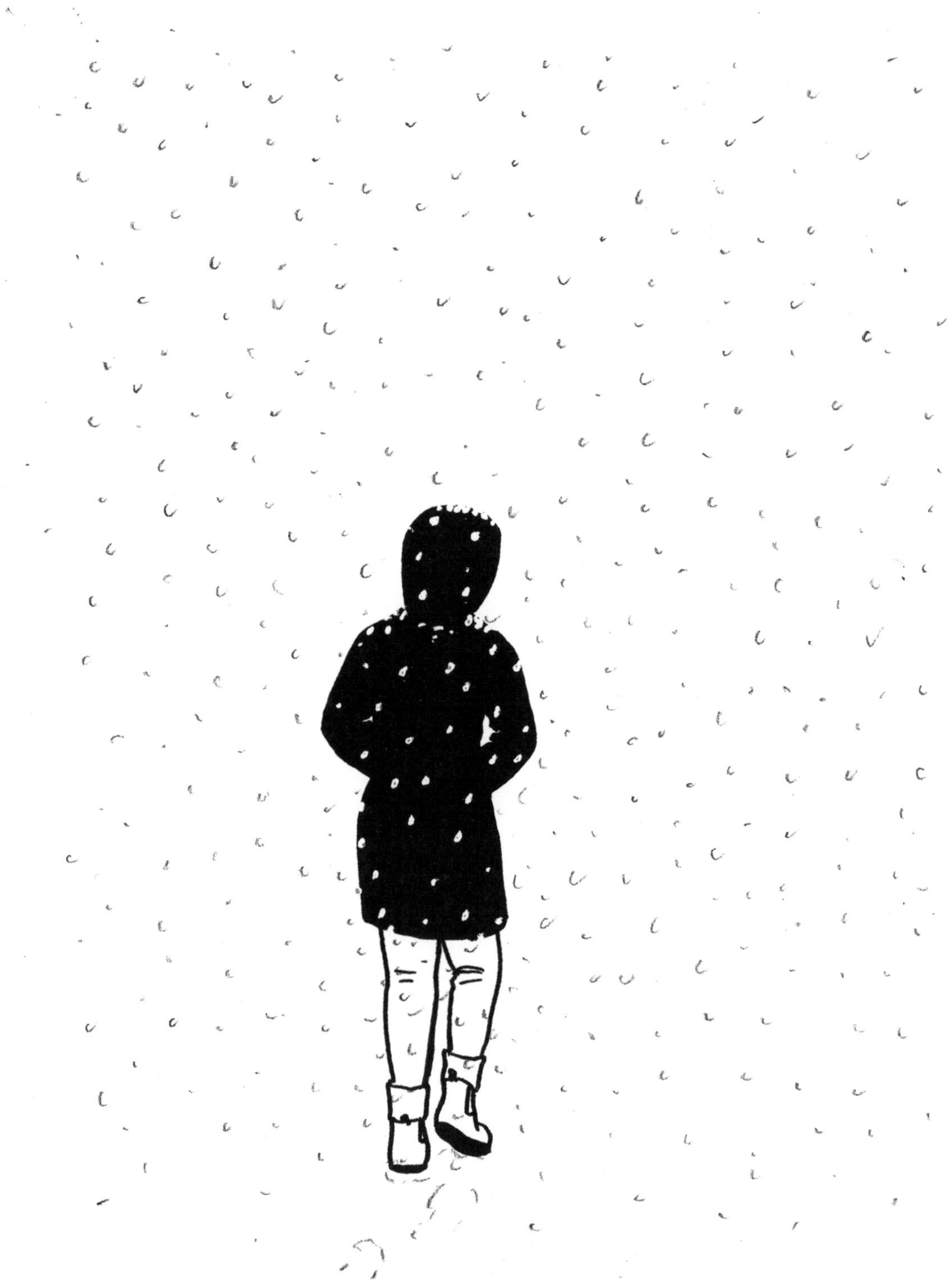

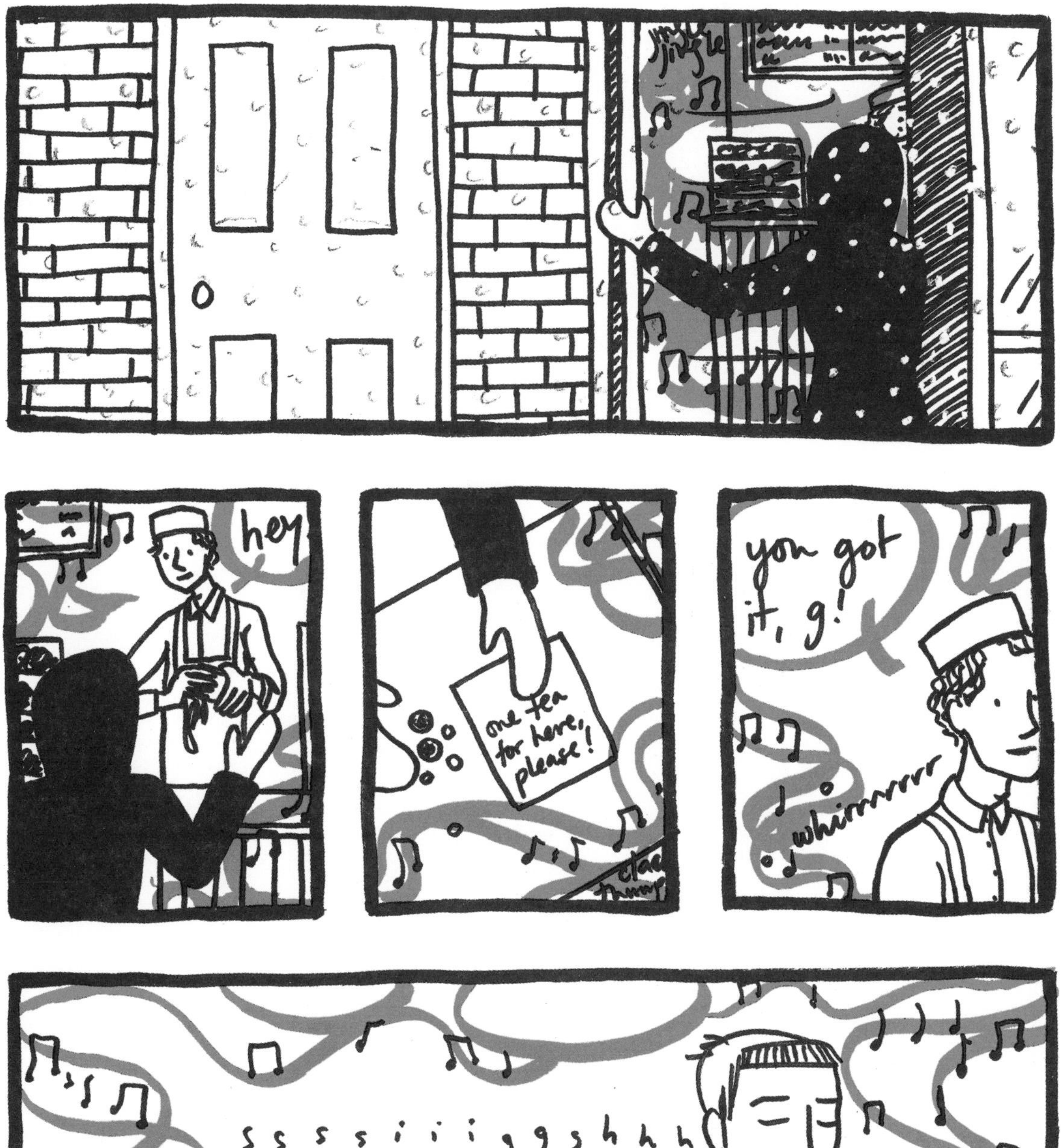
jingle
hey
one tea for here, please!
clac
you got it, g!
whirrrrrrr
ssssiiiigggshhhh

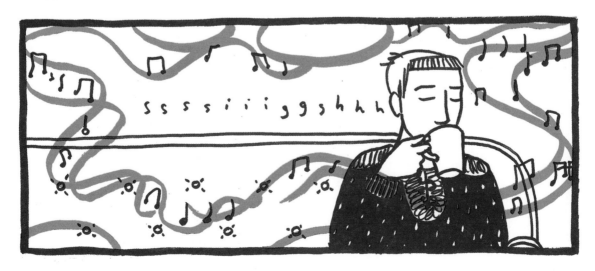

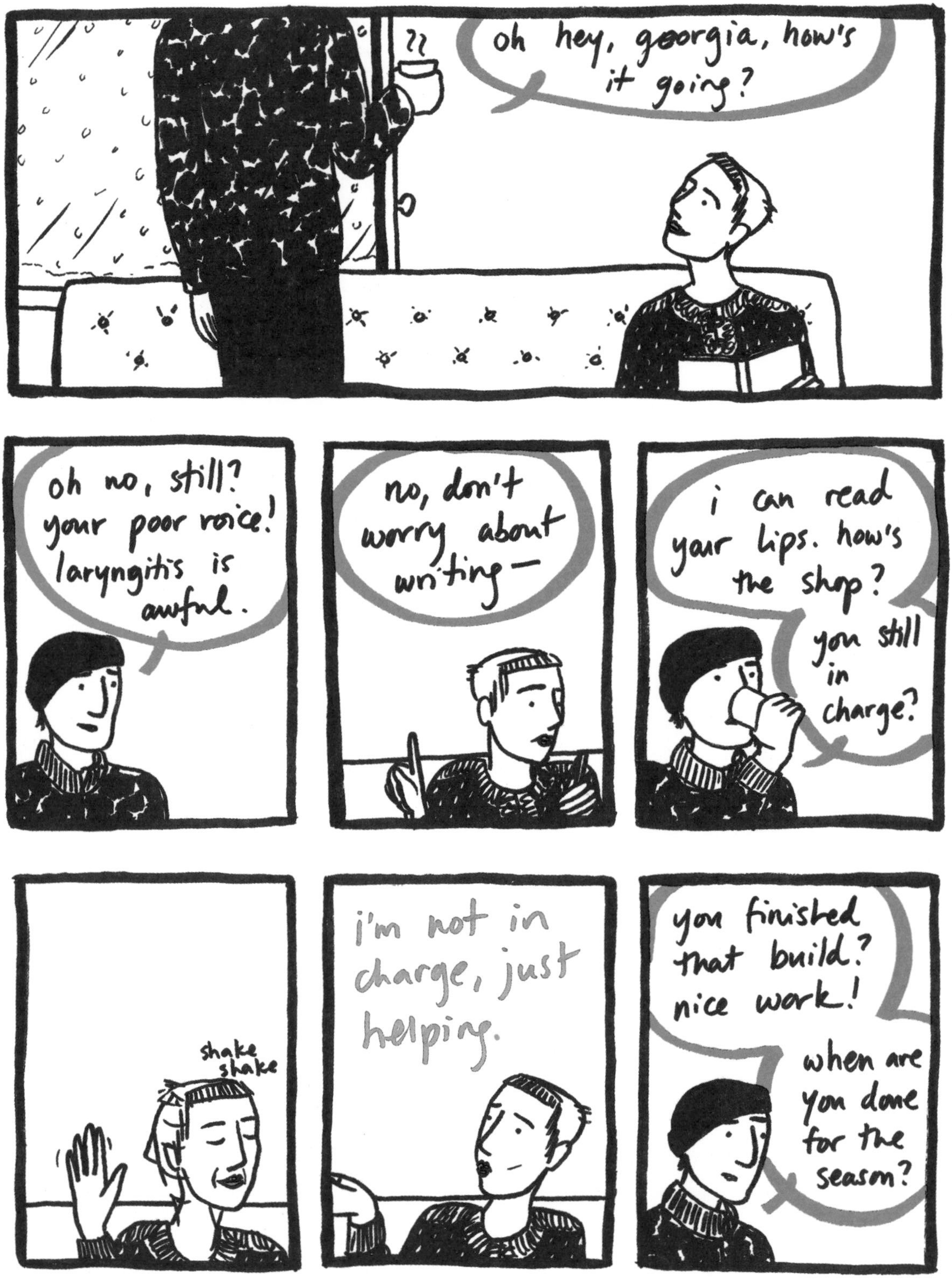

??
oh hey, georgia, how's it going?
oh no, still? your poor voice! laryngitis is awful.
no, don't worry about writing—
i can read your lips. how's the shop?
you still in charge?
shake shake
i'm not in charge, just helping.
you finished that build? nice work!
when are you done for the season?

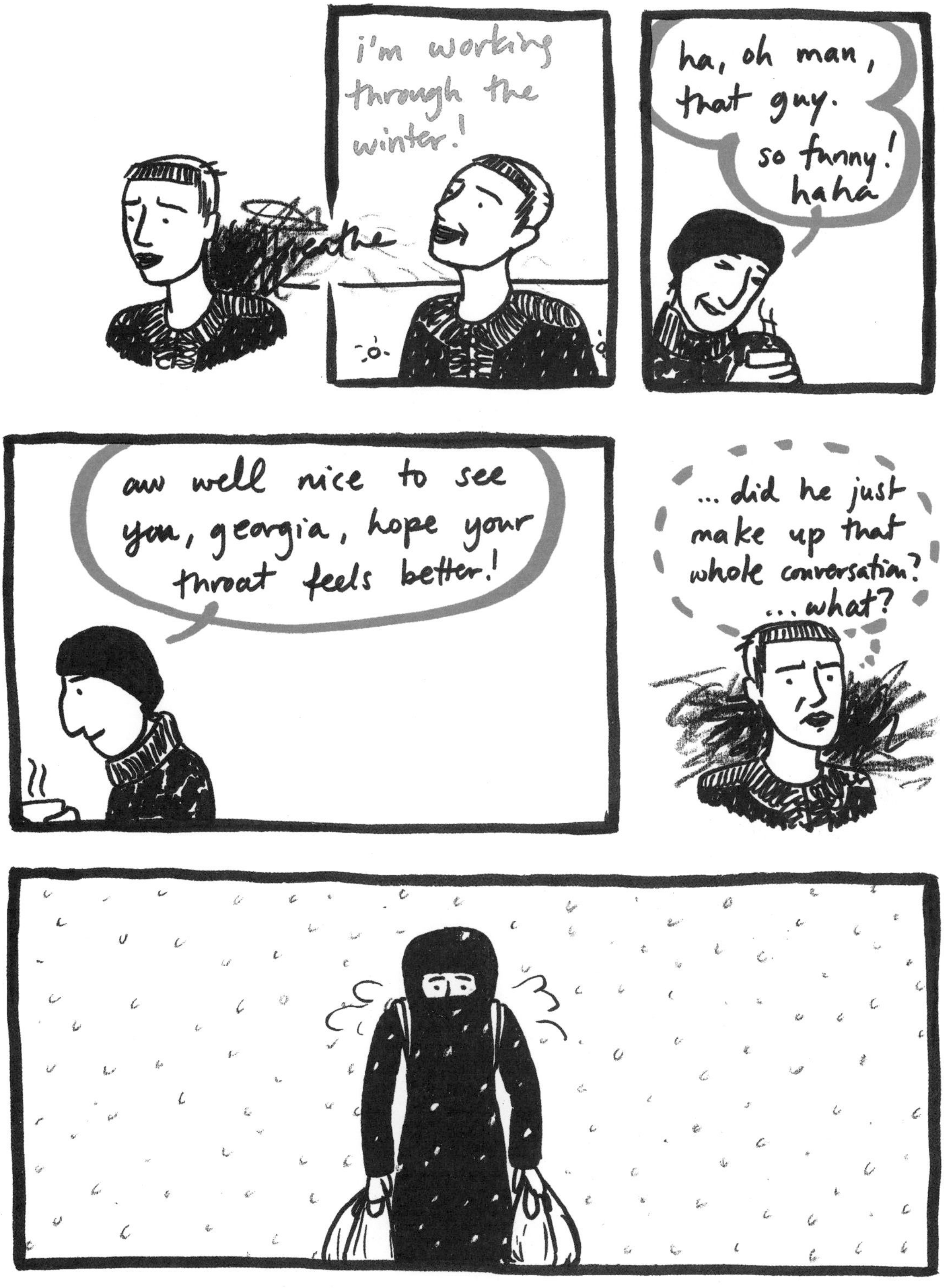

breathe
i'm working through the winter!
ha, oh man, that guy. so funny! haha
aw well nice to see you, georgia, hope your throat feels better!
... did he just make up that whole conversation? ... what?

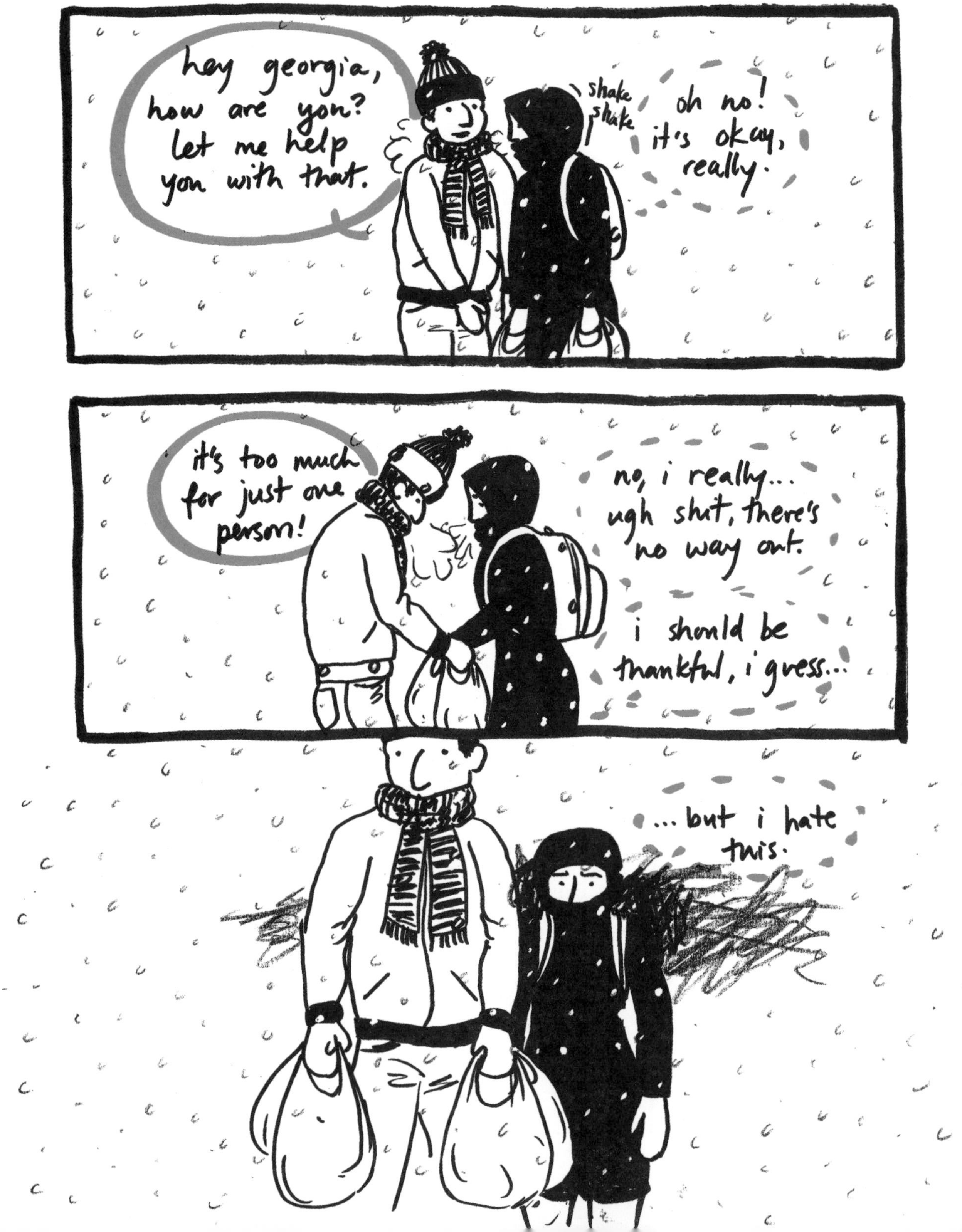
hey georgia, how are you? let me help you with that.
shake shake
oh no! it's okay, really.
it's too much for just one person!
no, i really... ugh shit, there's no way out.
i should be thankful, i guess...
...but i hate this.

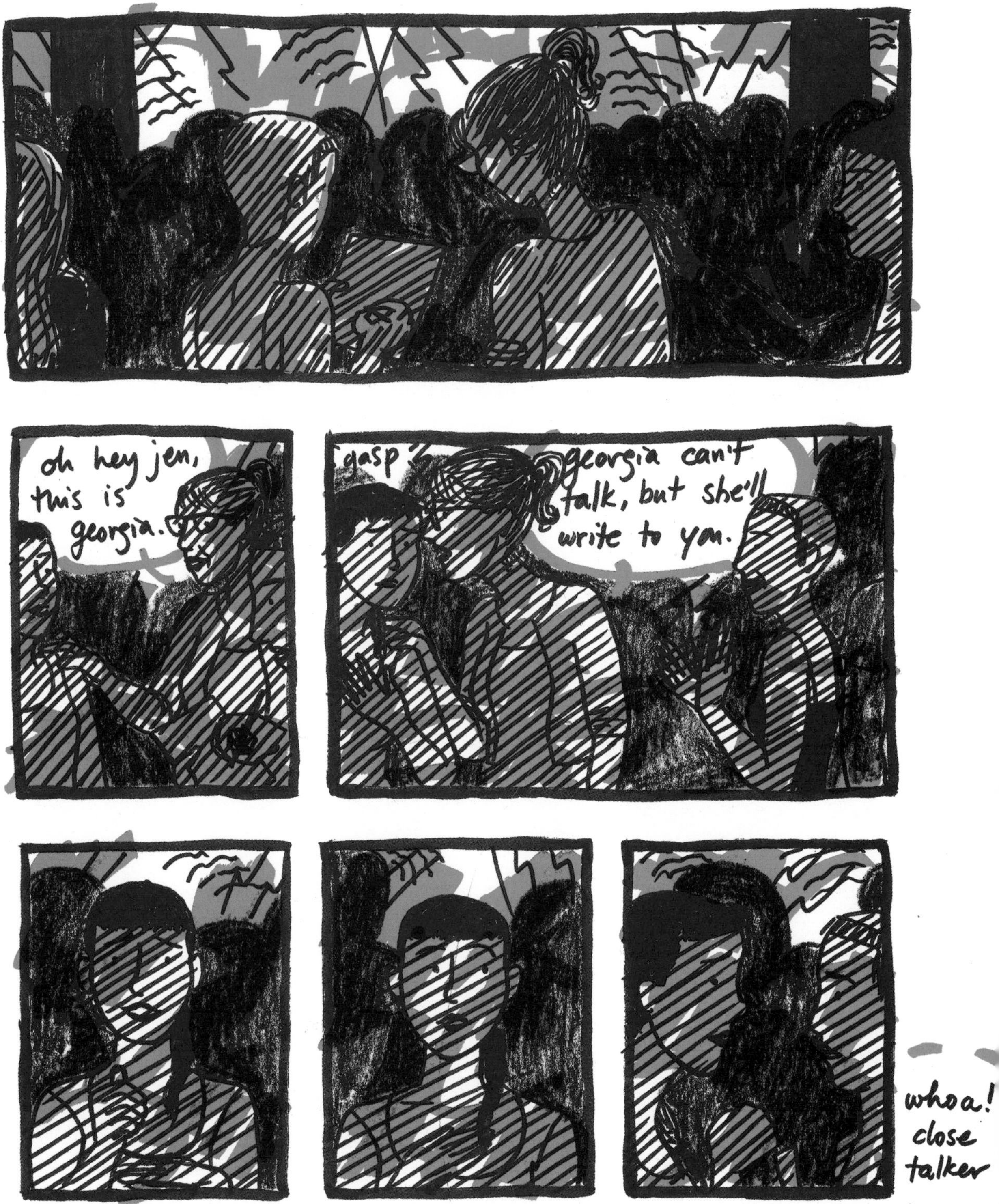
oh hey jen, this is georgia.
gasp
georgia can't talk, but she'll write to you.
whoa! close talker

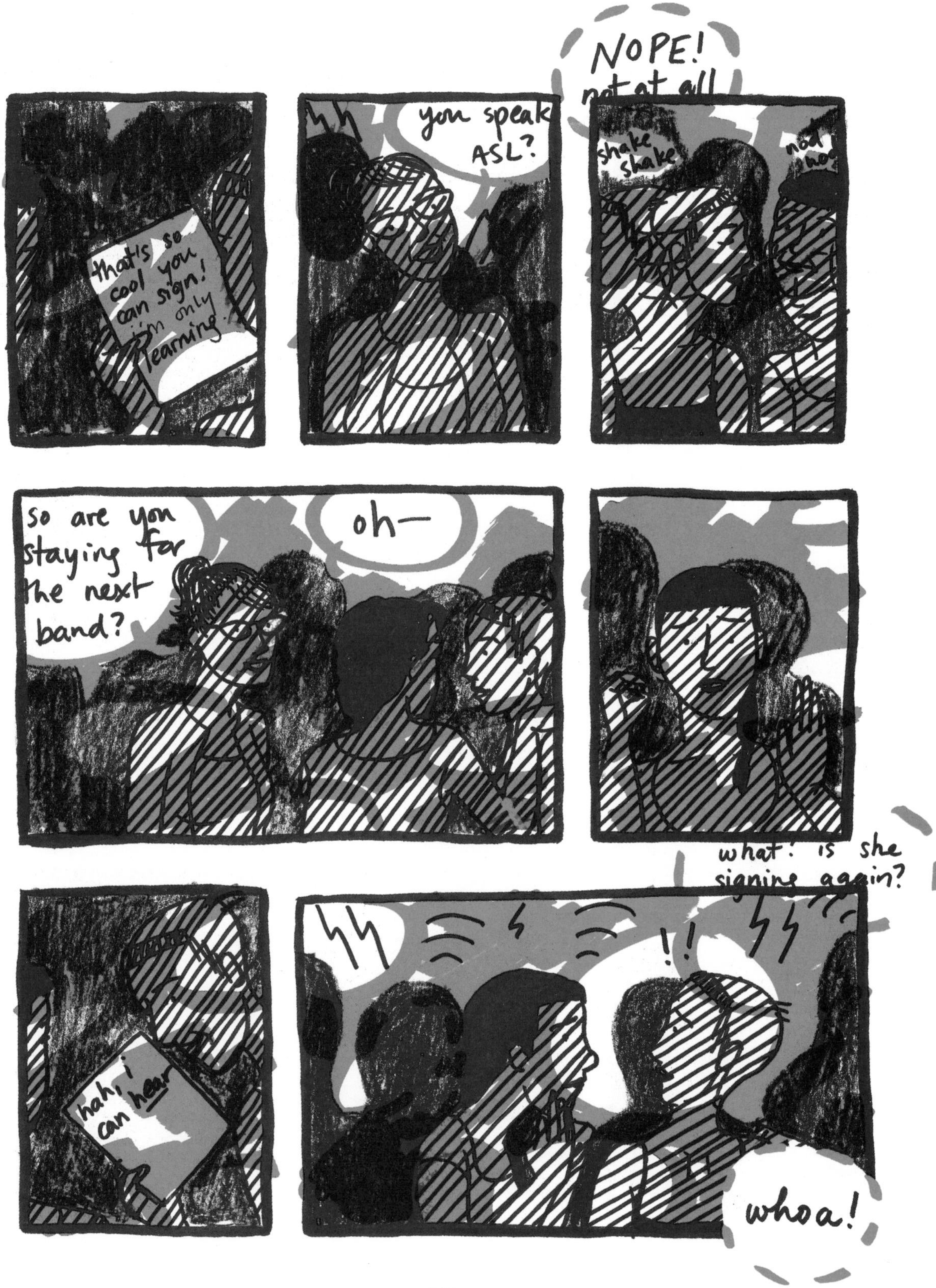
that's so cool you can sign! i'm only learning.
you speak ASL?
NOPE! not at all
shake shake
nod nod
so are you staying for the next band?
oh—
hah, i can hear
what! is she signing again?
!!
whoa!

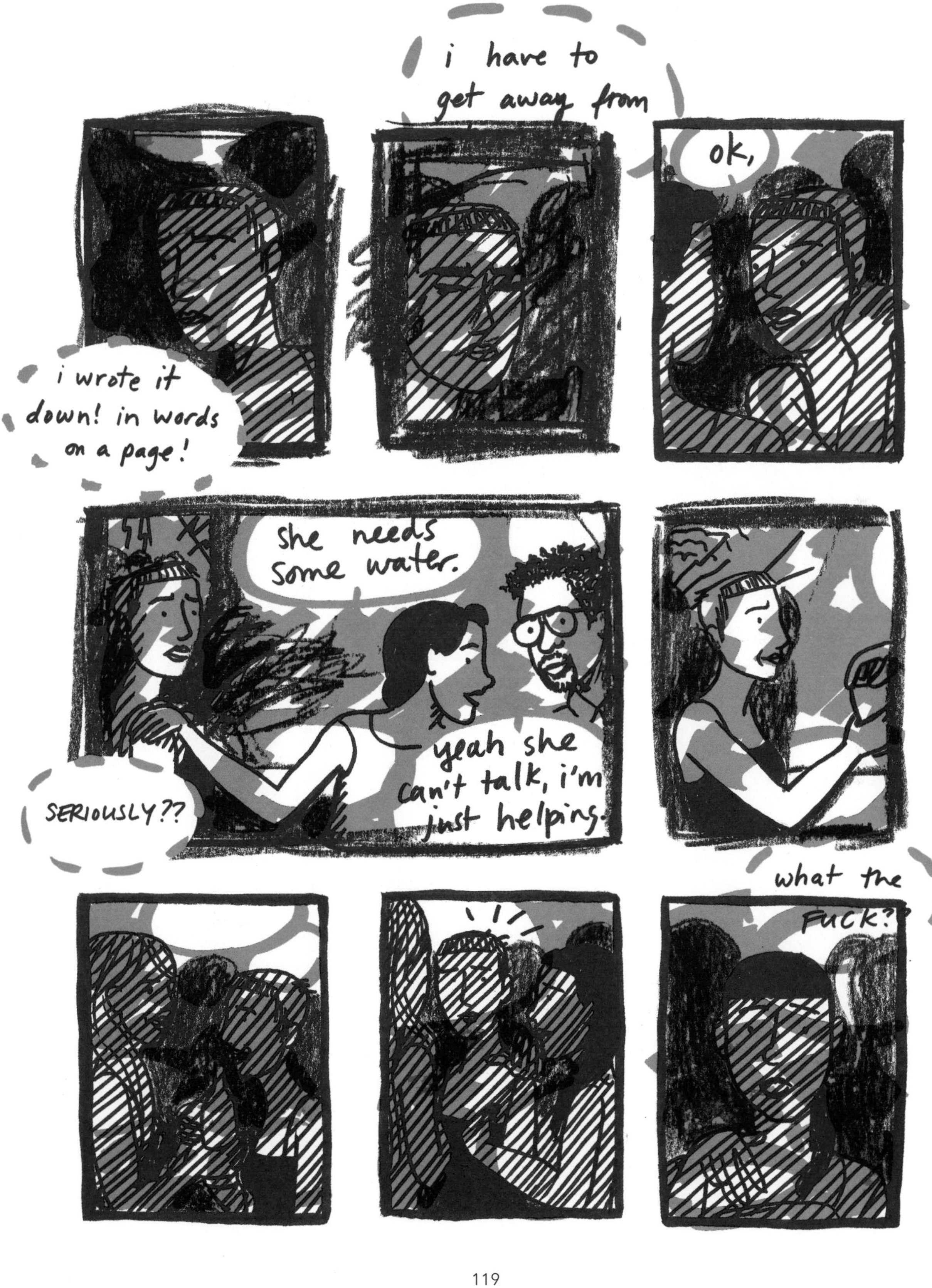
i have to get away from
ok,
i wrote it down! in words on a page!
she needs some water.
yeah she can't talk, i'm just helping.
SERIOUSLY??
what the FUCK??

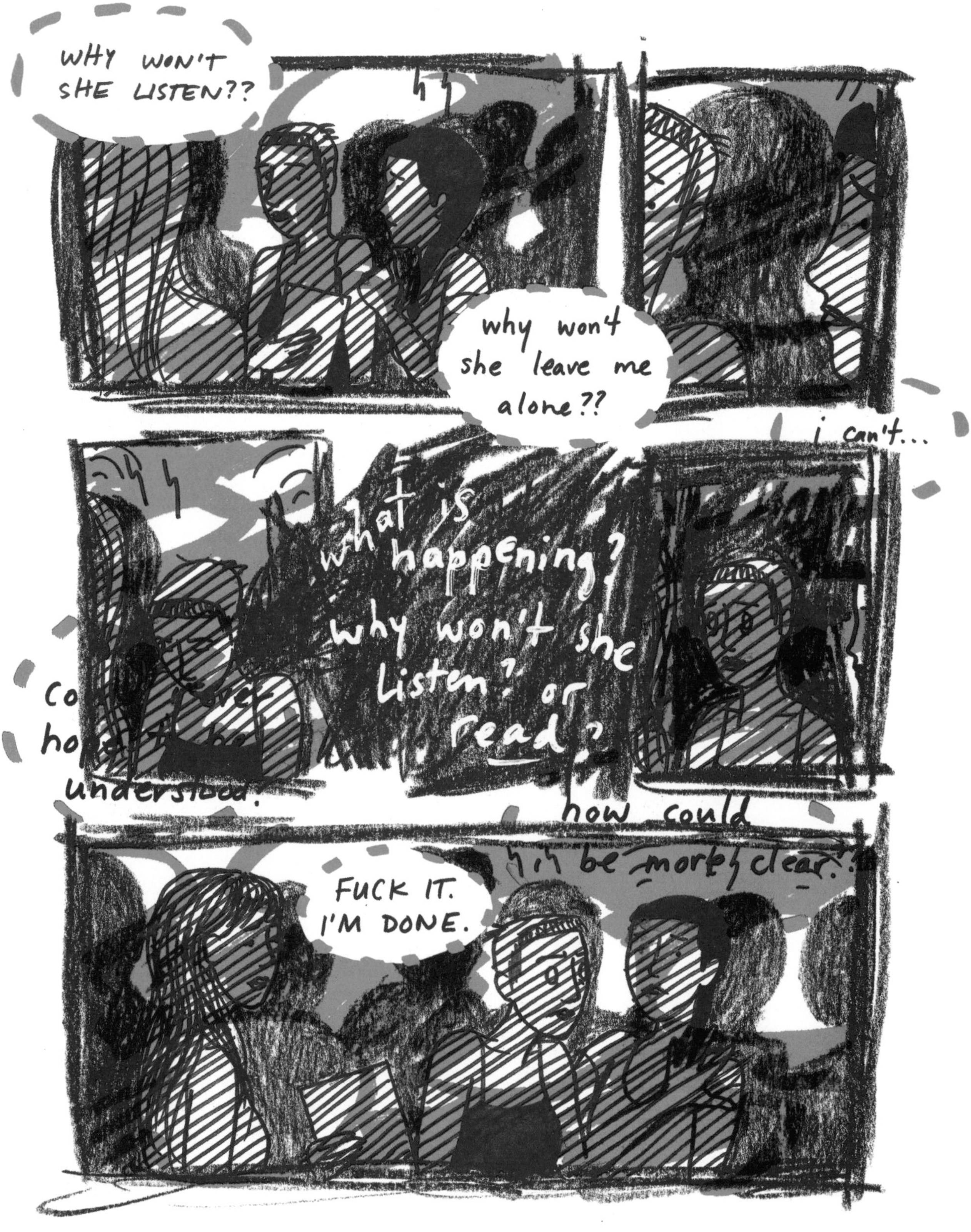
WHY WON'T SHE LISTEN??
why won't she leave me alone??
i can't...
what is happening? why won't she listen? or read?
how could
be more clear?!
FUCK IT. I'M DONE.

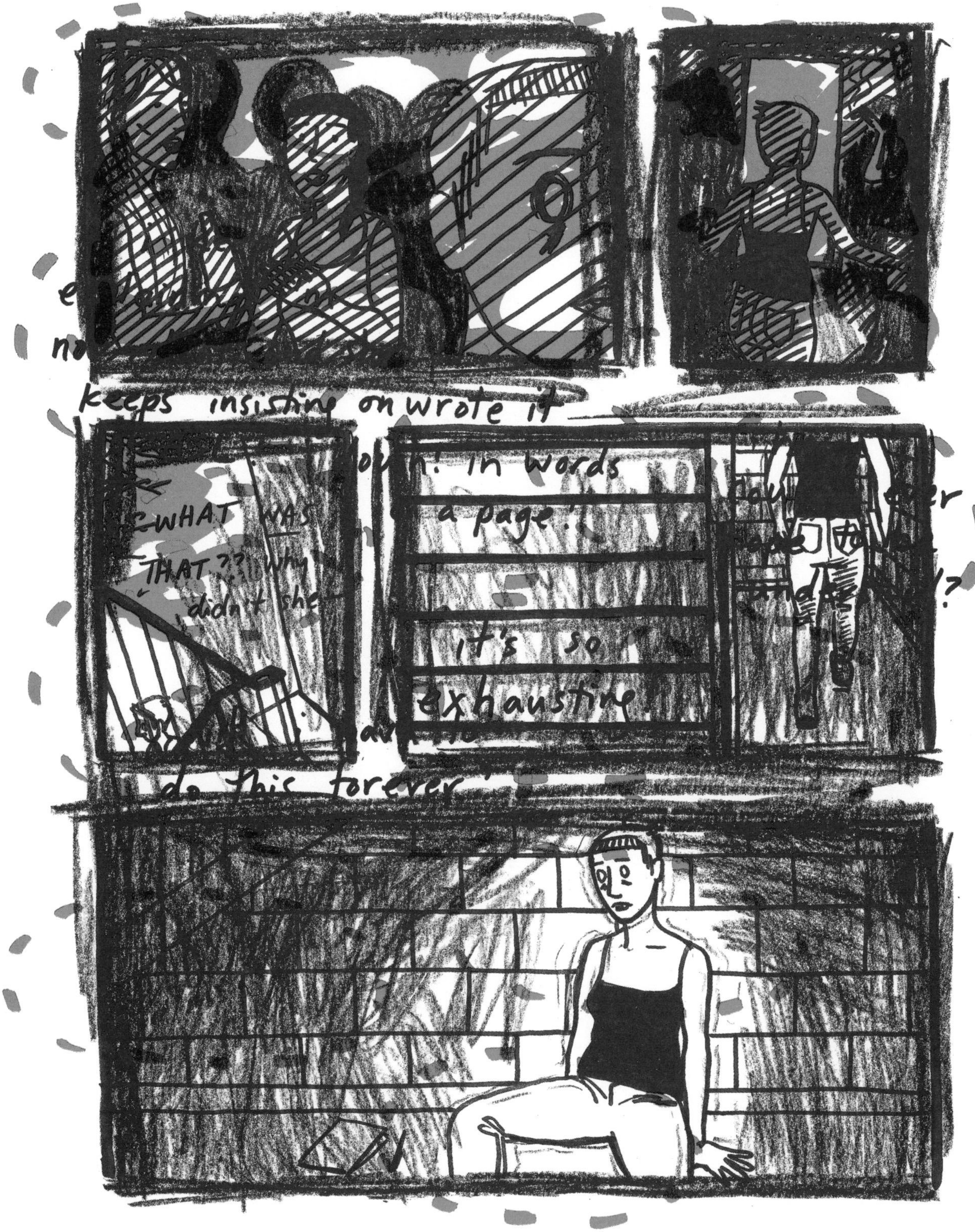
keeps insisting on wrote it
own! In words
a page!
WHAT WAS THAT?? Why didn't she
it's so exhaustive!
do this forever

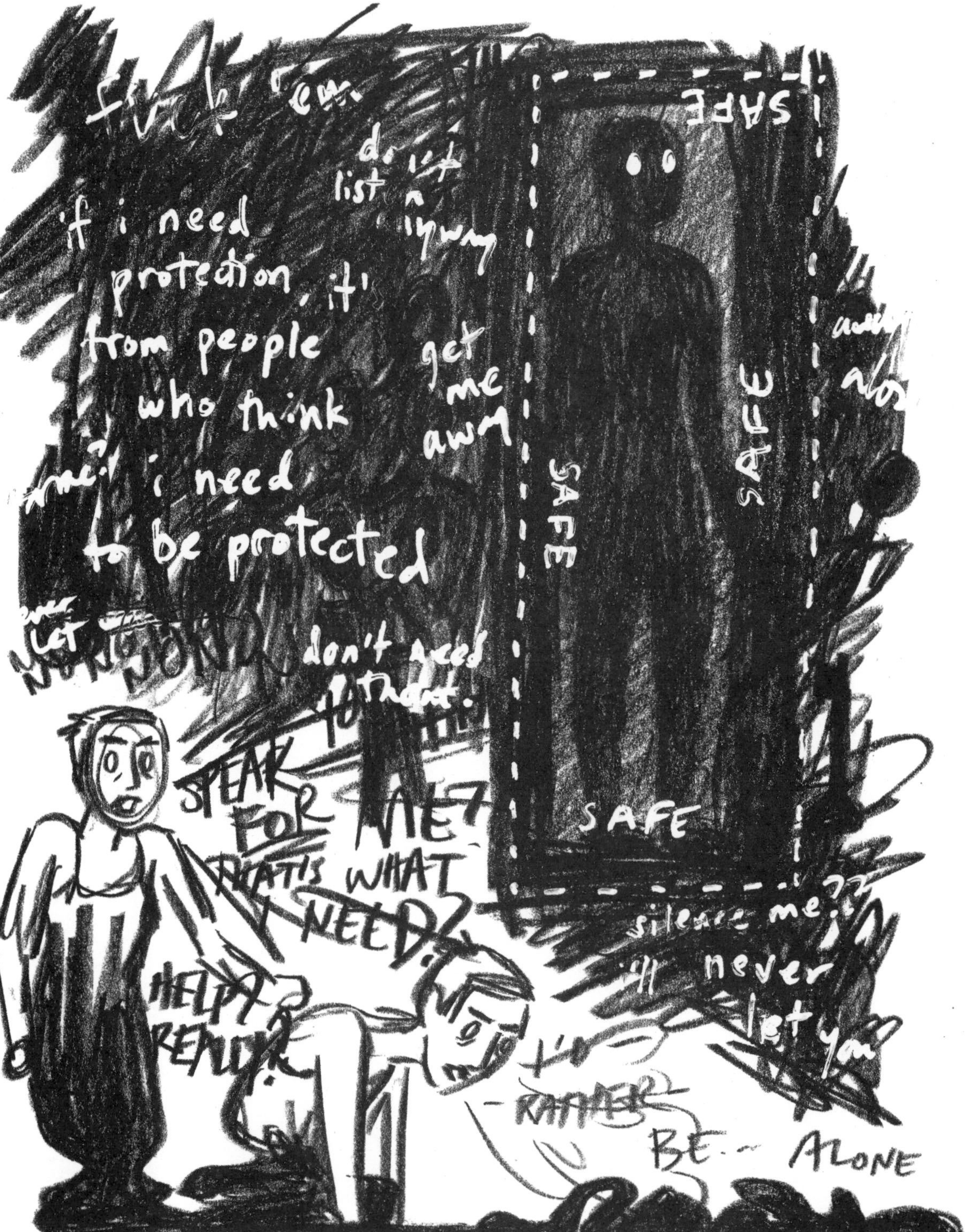
fuck 'em
don't listen anyway
if i need protection, it's from people who think i need to be protected
get me away
SAFE
SAFE
SAFE
SAFE
don't need them.
SPEAK FOR ME?
THAT IS WHAT I NEED.
silence me??
i'll never let you
I'D RATHER BE ALONE

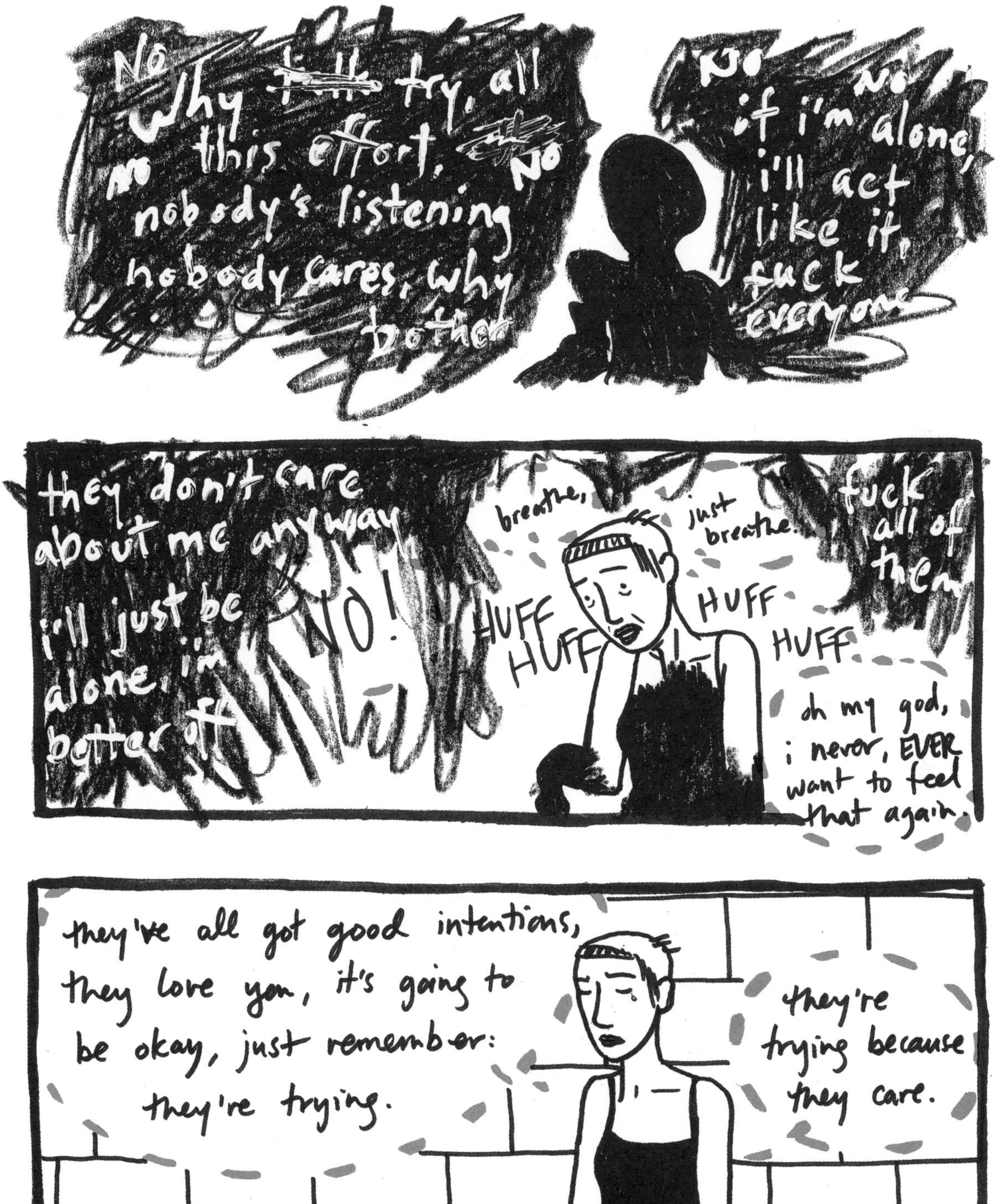
No why try, all
no this effort, No
nobody's listening
nobody cares, why bother
No No if i'm alone, i'll act like it, fuck everyone
they don't care about me anyway
i'll just be alone, i'm better off
NO!
breathe, just breathe.
HUFF HUFF
HUFF HUFF
fuck all of them
oh my god, i never, EVER want to feel that again.
they've all got good intentions, they love you, it's going to be okay, just remember: they're trying.
they're trying because they care.

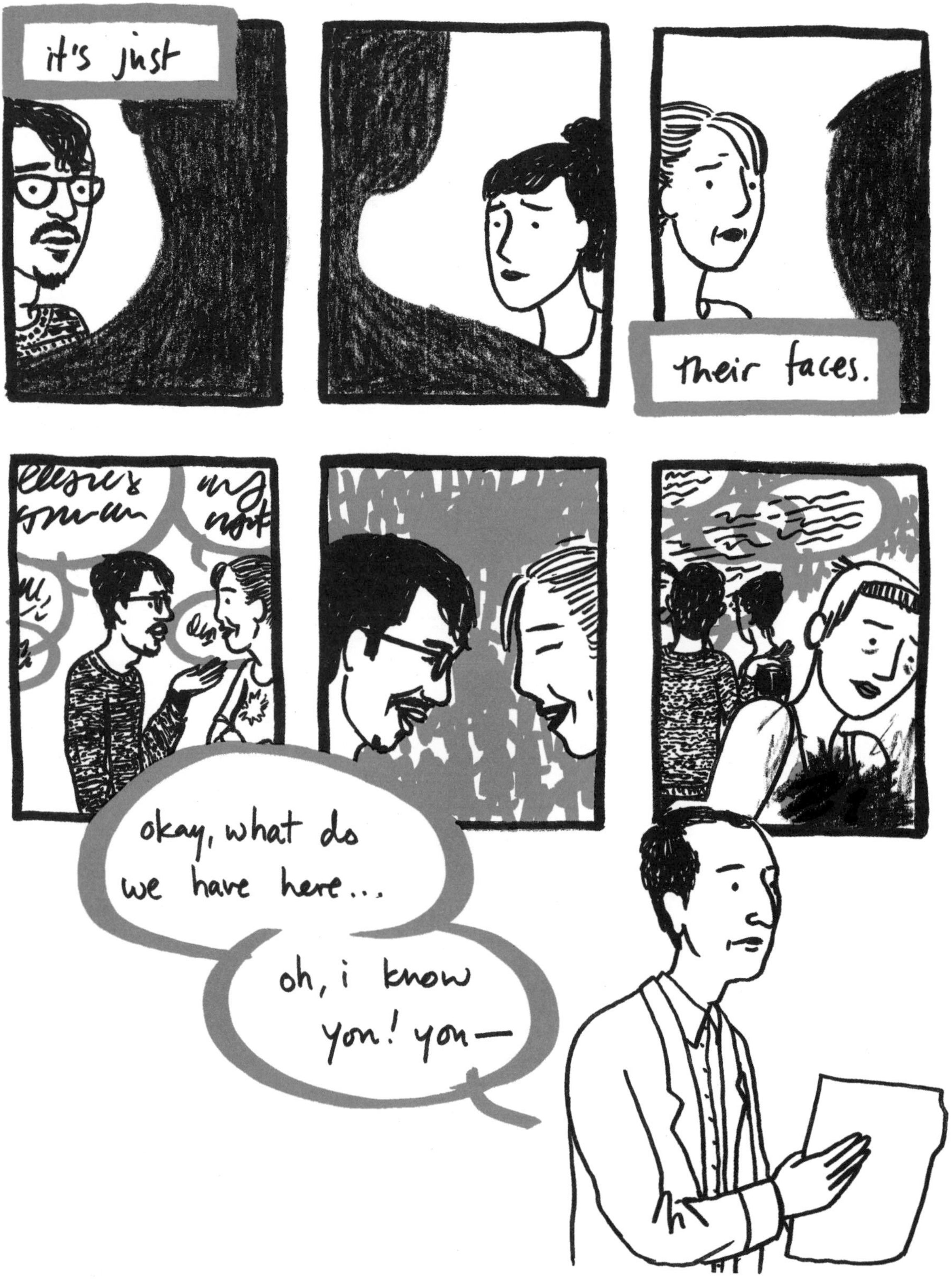
it's just
their faces.
okay, what do we have here...
oh, i know you! you—

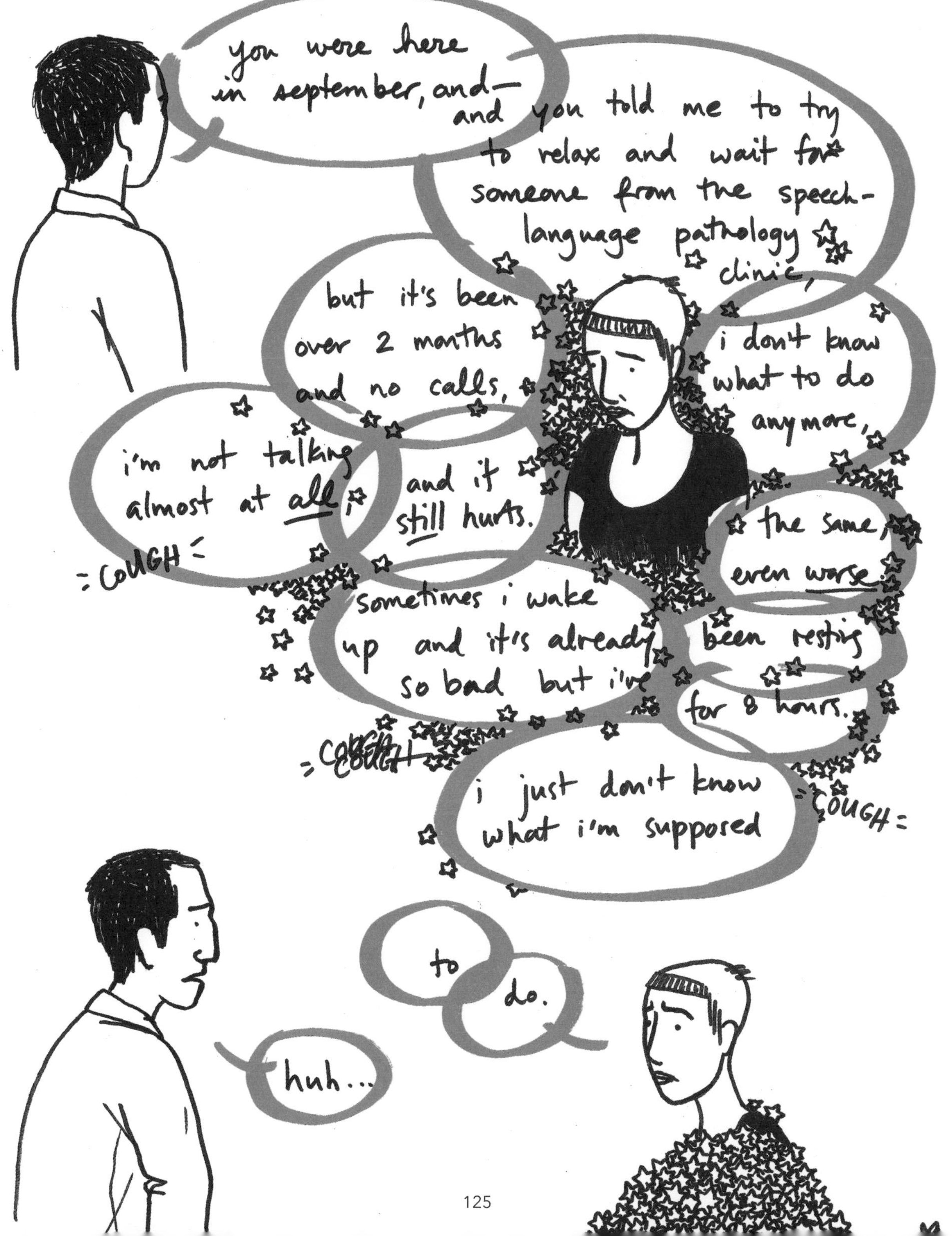
you were here in september, and—
and you told me to try to relax and wait for someone from the speech-language pathology clinic,
but it's been over 2 months and no calls,
i'm not talking almost at all,
=COUGH=
and it still hurts.
i don't know what to do anymore,
the same,
even worse.
sometimes i wake up and it's already so bad but i've
been resting for 8 hours.
=COUGH COUGH
i just don't know what i'm supposed
=COUGH=
to
do.
huh...

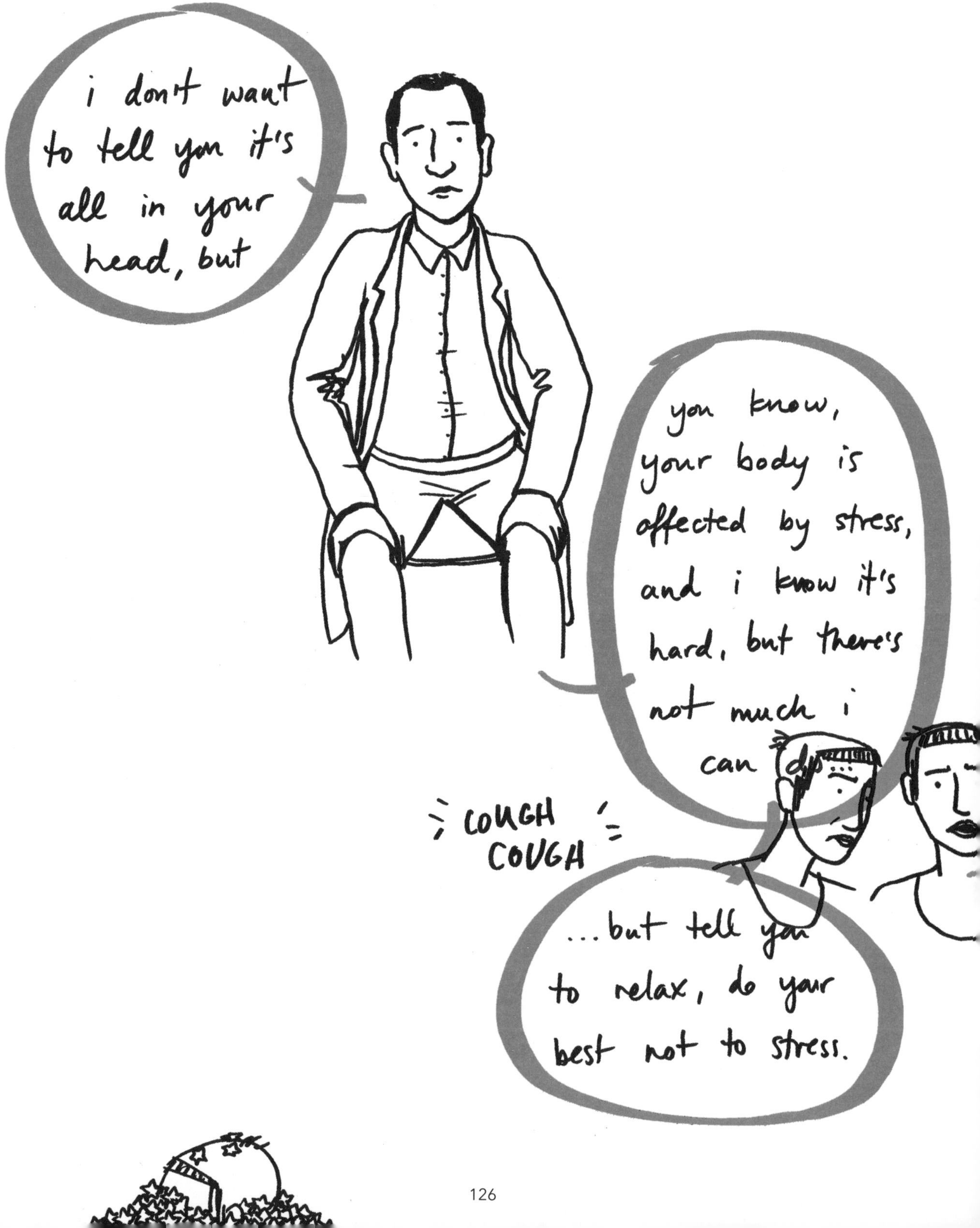
i don't want to tell you it's all in your head, but
you know, your body is affected by stress, and i know it's hard, but there's not much i can
COUGH COUGH
...but tell you to relax, do your best not to stress.

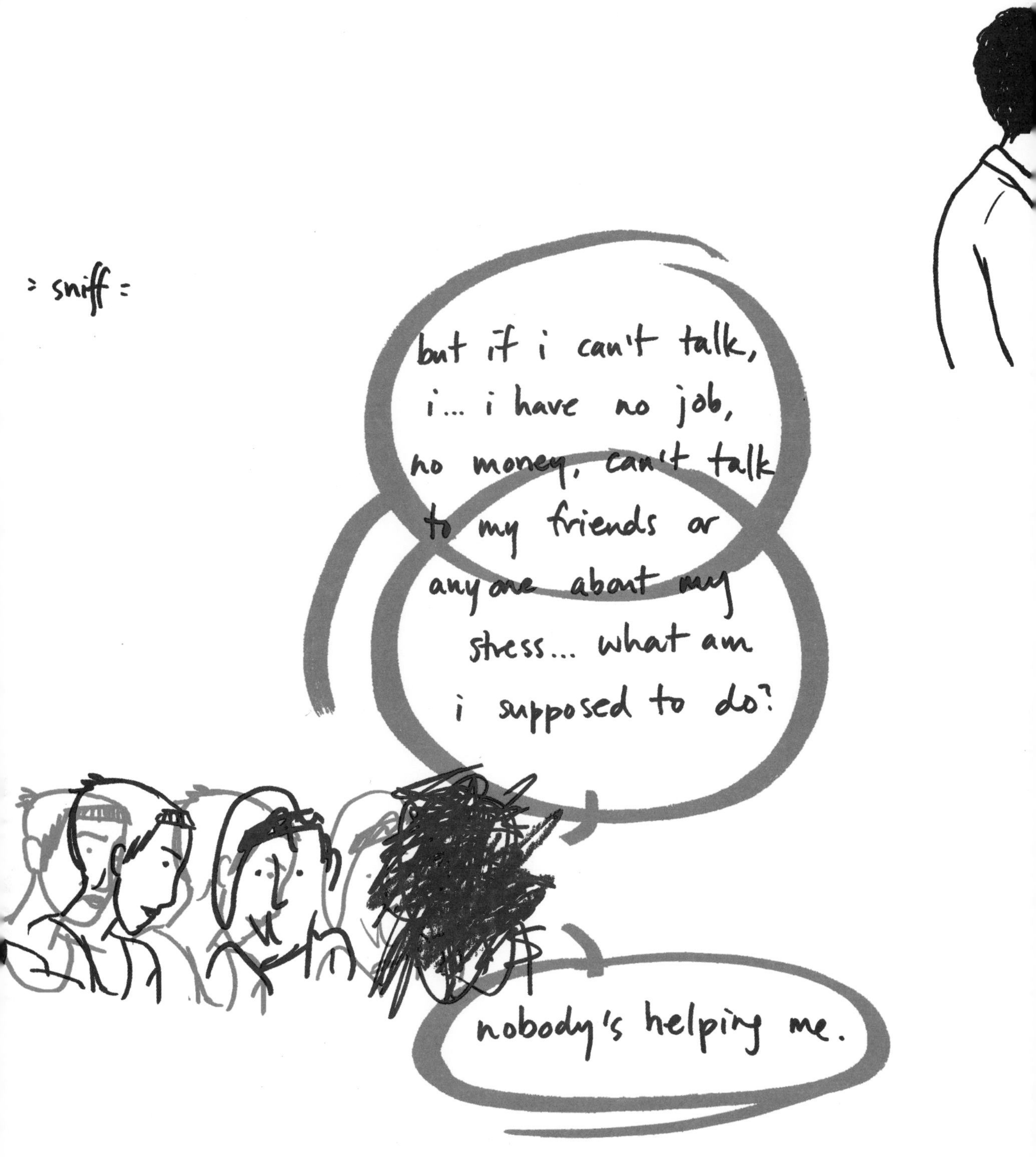
= sniff =
but if i can't talk, i... i have no job, no money, can't talk to my friends or anyone about my stress... what am i supposed to do?
nobody's helping me.

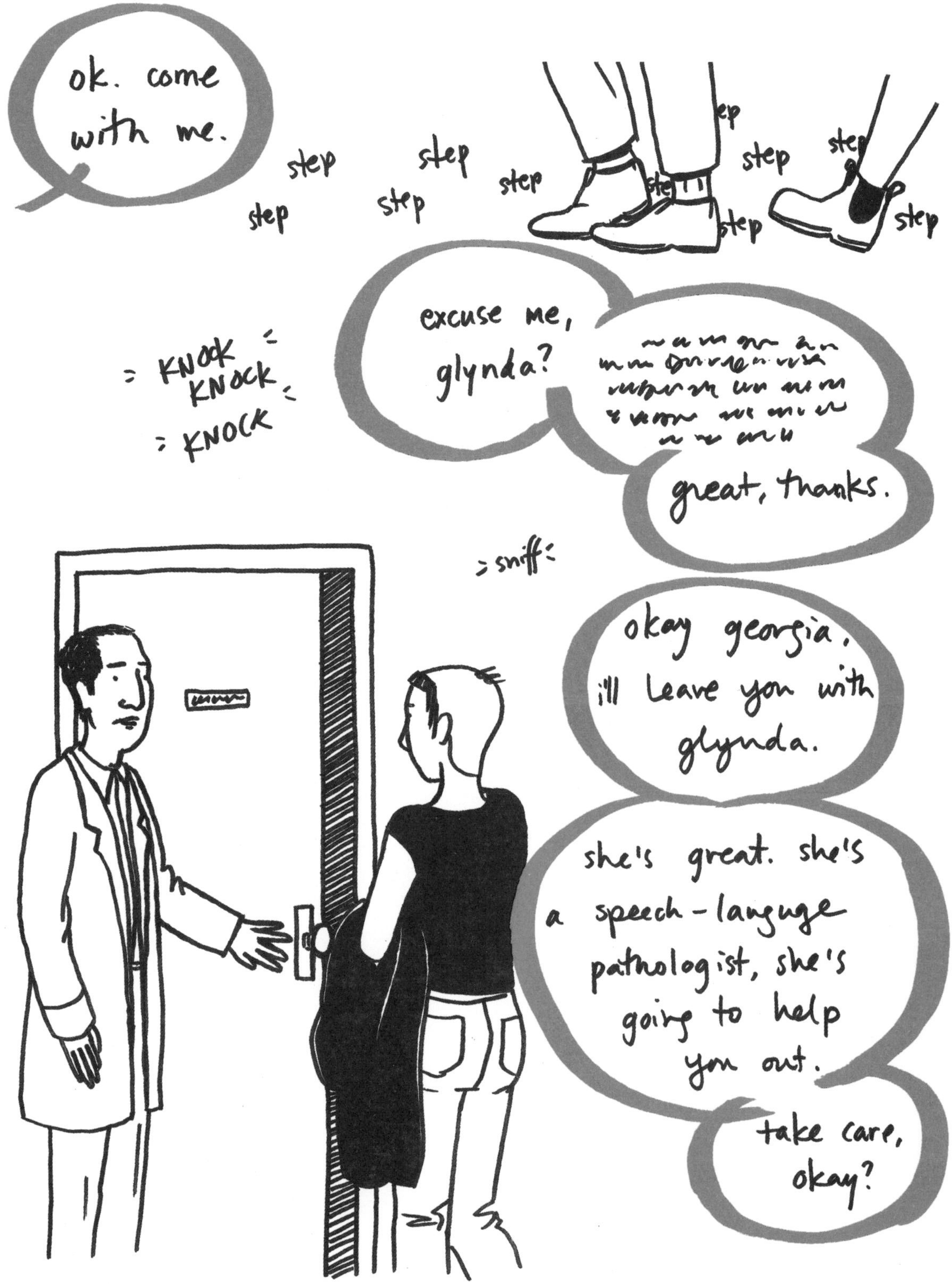
ok. come with me.
step step step step step
step step step step step
KNOCK KNOCK KNOCK
excuse me, glynda?
great, thanks.
sniff
okay georgia. i'll leave you with glynda.
she's great. she's a speech-languge pathologist, she's going to help you out.
take care, okay?

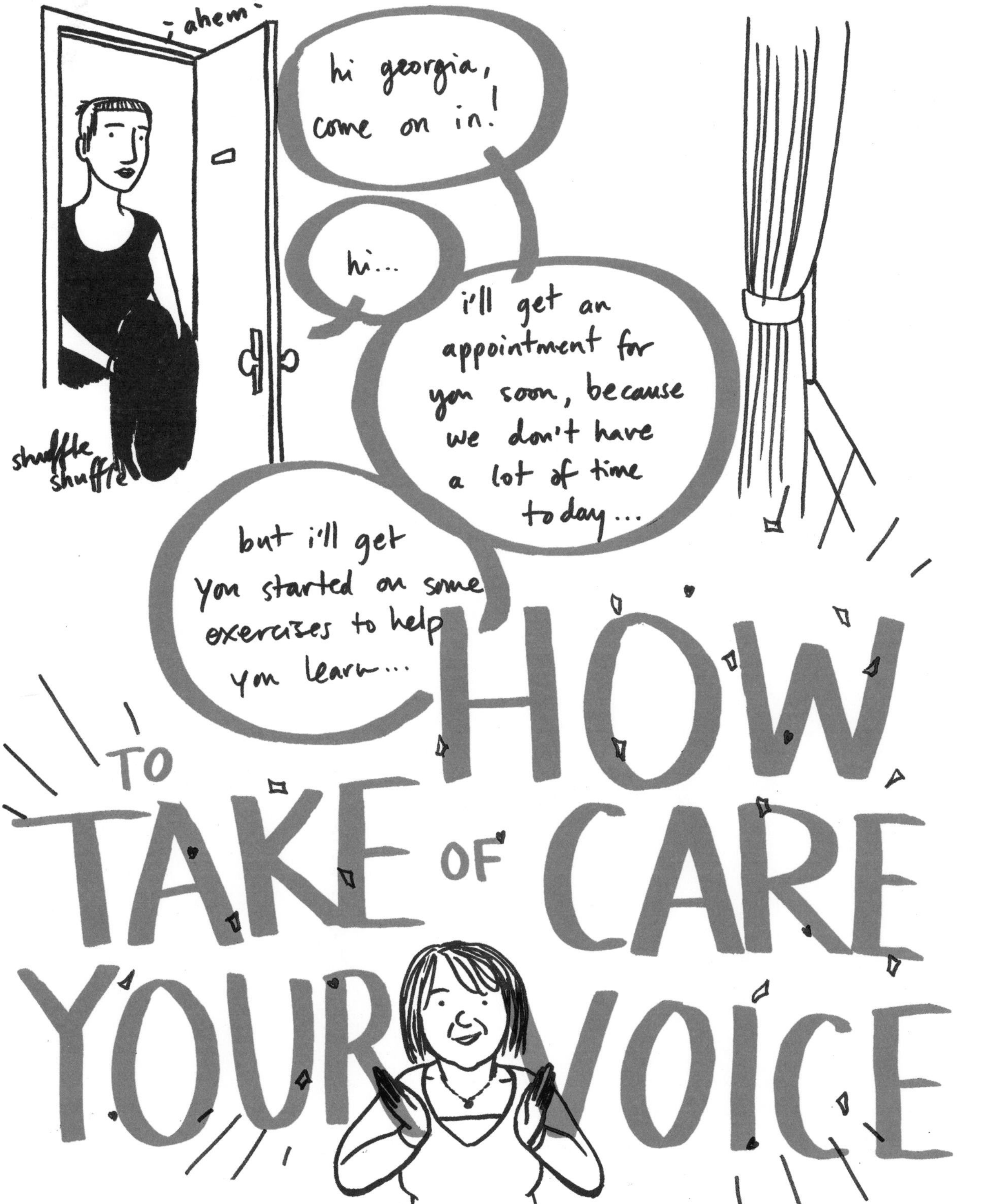
:ahem:
hi georgia, come on in!
hi...
i'll get an appointment for you soon, because we don't have a lot of time today...
but i'll get you started on some exercises to help you learn...
HOW TO TAKE CARE OF YOUR VOICE
shuffle shuffle

okay let's get your voice on here
gosh, well if this computer is gonna work for me today! okay, wait, here it is.
now take this, i'm just...
tap tap tap tap
rustle rustle
SHOVE
ah, hm, okay... ya, let's get you to sing for one full breath.

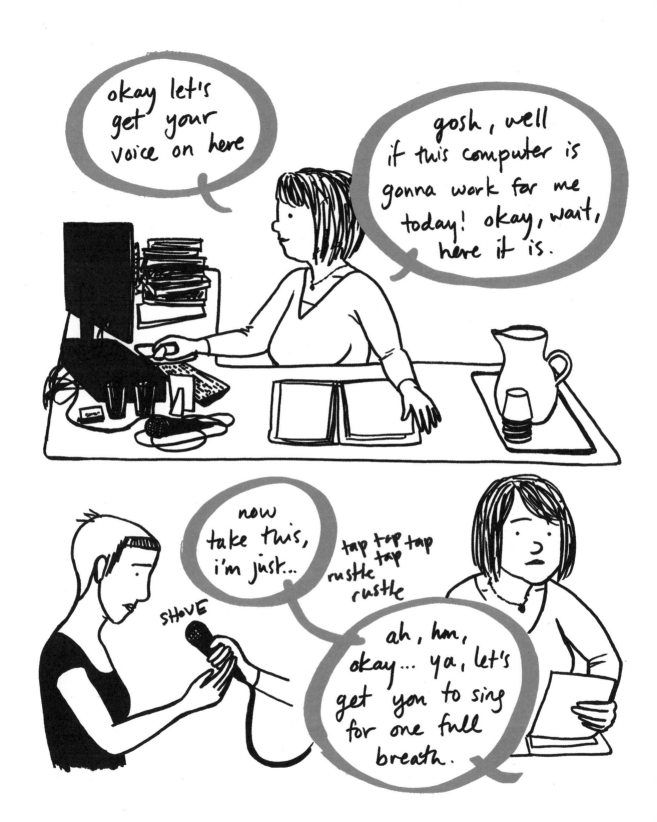

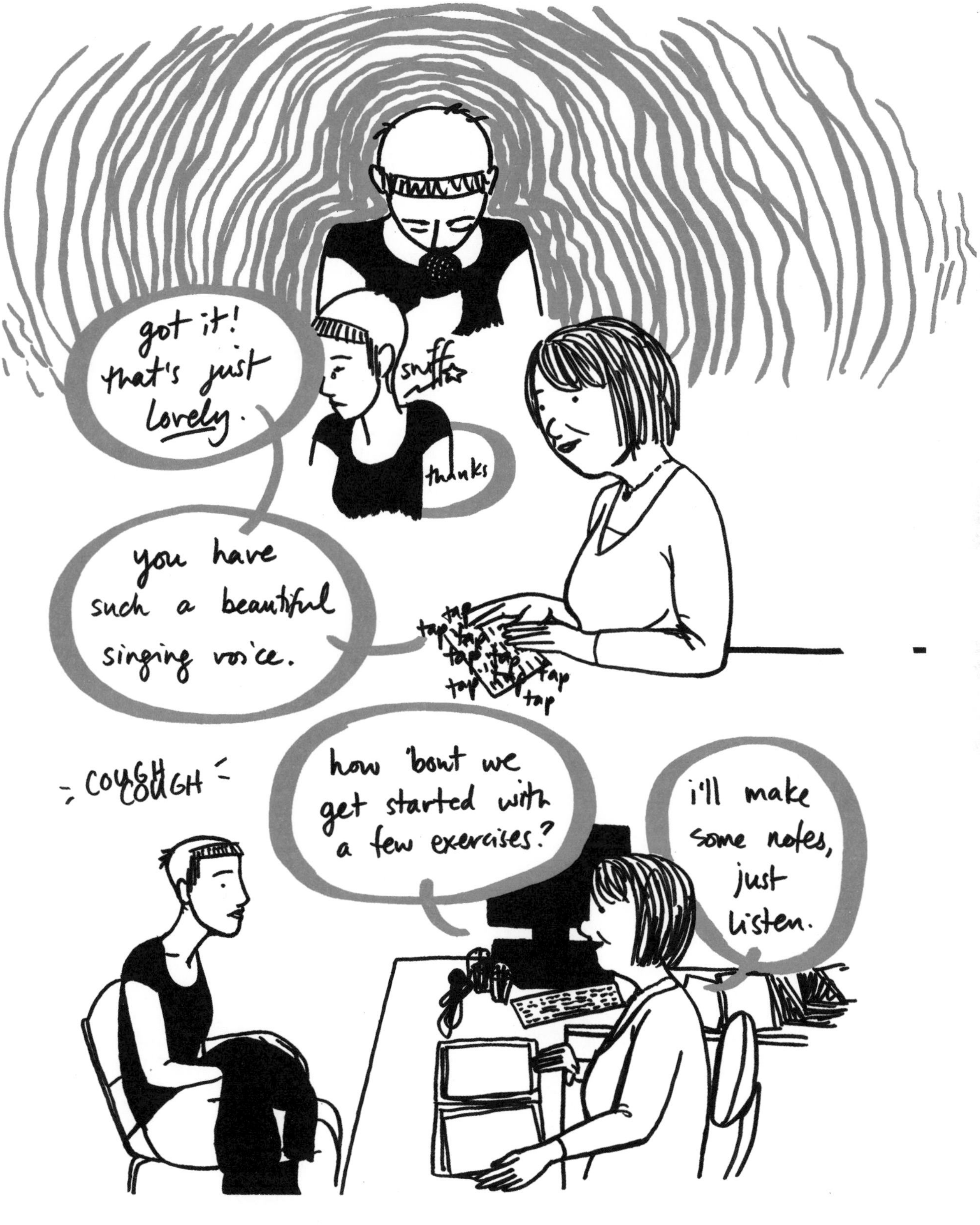
got it! that's just lovely.
sniff
thanks
you have such a beautiful singing voice.
tap tap tap tap tap tap tap tap tap
COUGH COUGH
how 'bout we get started with a few exercises?
i'll make some notes, just listen.

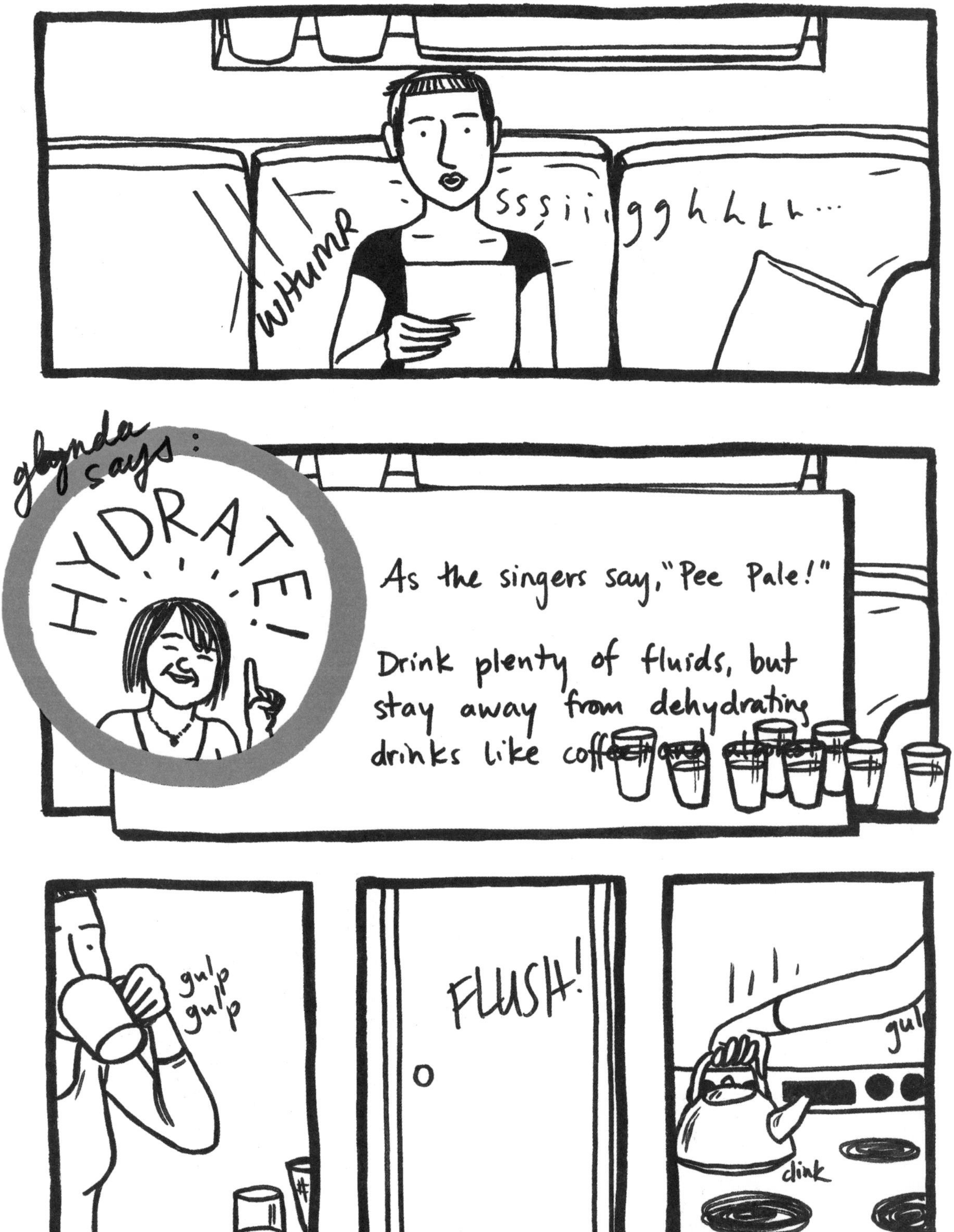
WHUMP
sssiiigghhhh...
glynda says:
HYDRATE!
As the singers say, "Pee Pale!"
Drink plenty of fluids, but stay away from dehydrating drinks like co
gulp gulp
FLUSH!
gul
clink

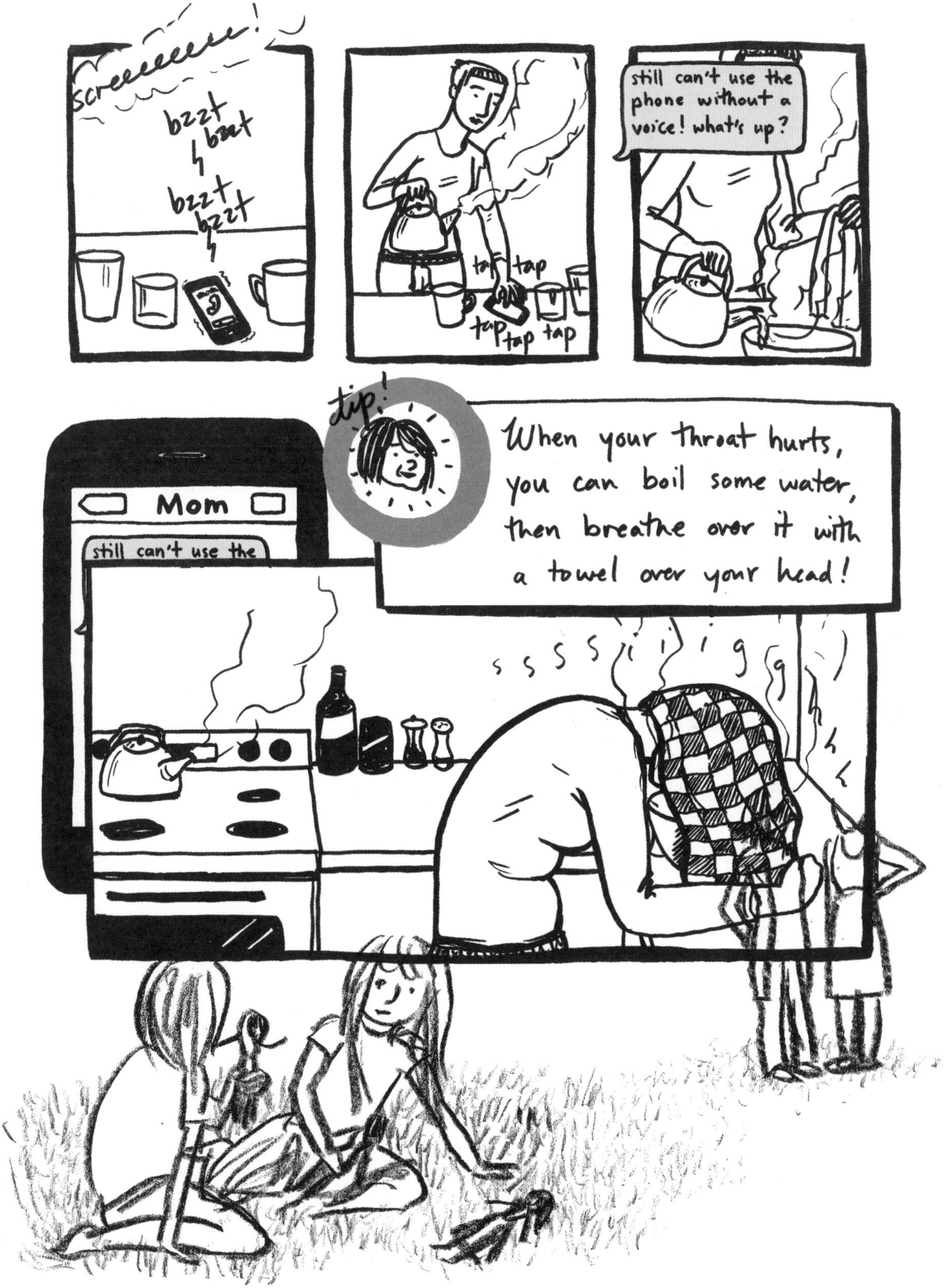
screeeeeeee!
bzzt bzzt
bzzt bzzt
tap tap
tap tap tap
still can't use the phone without a voice! what's up?
tip!
Mom
still can't use the
When your throat hurts, you can boil some water, then breathe over it with a towel over your head!
sssssiiigg

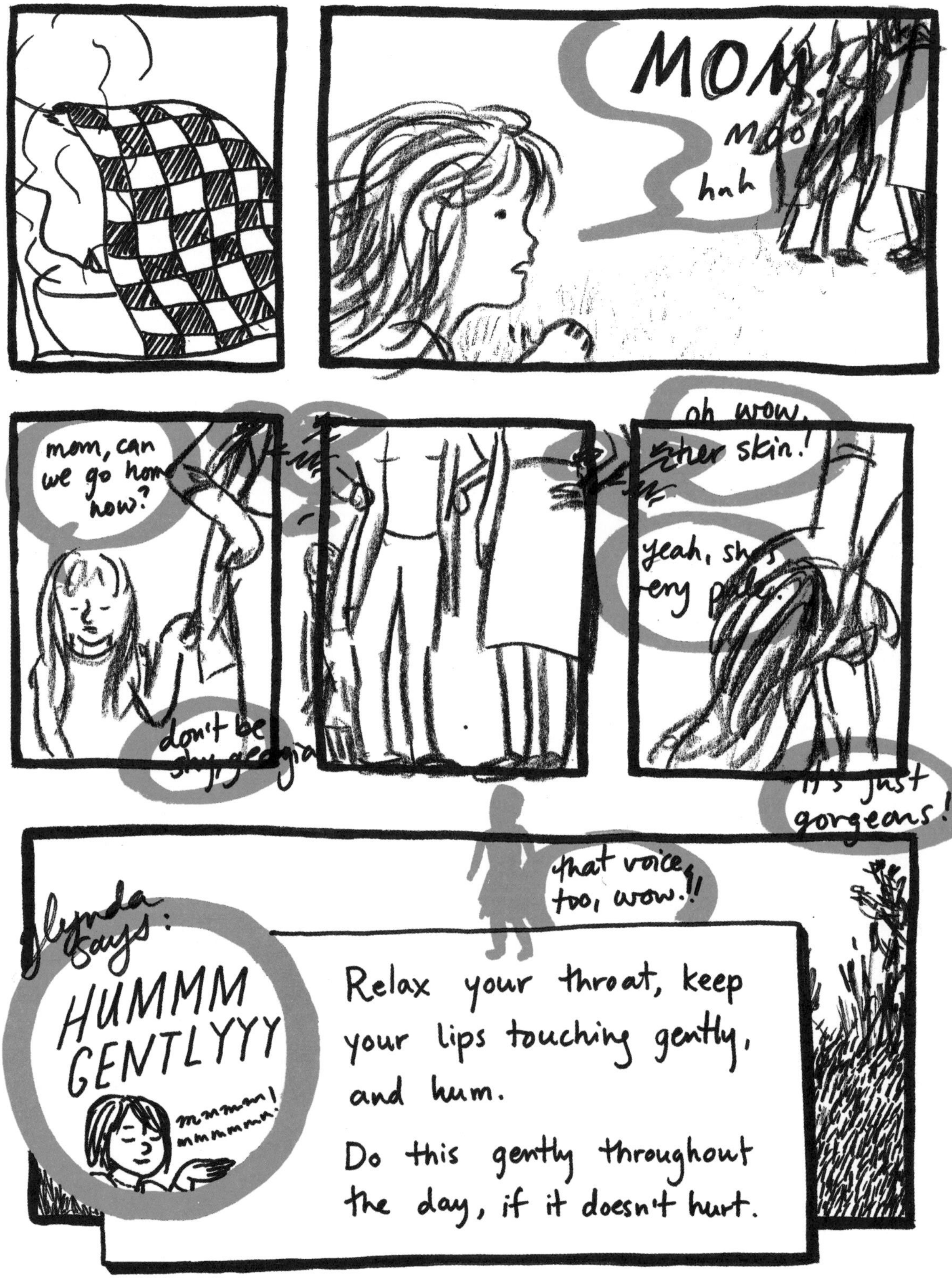
MOM!
MOM
hah
mom, can we go hom now?
don't be shy, georgia
oh wow, her skin!
yeah, she's very pale.
it's just gorgeous!
that voice, too, wow!!
glynda says:
HUMMM GENTLYYY
mmmmm! mmmmmm!
Relax your throat, keep your lips touching gently, and hum.
Do this gently throughout the day, if it doesn't hurt.

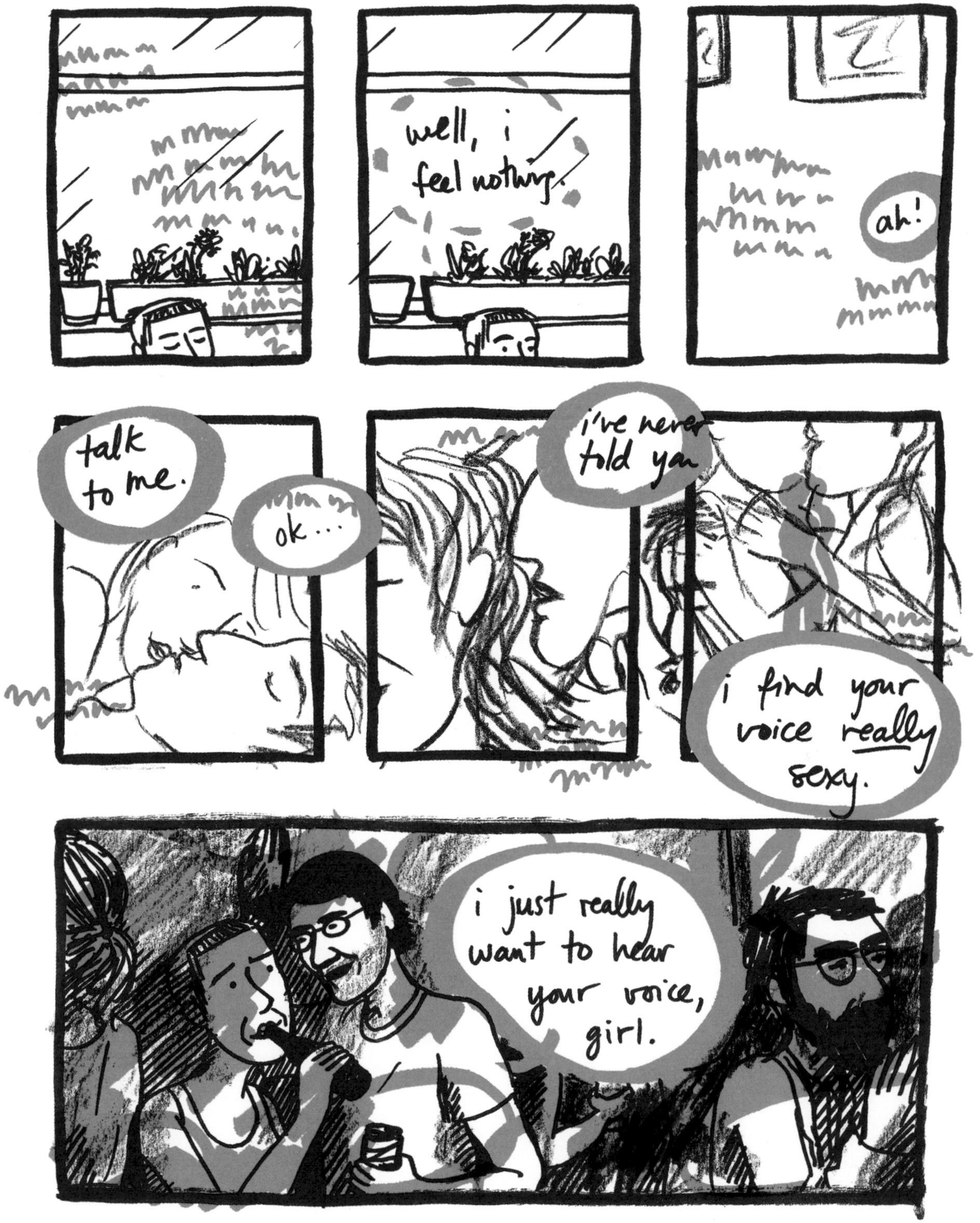
well, i feel nothing.
ah!
talk to me.
ok...
i've never told you
i find your voice really sexy.
i just really want to hear your voice, girl.

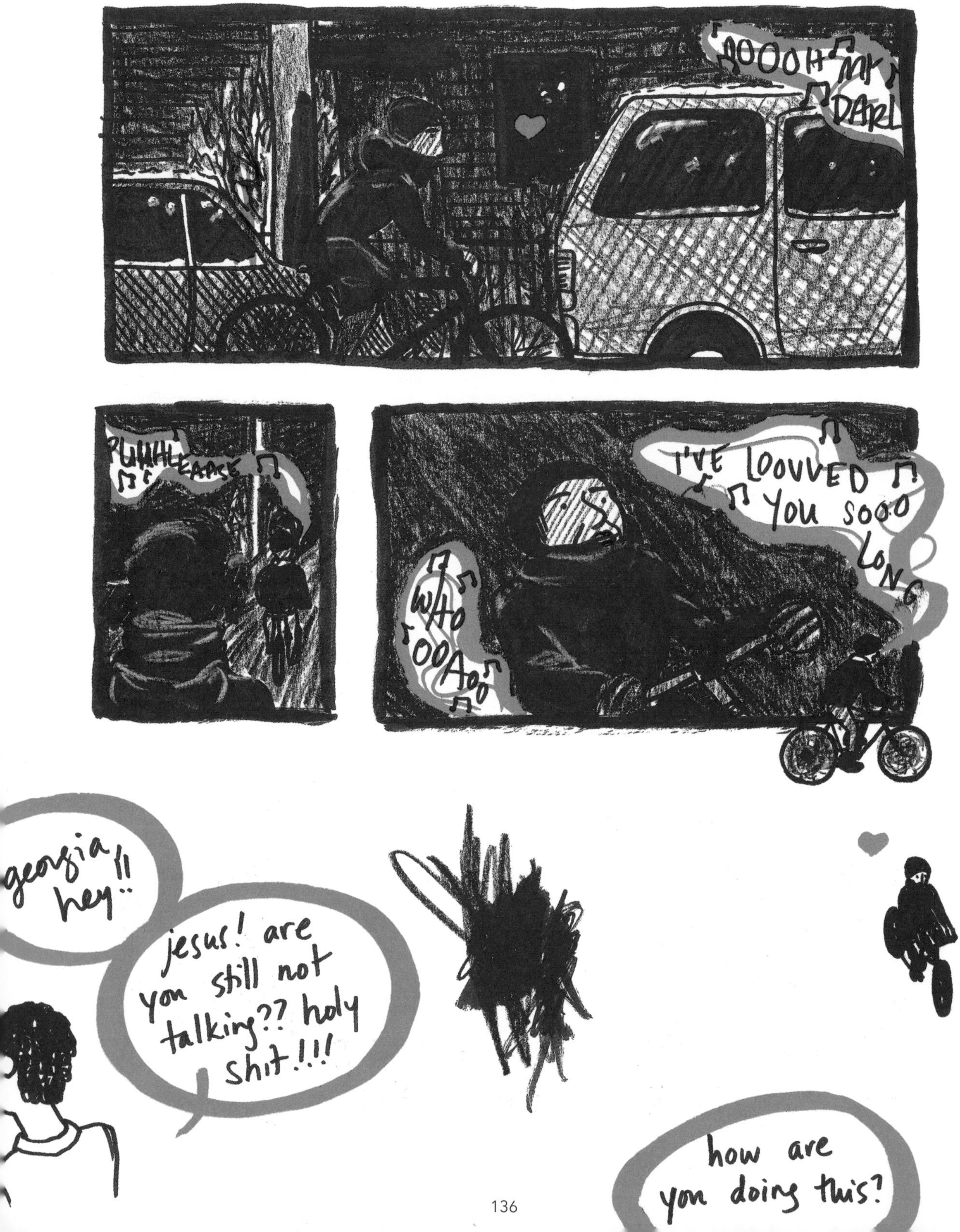
OOOOH MY DARL
PUHHLEAPSE
I'VE LOOVVED YOU SOOO LONG
WHO OOAOO
georgia hey!!
jesus! are you still not talking?? holy shit!!!
how are you doing this?

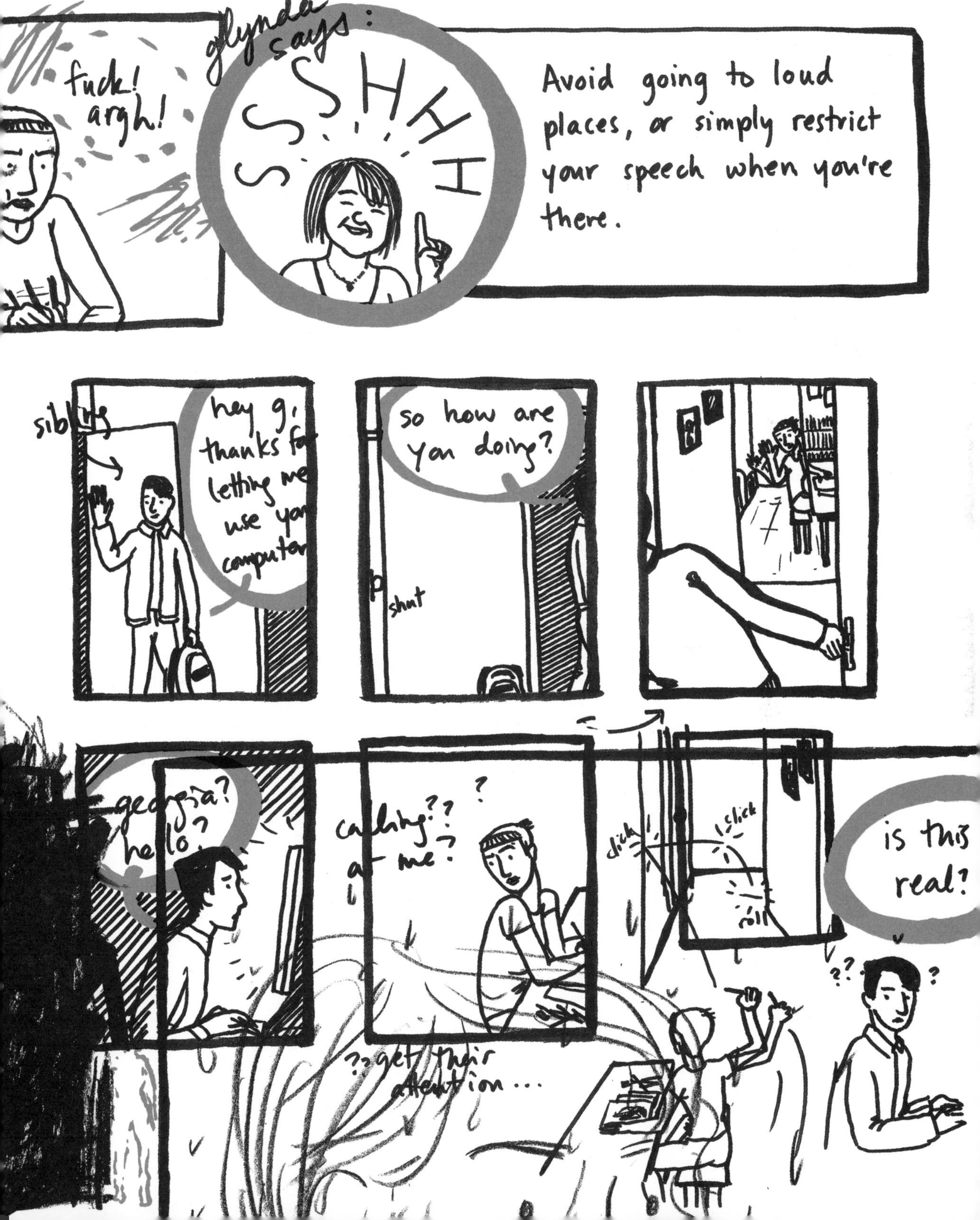
fuck! argh!
glynda says:
SSHHH
Avoid going to loud places, or simply restrict your speech when you're there.
sibling
hey g, thanks fo letting me use yo computer
so how are you doing?
shut
georgia? hello?
calling?? at me?
?
click
click
roll
is this real?
??get their attention...

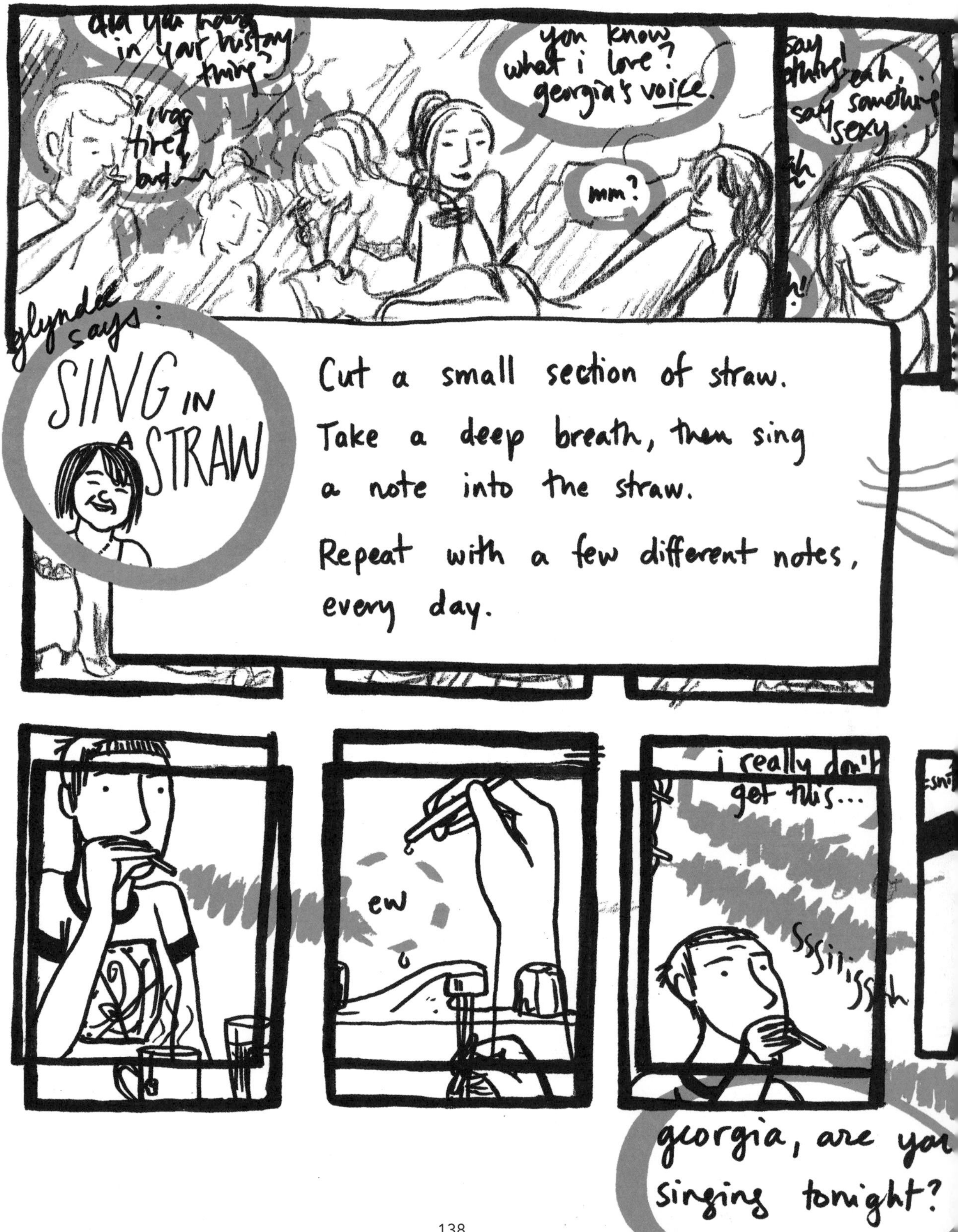
did you have in your history thing?
i was tired but—
you know what i love? georgia's voice.
mm?
yeah, say something sexy.
glynda says:
SING IN A STRAW
Cut a small section of straw.
Take a deep breath, then sing a note into the straw.
Repeat with a few different notes, every day.
ew
i really don't get this...
Sssiiissssh
georgia, are you singing tonight?

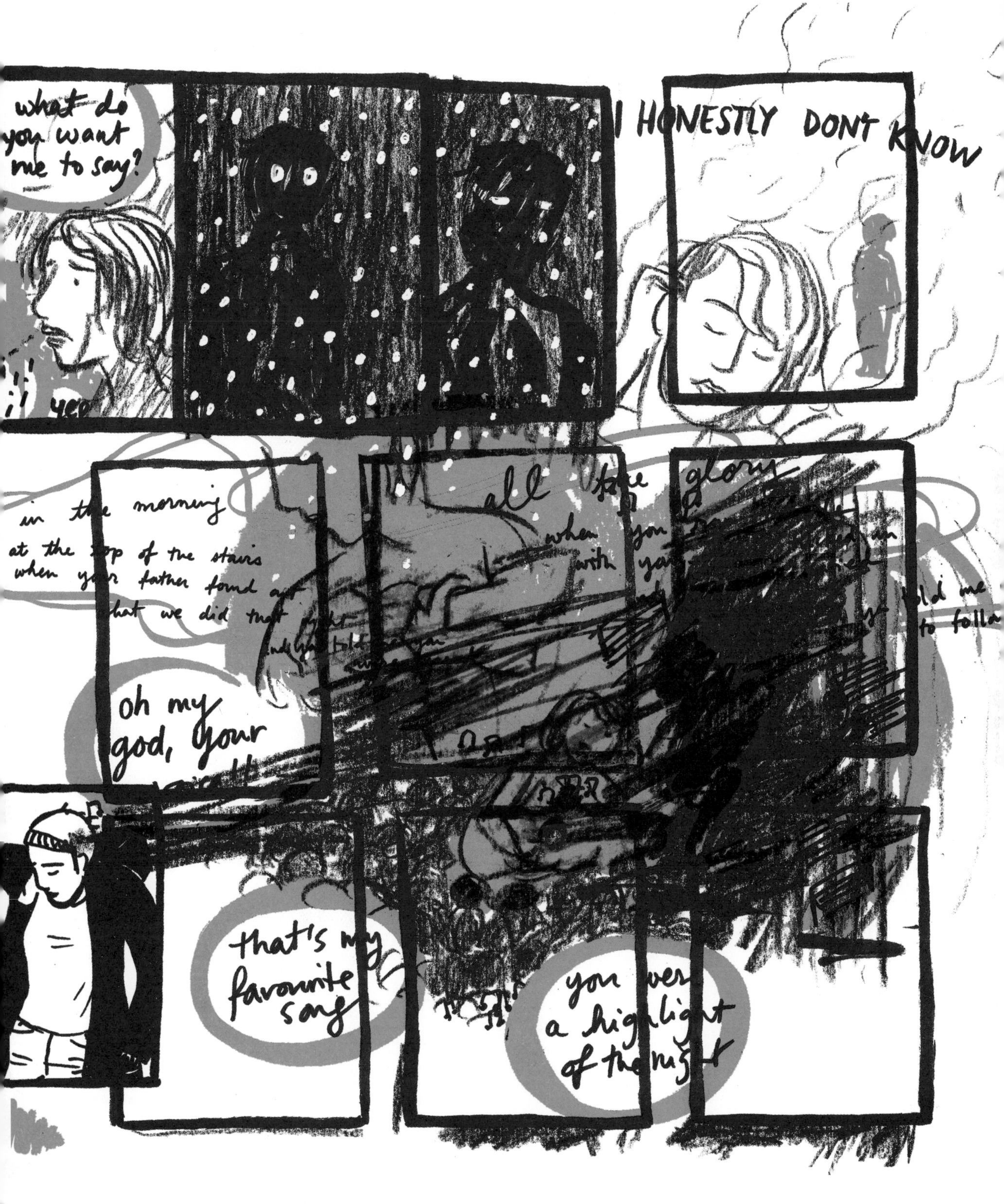
what do you want me to say?
yep
I HONESTLY DONT KNOW
in the morning
at the top of the stairs
when your father found out
what we did that night
all the glory
oh my god, your
that's my favourite song
you wer
a highlight
of the night

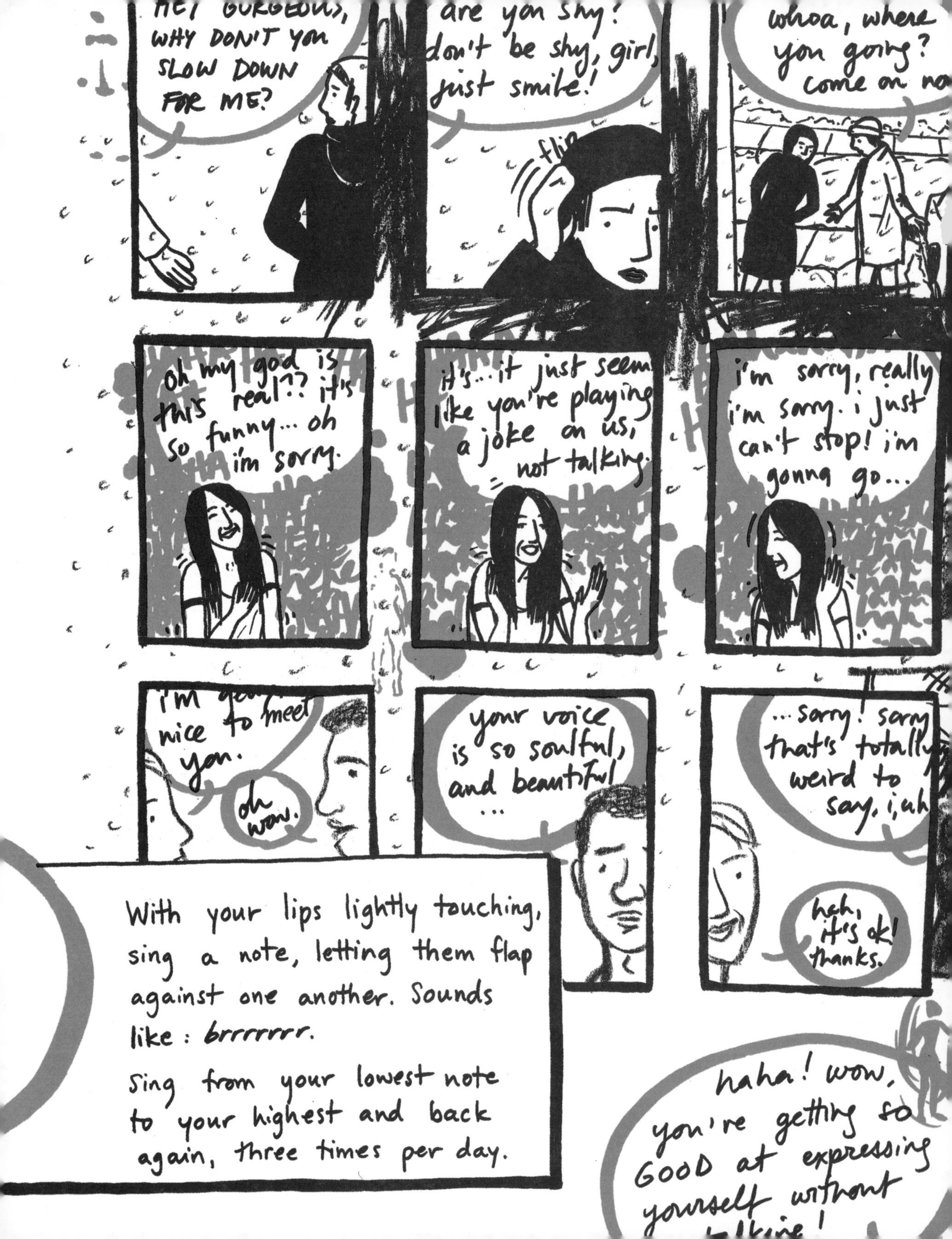

WHY DON'T YOU SLOW DOWN FOR ME?
are you shy? don't be shy, girl, just smile!
whoa, where you going? come on no
oh my god is this real?? it's so funny... oh i'm sorry
it's... it just seem like you're playing a joke on us, not talking.
i'm sorry, really i'm sorry. i just can't stop! i'm gonna go...
nice to meet you.
oh wow.
your voice is so soulful, and beautiful ...
...sorry! sorry that's totally weird to say. i, uh
hah, it's ok! thanks.
With your lips lightly touching, sing a note, letting them flap against one another. Sounds like : *brrrrrrr.*
Sing from your lowest note to your highest and back again, three times per day.
haha! wow, you're getting so GOOD at expressing yourself without

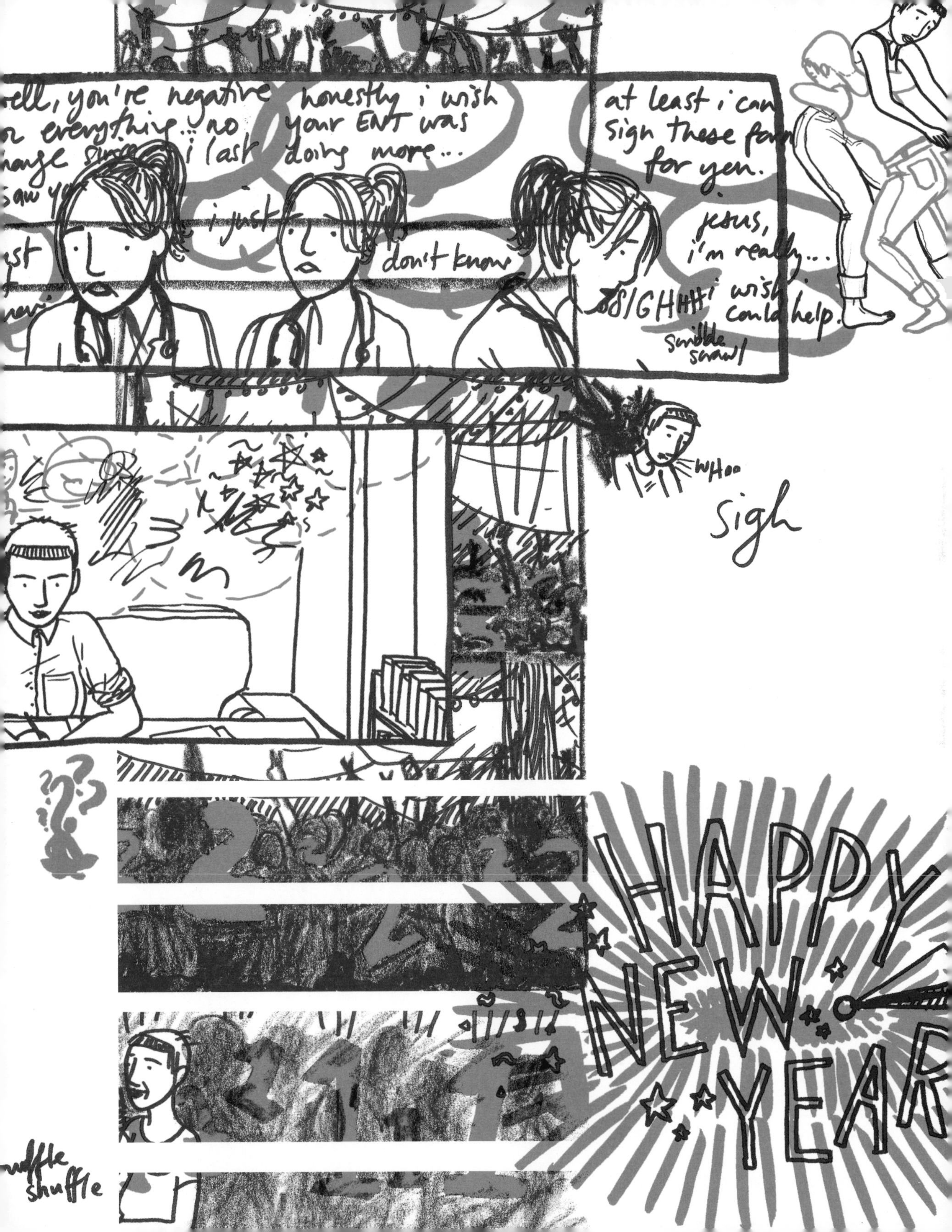
ell, you're negative
r everything... no
hange since i last
aw y
honestly i wish
your ENT was
doing more...
i just
don't know
at least i can
sign these for
for you.
jesus,
i'm really...
SIGHHH
i wish
could help.
scribble
scrawl
WHoo
sigh
shuffle
shuffle
HAPPY
NEW
YEAR

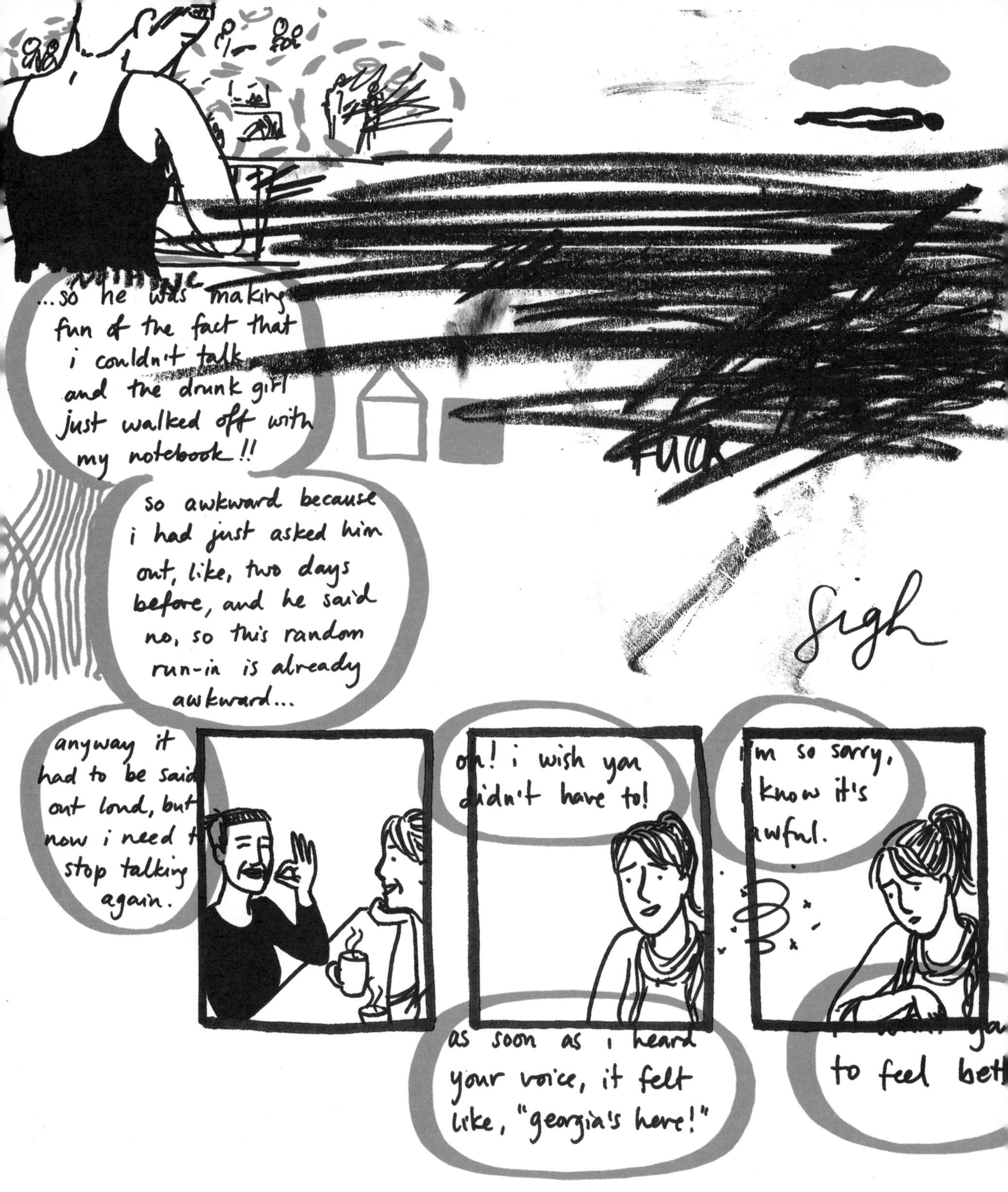
...so he was making fun of the fact that i couldn't talk and the drunk girl just walked off with my notebook!!
so awkward because i had just asked him out, like, two days before, and he said no, so this random run-in is already awkward...
Sigh
anyway it had to be said out loud, but now i need to stop talking again.
oh! i wish you didn't have to!
as soon as i heard your voice, it felt like, "georgia's here!"
i'm so sorry, i know it's awful.
to feel bet

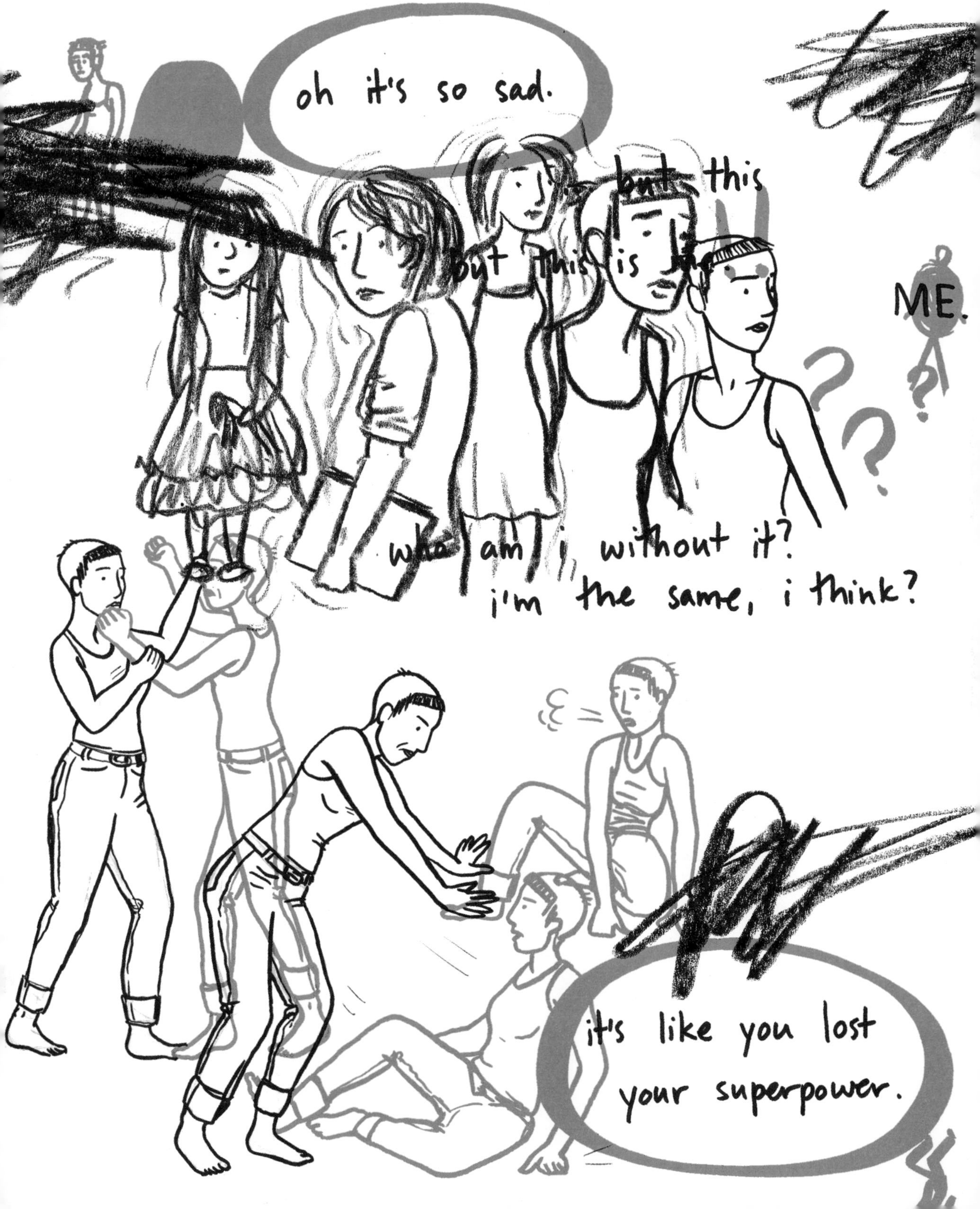
oh it's so sad.
but this
but this is
ME.
who am i without it?
i'm the same, i think?
it's like you lost your superpower.

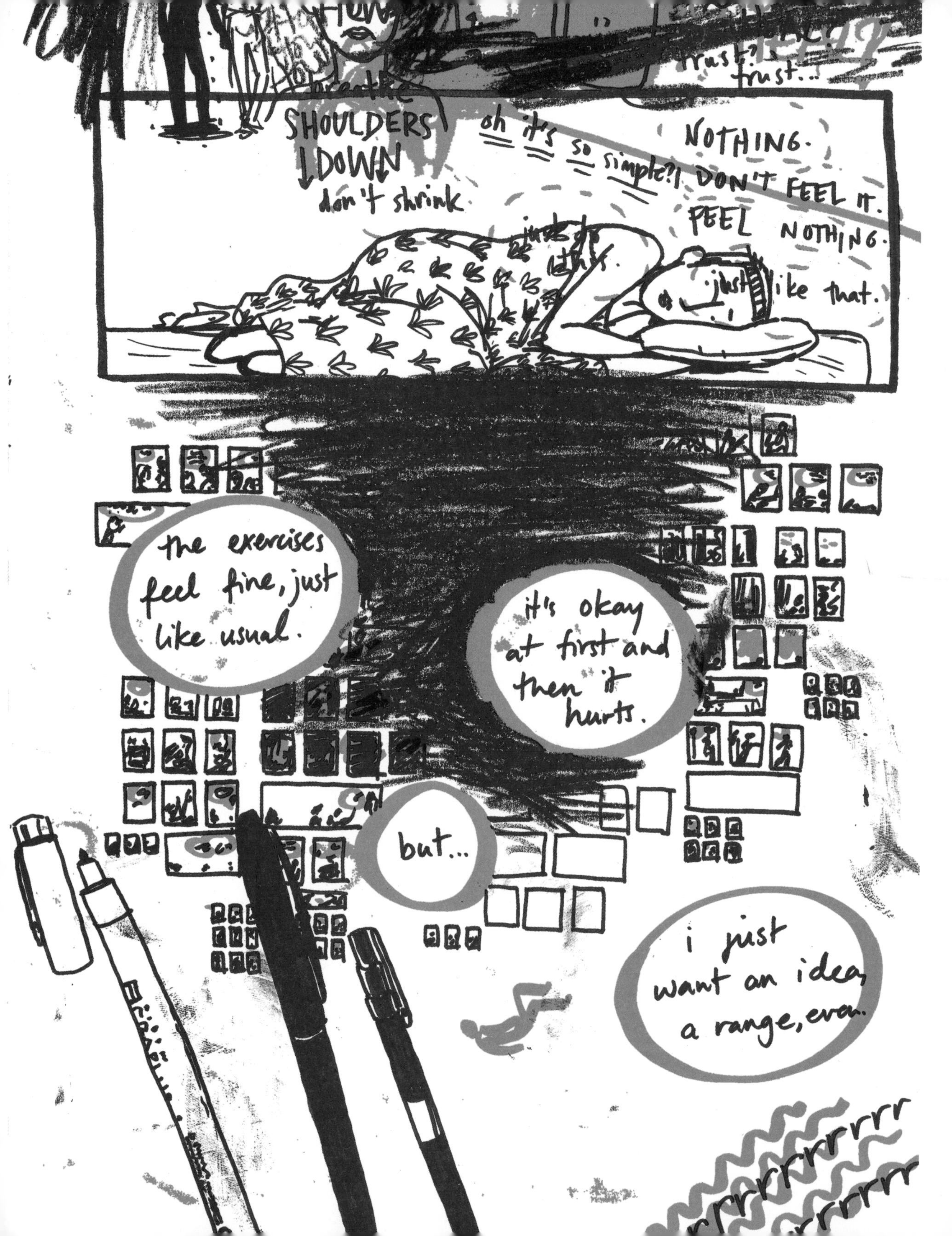

trust?, trust...
breathe
SHOULDERS DOWN
don't shrink
oh it's so simple?!
NOTHING. DON'T FEEL IT. FEEL NOTHING.
just do this.
just like that.
the exercises feel fine, just like usual.
it's okay at first and then it hurts.
but...
i just want an idea, a range, even.
rrrrrrrrrr
rrrrrrrrrr

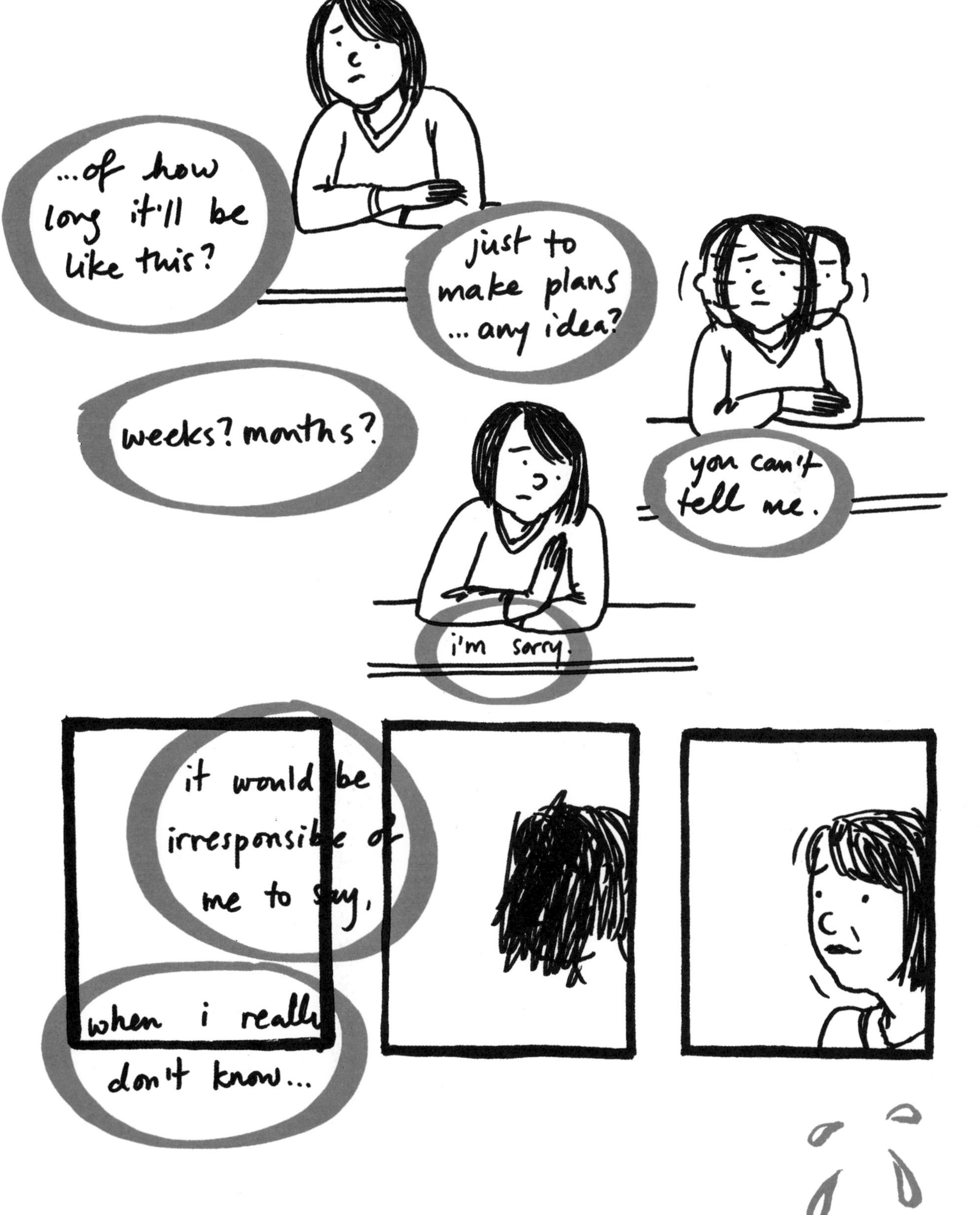
...of how long it'll be like this?
just to make plans ...any idea?
weeks? months?
you can't tell me.
i'm sorry.
it would be irresponsible of me to say,
when i really don't know...

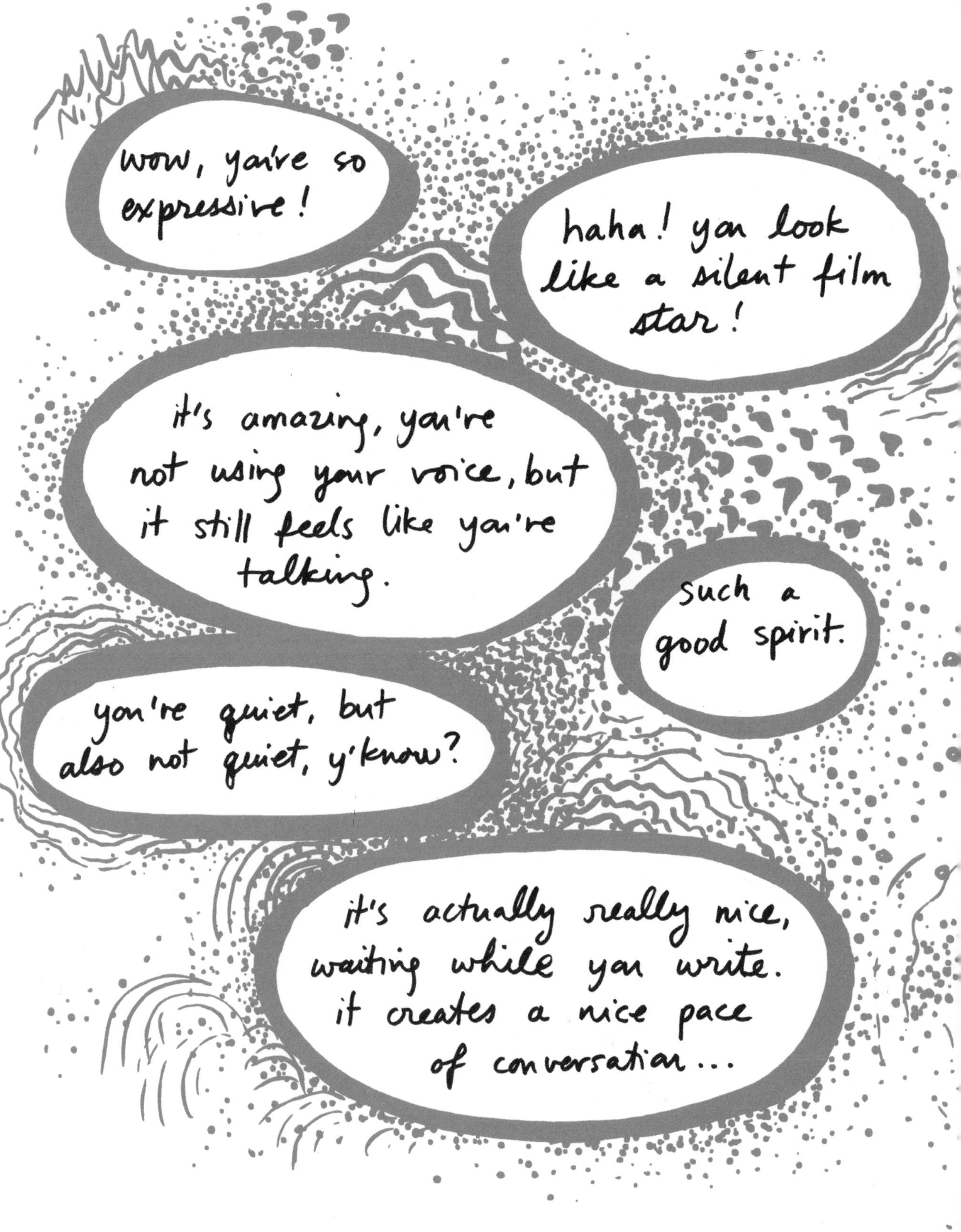
wow, you're so expressive!
haha! you look like a silent film star!
it's amazing, you're not using your voice, but it still feels like you're talking.
such a good spirit.
you're quiet, but also not quiet, y'know?
it's actually really nice, waiting while you write. it creates a nice pace of conversation...

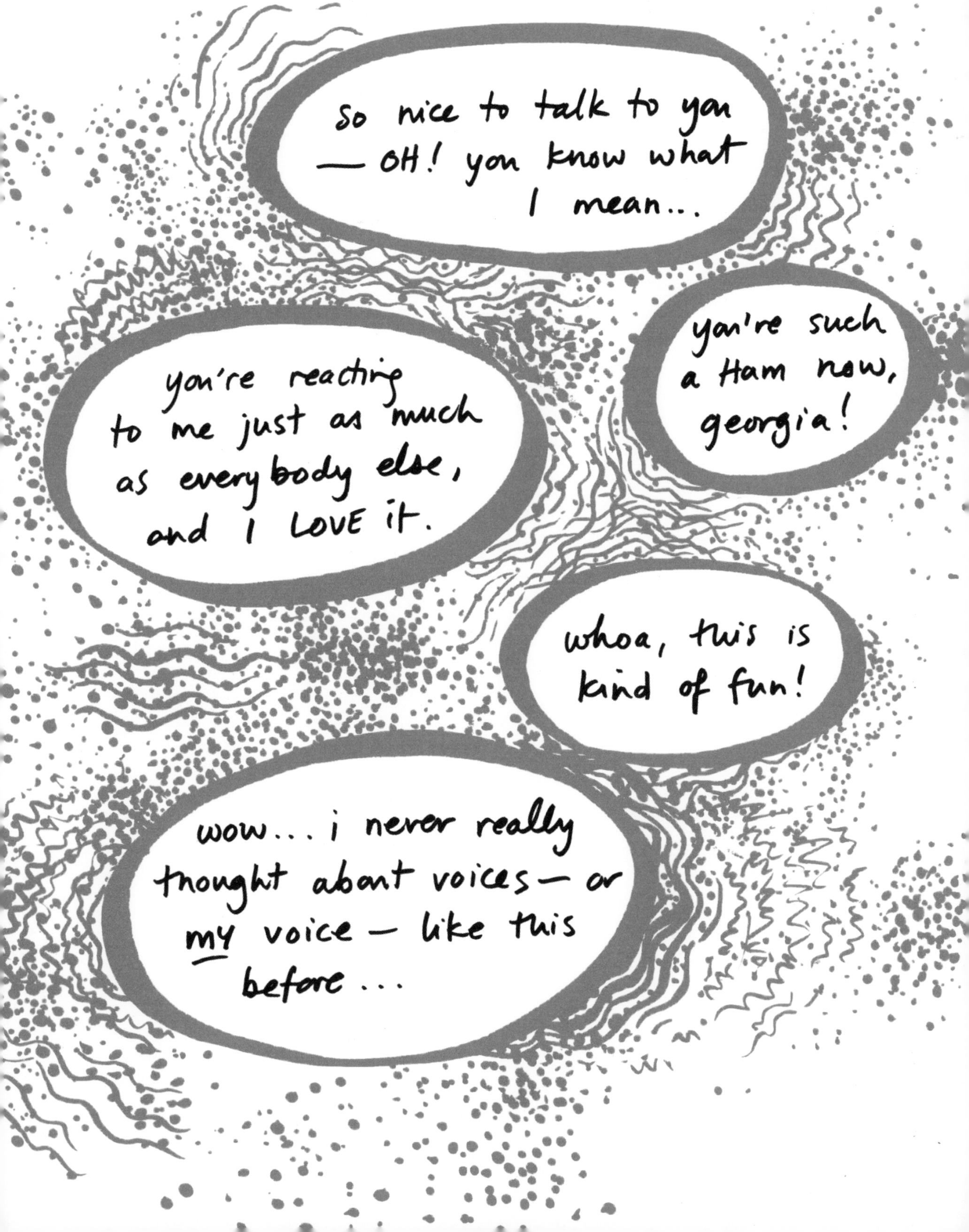
so nice to talk to you — OH! you know what I mean...
you're reacting to me just as much as everybody else, and I LOVE it.
you're such a Ham now, georgia!
whoa, this is kind of fun!
wow... i never really thought about voices — or MY voice — like this before...

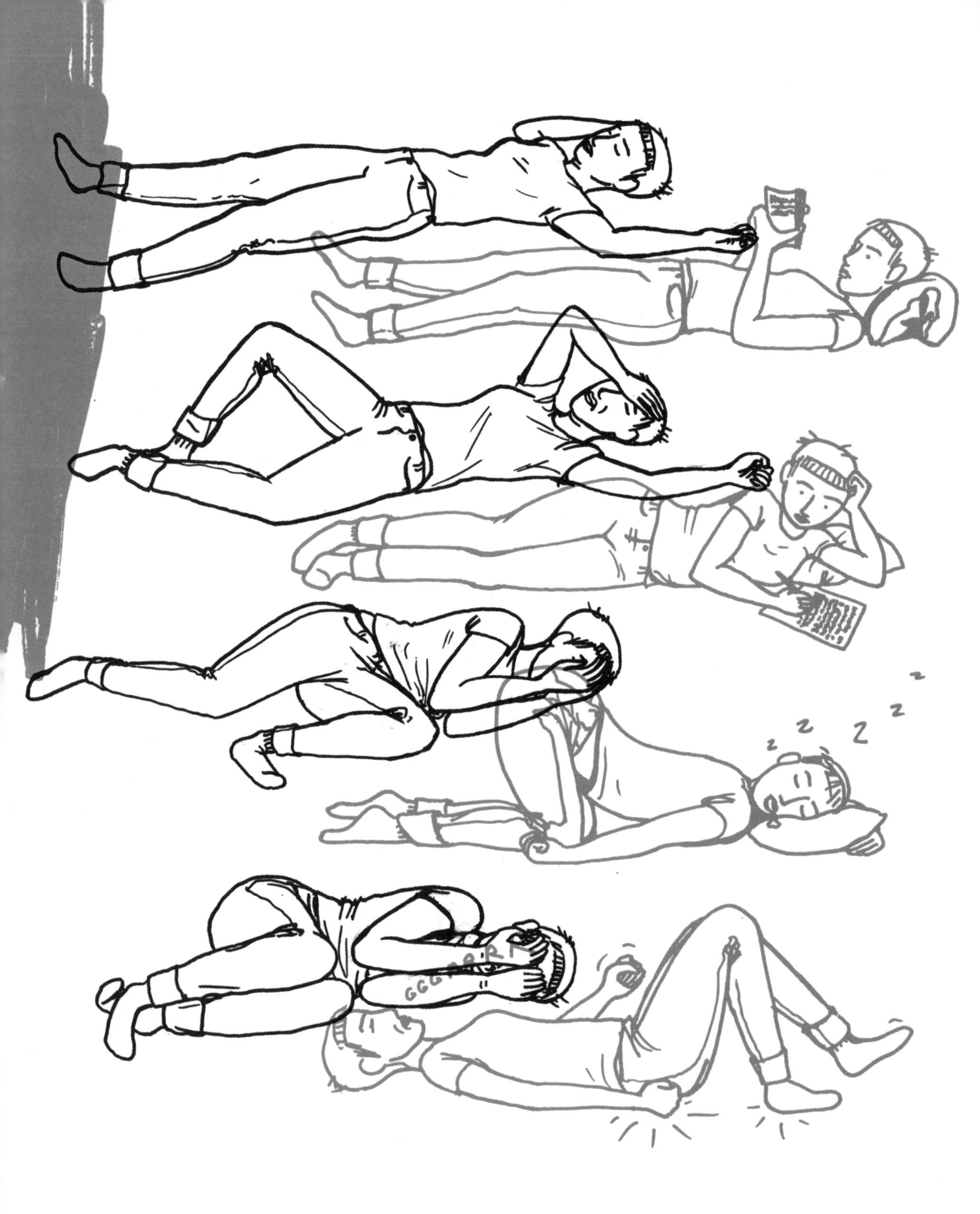

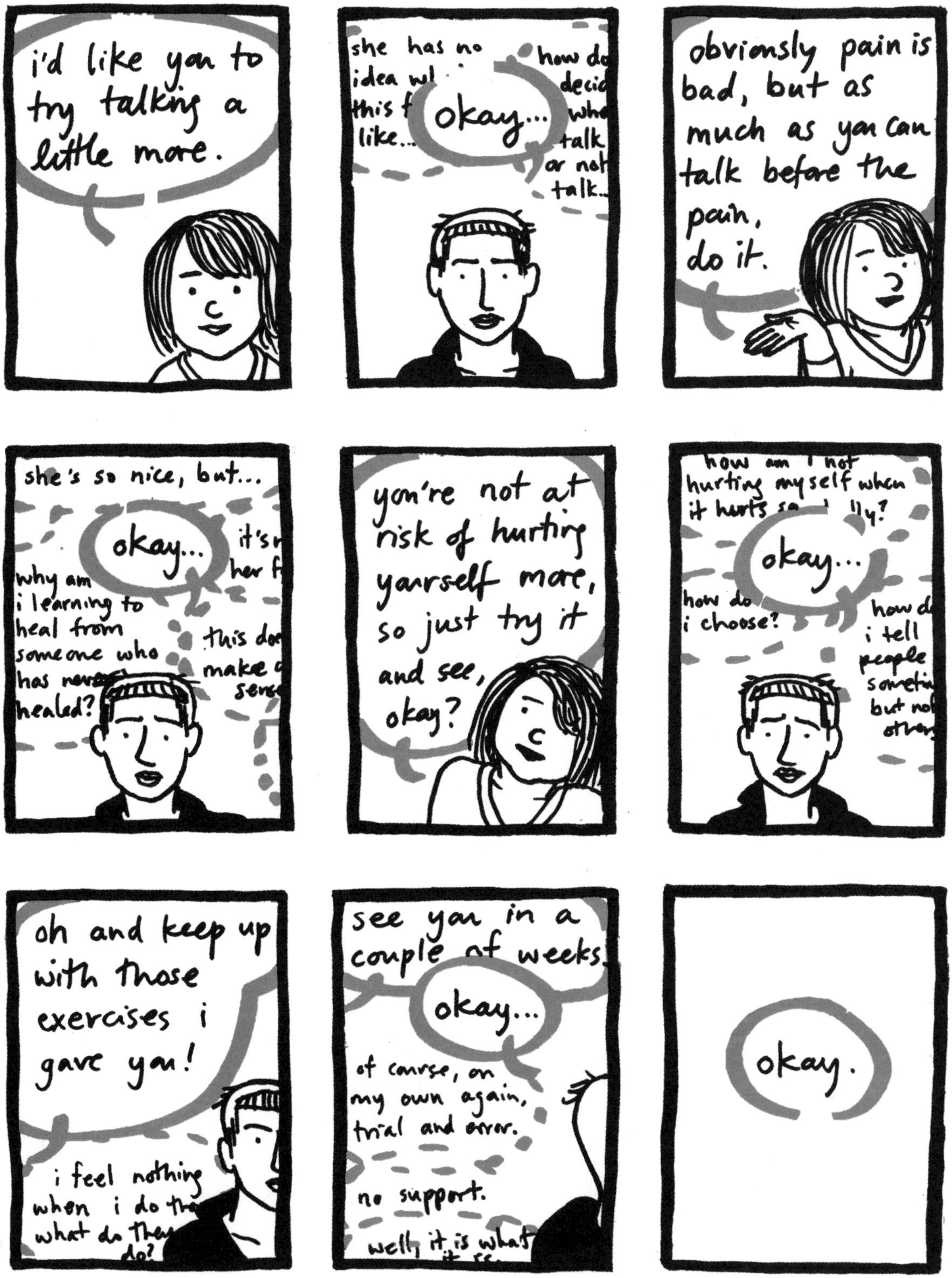
i'd like you to try talking a little more.
she has no idea
this
like...
okay...
how do
decid
talk
or not
talk...
obviously pain is bad, but as much as you can talk before the pain, do it.
she's so nice, but...
okay...
it's
her f
why am i learning to heal from someone who has never healed?
this do
make
sense
you're not at risk of hurting yourself more, so just try it and see, okay?
how am i not hurting myself when it hurts
okay...
how do i choose?
how d
i tell
people
someti
but no
other
oh and keep up with those exercises i gave you!
i feel nothing
when i do th
what do the
do?
see you in a couple of weeks.
okay...
of course, on my own again, trial and error.
no support.
well, it is what
okay.

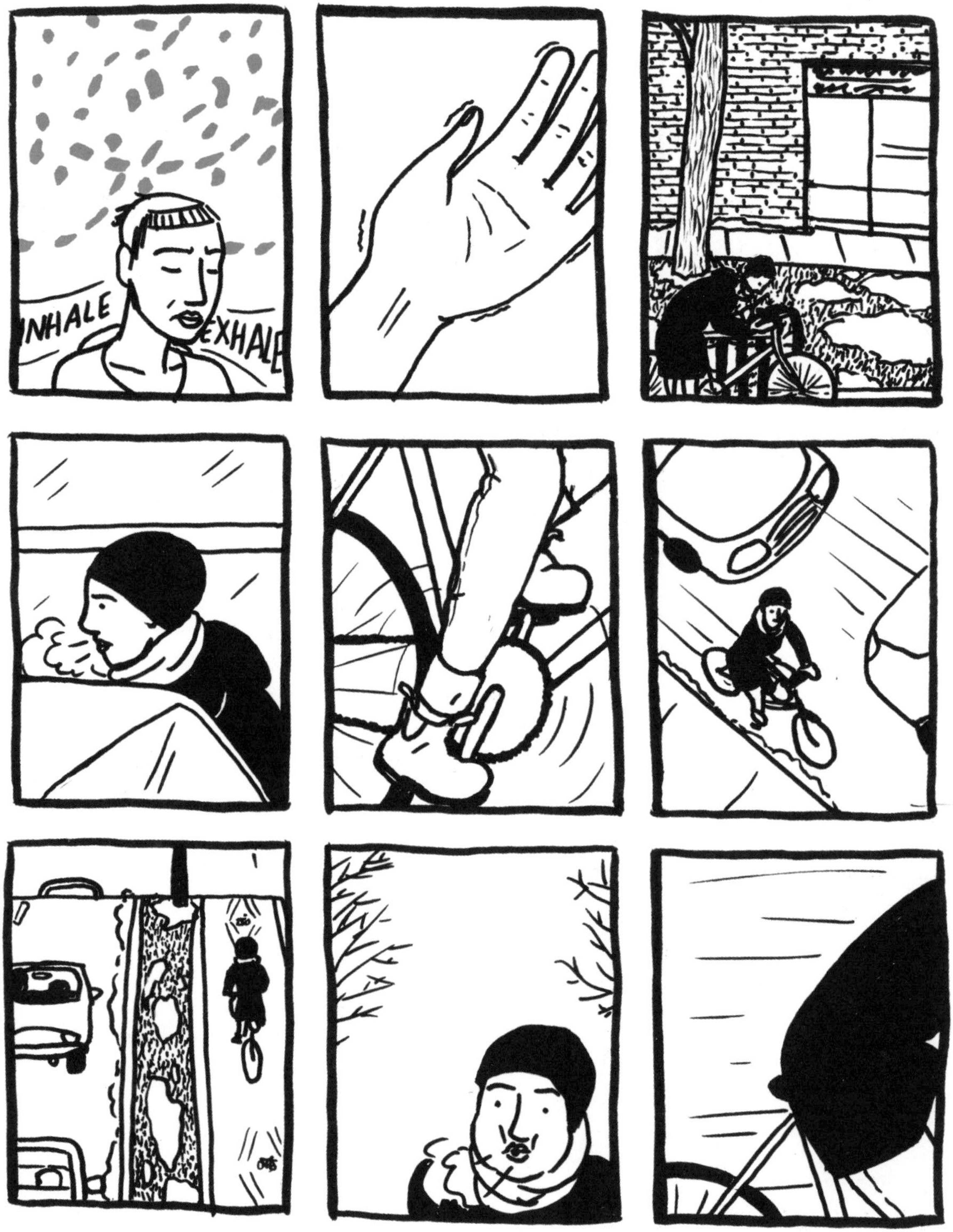
INHALE
EXHALE

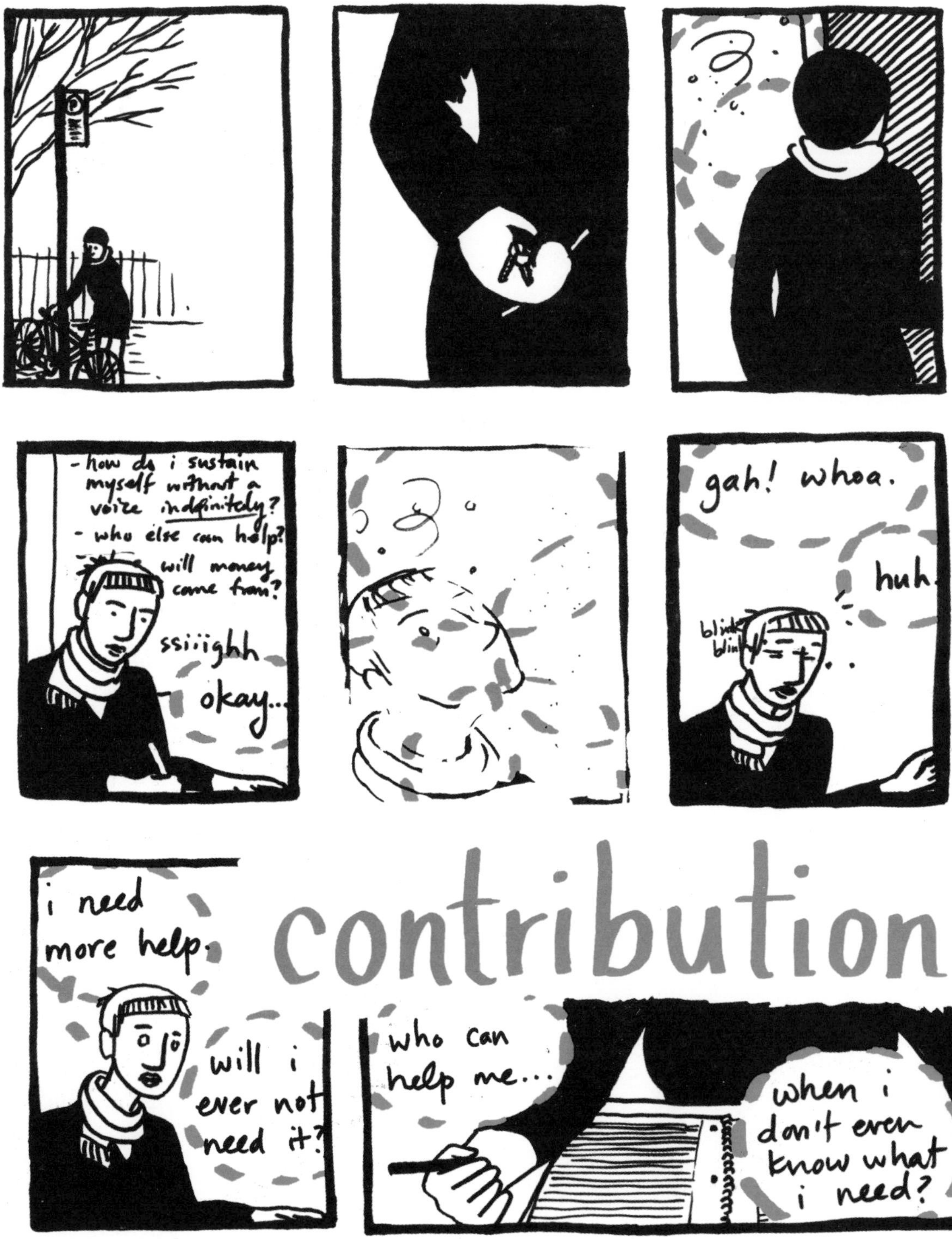

-how do i sustain myself without a voice indefinitely?
- who else can help?
will money come from?
ssiiighh
okay...
gah! whoa.
huh.
blink blink
i need more help.
contribution
will i ever not need it?
who can help me...
when i don't even know what i need?

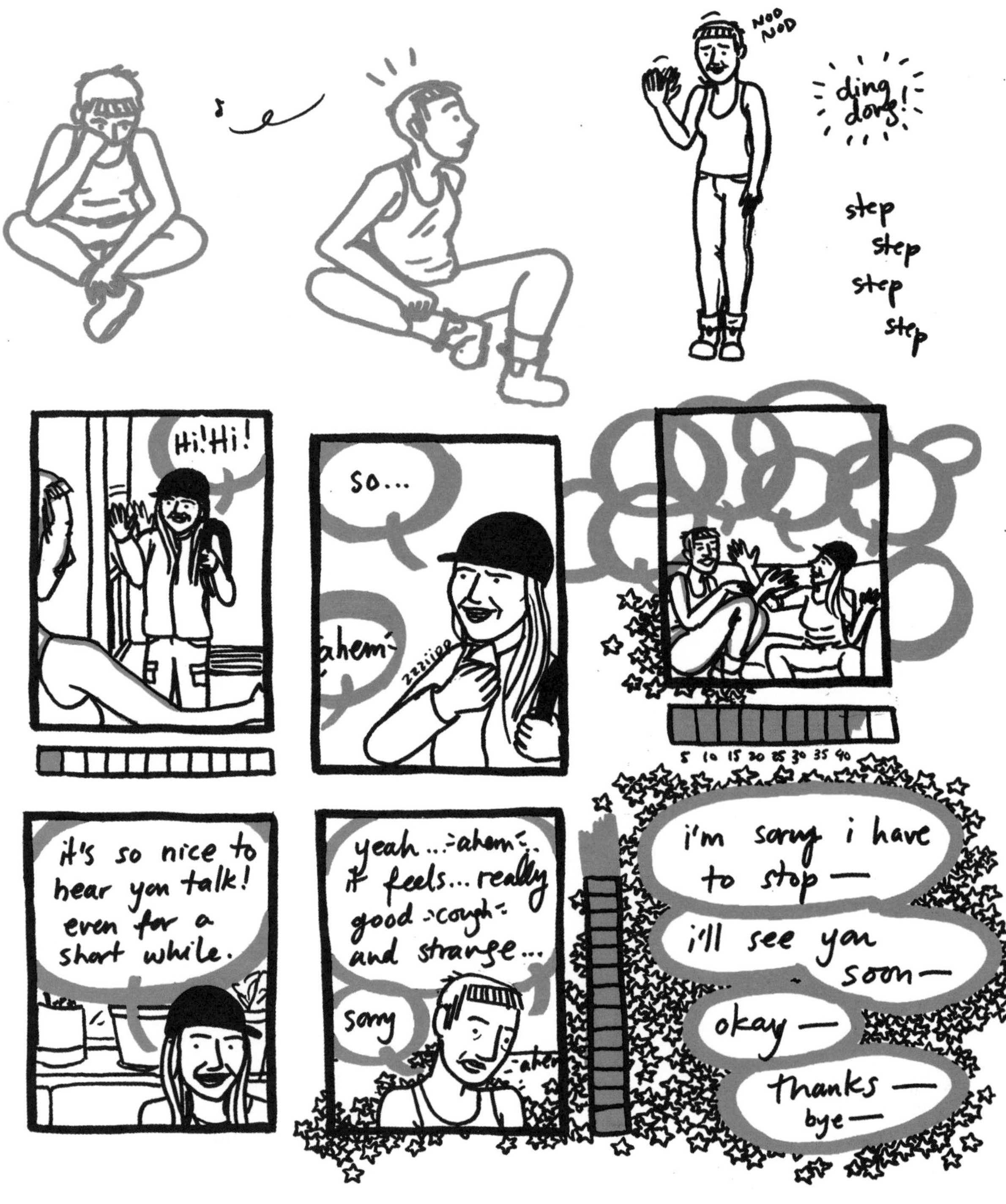
NOD NOD
ding dong!
step step step step
Hi! Hi!
so...
ahem
zzziipp
5 10 15 20 25 30 35 40
it's so nice to hear you talk! even for a short while.
yeah... ahem... it feels... really good cough and strange...
sorry
ahem
i'm sorry i have to stop—
i'll see you soon—
okay—
thanks—
bye—

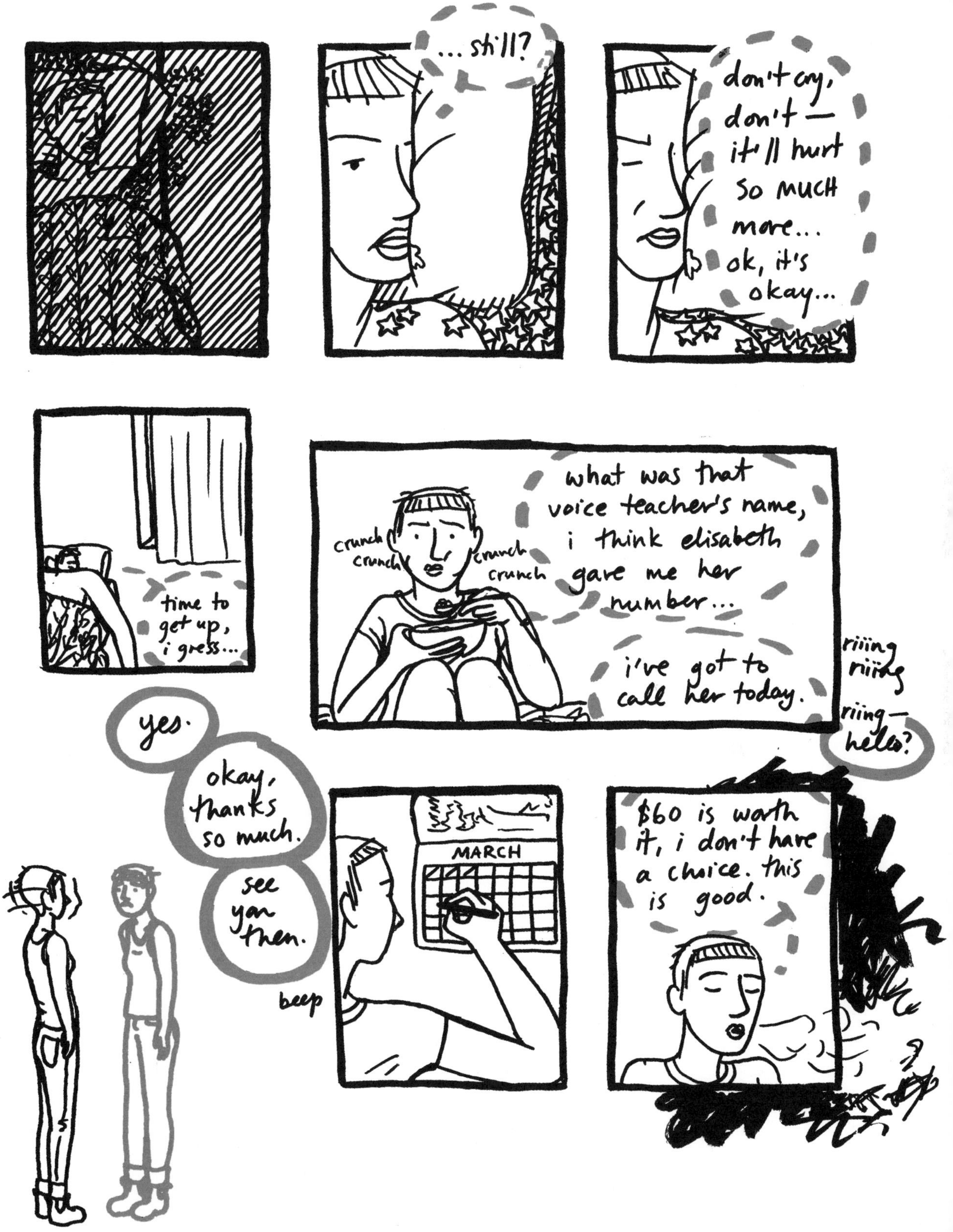
... still?
don't cry, don't — it'll hurt so MUCH more... ok, it's okay...
time to get up, i guess...
crunch crunch
crunch crunch
what was that voice teacher's name, i think elisabeth gave me her number...
i've got to call her today.
riiing riiing
riiing—
hello?
yes.
okay, thanks so much.
see you then.
beep
MARCH
$60 is worth it, i don't have a choice. this is good.

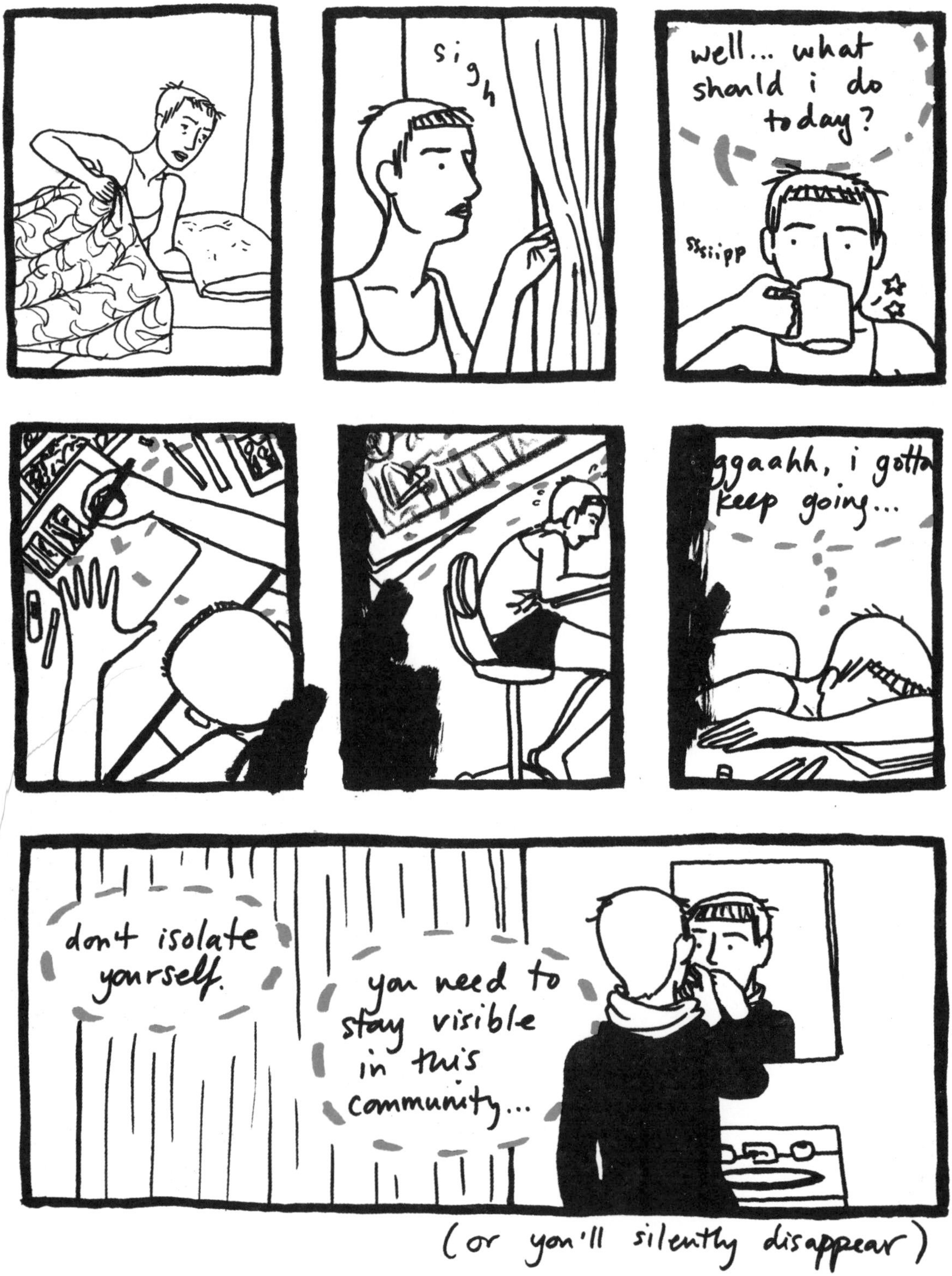
sigh
well... what should i do today?
sssiipp
ggaahh, i gotta keep going...
don't isolate yourself.
you need to stay visible in this community...
(or you'll silently disappear)

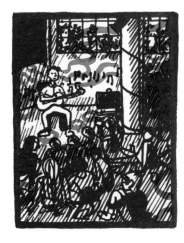

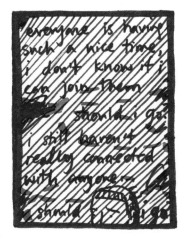

everyone is having
such a nice time
i don't know if i
can join them

should i go
i still haven't
really connected
with anyone...

should i...

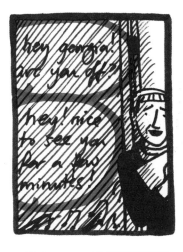

hey georgia!
are you off?

hey! nice
to see you
for a few
minutes!

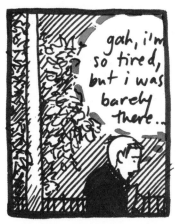

gah, i'm
so tired,
but i was
barely
there...

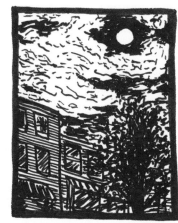

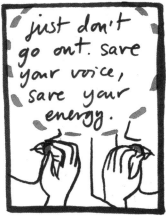

just don't
go out. save
your voice,
save your
energy.

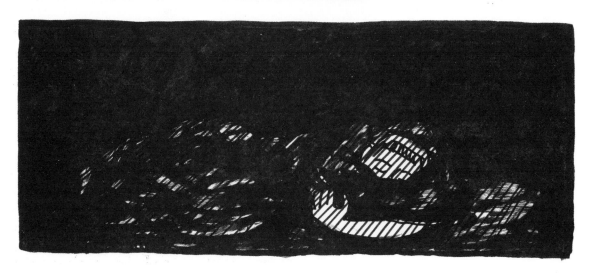

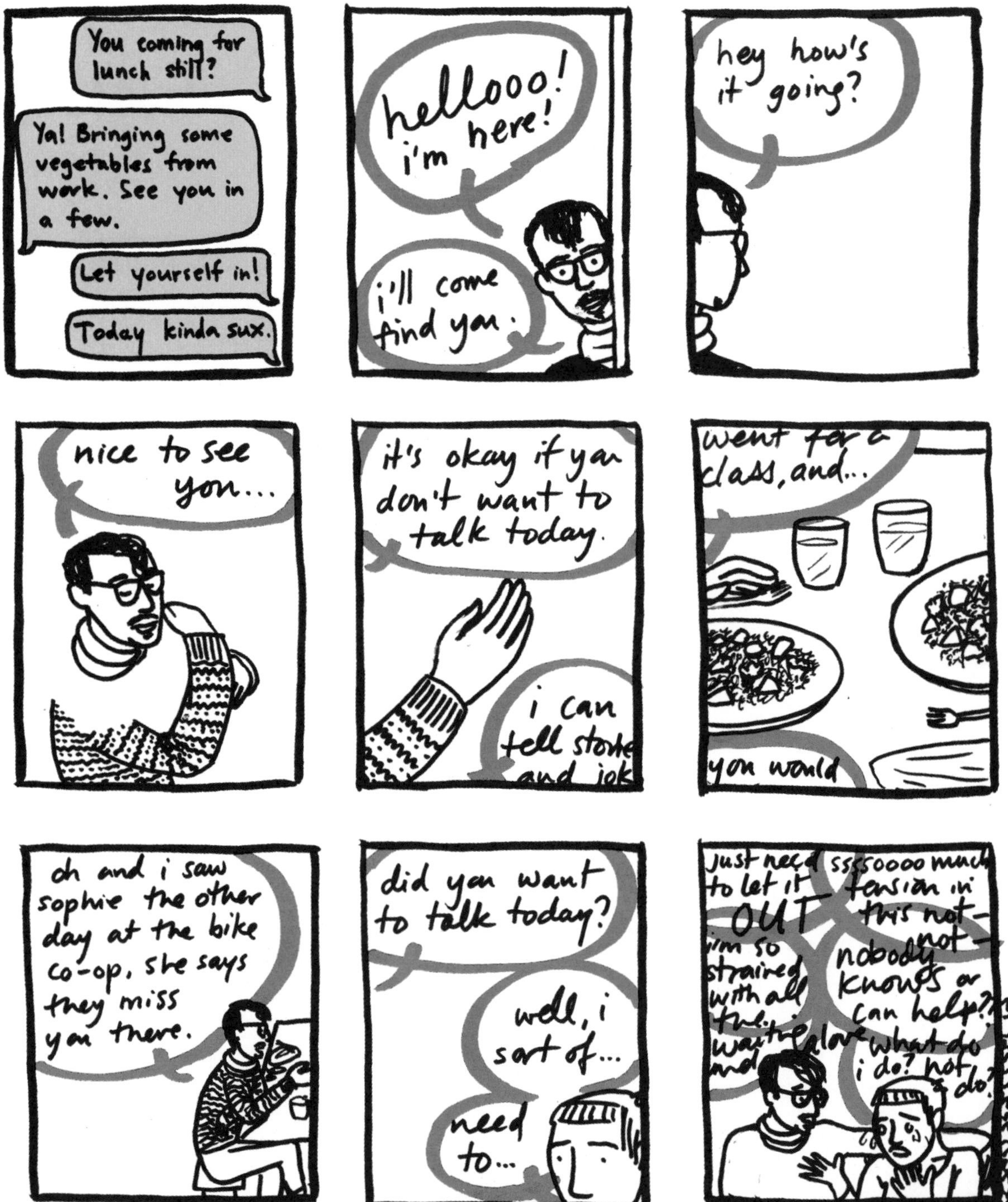
You coming for lunch still?
Ya! Bringing some vegetables from work. See you in a few.
Let yourself in!
Today kinda sux.
hellooo! i'm here!
i'll come find you.
hey how's it going?
nice to see you...
it's okay if you don't want to talk today.
i can tell storie and jok
went for a class, and...
you would
oh and i saw sophie the other day at the bike co-op, she says they miss you there.
did you want to talk today?
well, i sort of...
need to...
just need to let it OUT
ssssoooo much tension in this not— not—
i'm so strained with all the
nobody knows or can help??
what do i do? not do?

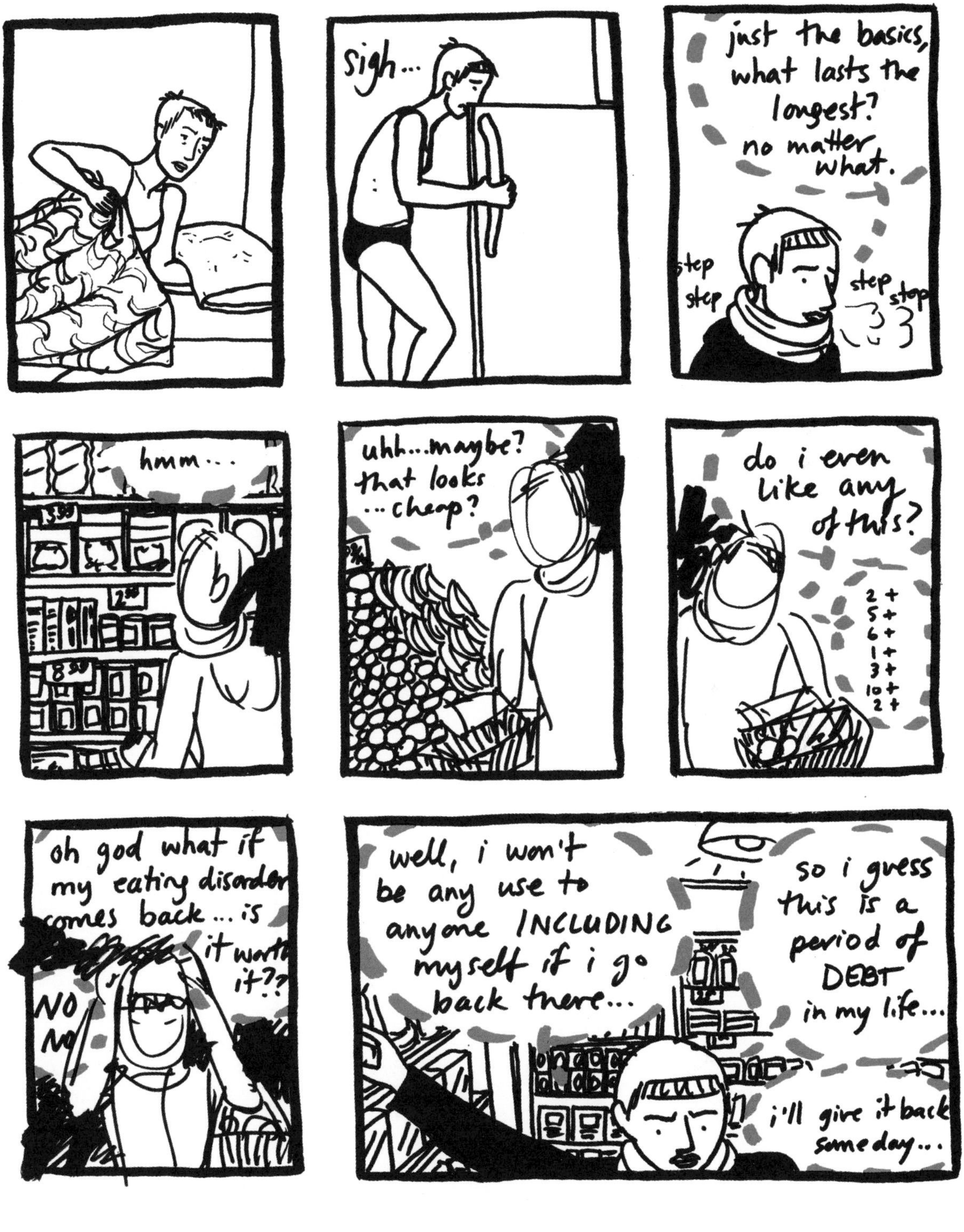

sigh...
just the basics, what lasts the longest? no matter what.
step step
step step
hmm...
uhh... maybe? that looks ...cheap?
do i even like any of this?
2 + 5 + 6 + 1 + 3 + 10 + 2 +
oh god what if my eating disorder comes back... is it worth it??
NO NO
well, i won't be any use to anyone INCLUDING myself if i go back there...
so i guess this is a period of DEBT in my life...
i'll give it back someday...

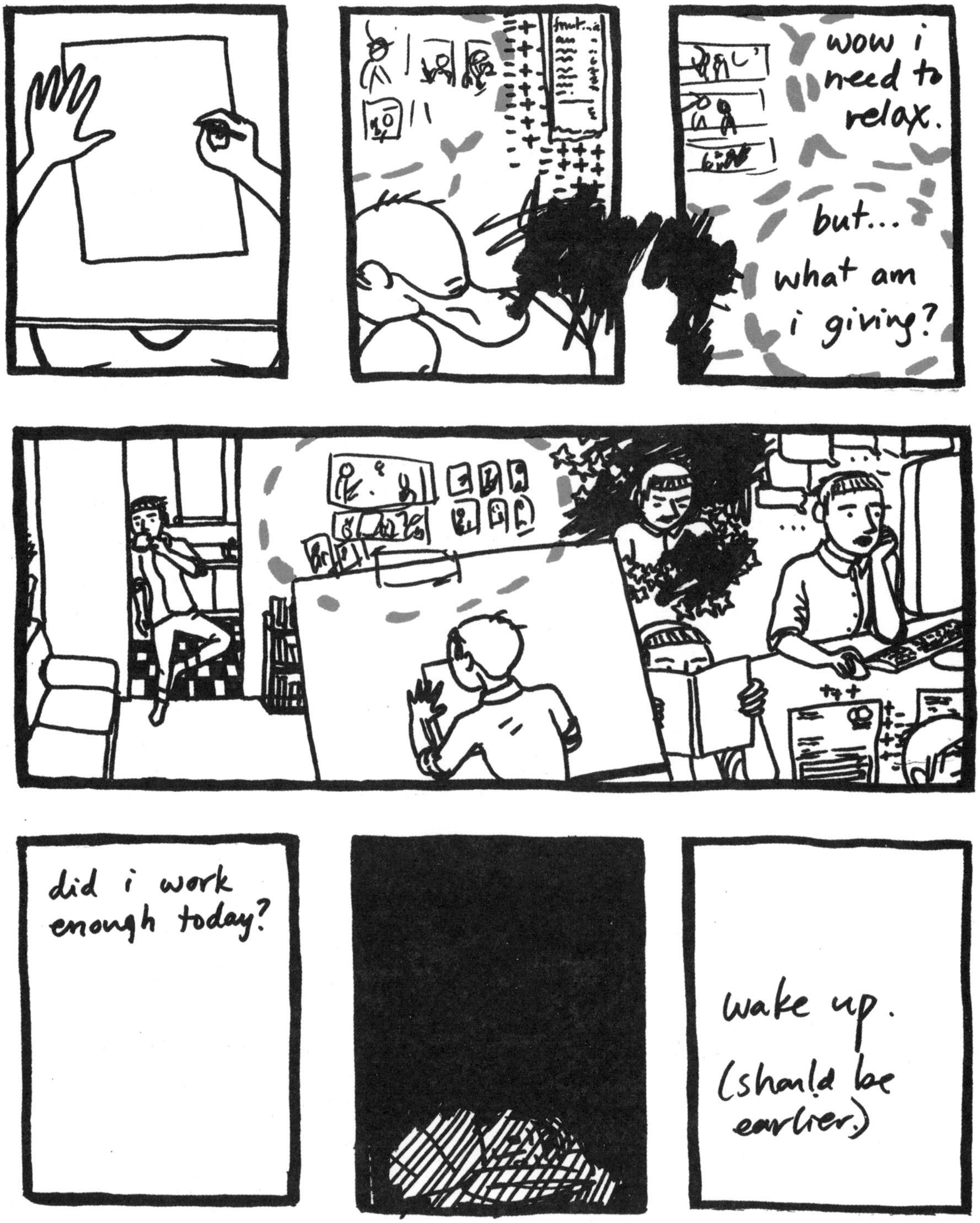
wow i need to relax.
but... what am i giving?
did i work enough today?
wake up.
(should be earlier.)

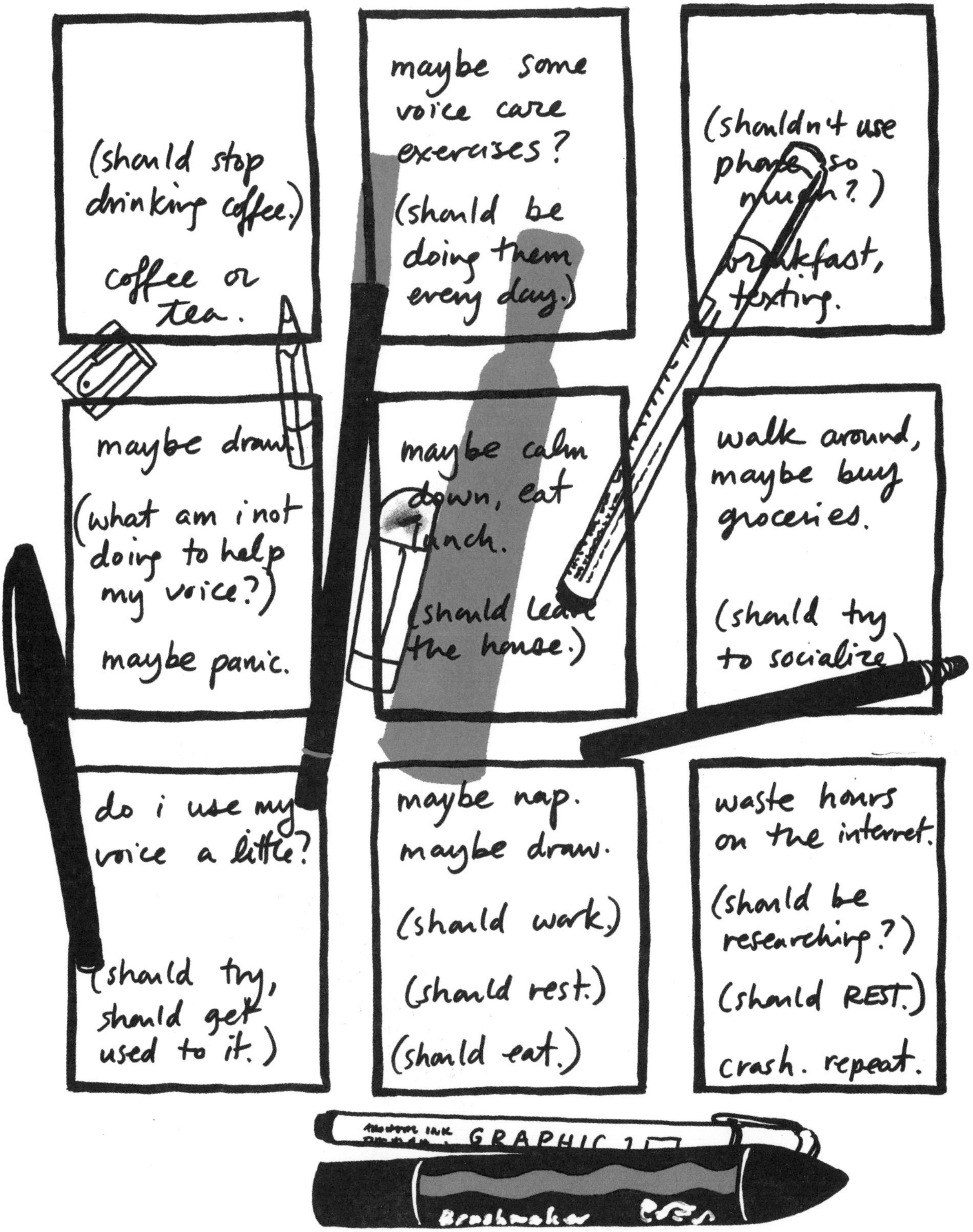

(should stop drinking coffee.)

coffee or tea.

maybe some voice care exercises?

(should be doing them every day.)

(shouldn't use phone so much?)

breakfast, texting.

maybe draw.

(what am i not doing to help my voice?)

maybe panic.

maybe calm down, eat lunch.

(should leave the house.)

walk around, maybe buy groceries.

(should try to socialize.)

do i use my voice a little?

(should try, should get used to it.)

maybe nap.
maybe draw.
(should work.)
(should rest.)
(should eat.)

waste hours on the internet.

(should be researching?)

(should REST.)

crash. repeat.

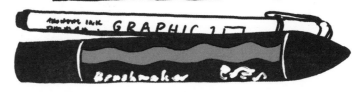

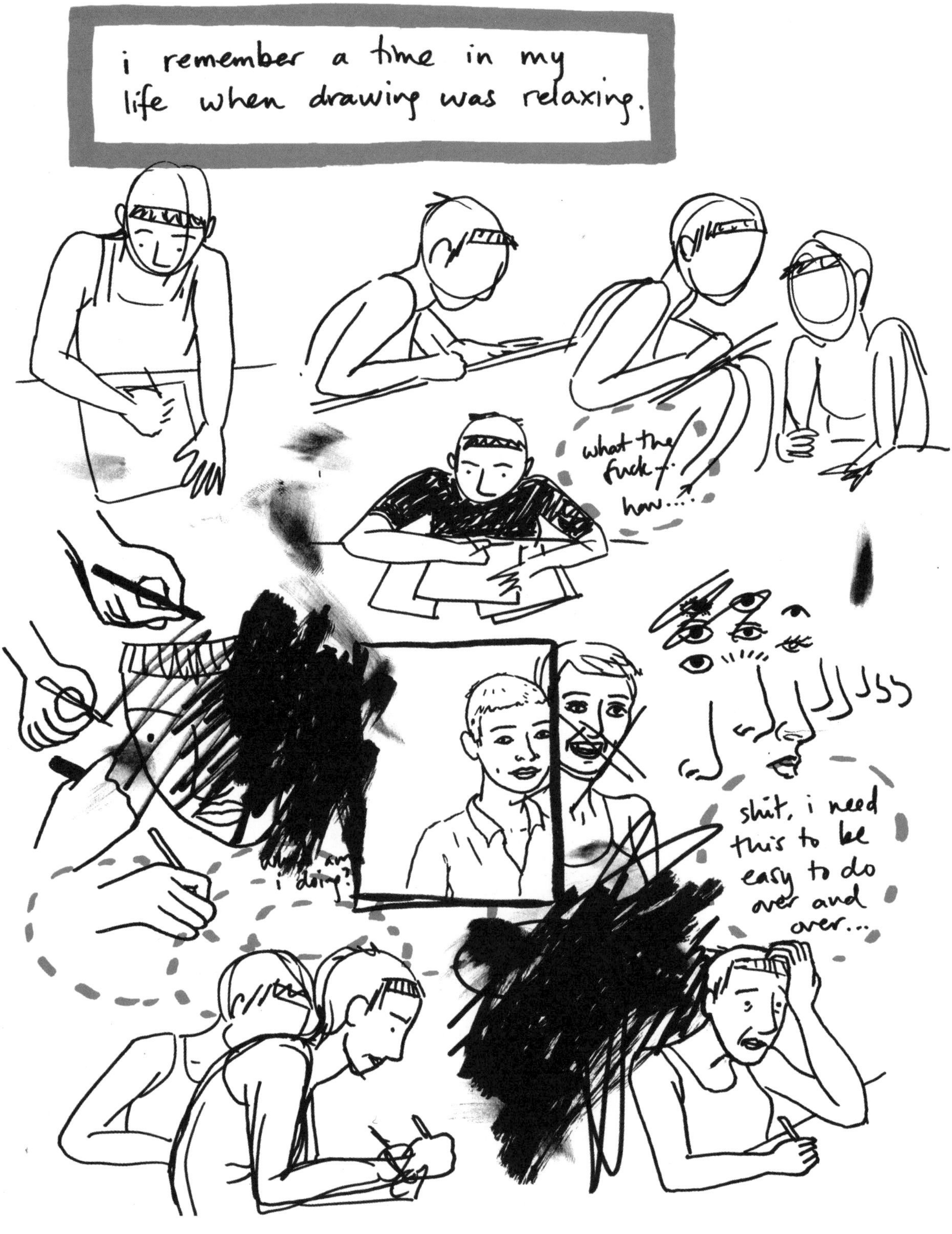
i remember a time in my life when drawing was relaxing.
what the fuck... how....
am i doing?
shit, i need this to be easy to do over and over...

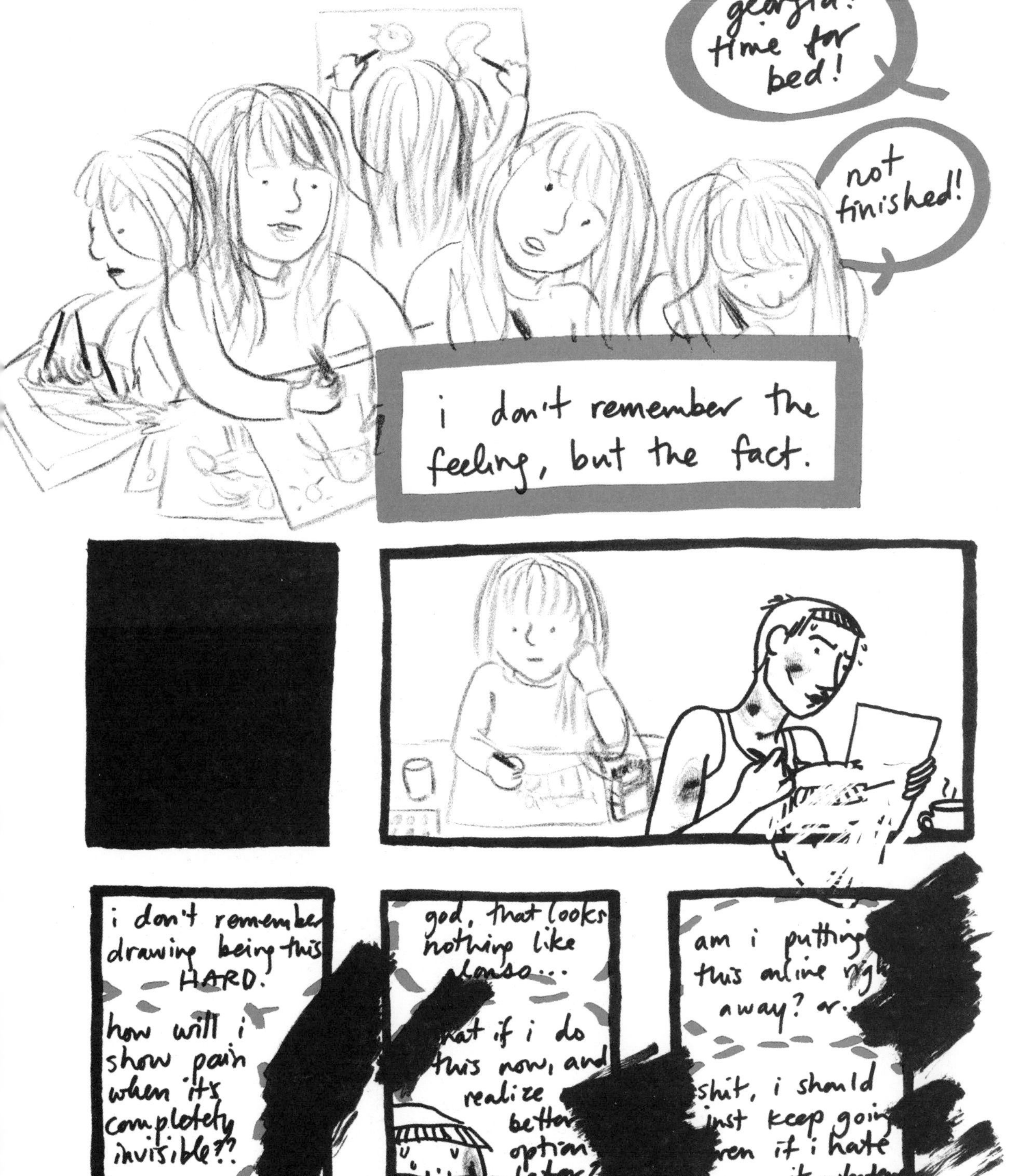
georgia! time for bed!
not finished!
i don't remember the feeling, but the fact.
i don't remember drawing being this HARD.
how will i show pain when it's completely invisible?!?
god, that looks nothing like
if i do this now, and realize
later?
am i putting this online
away?
shit, i should
keep going
if i hate it, whatever

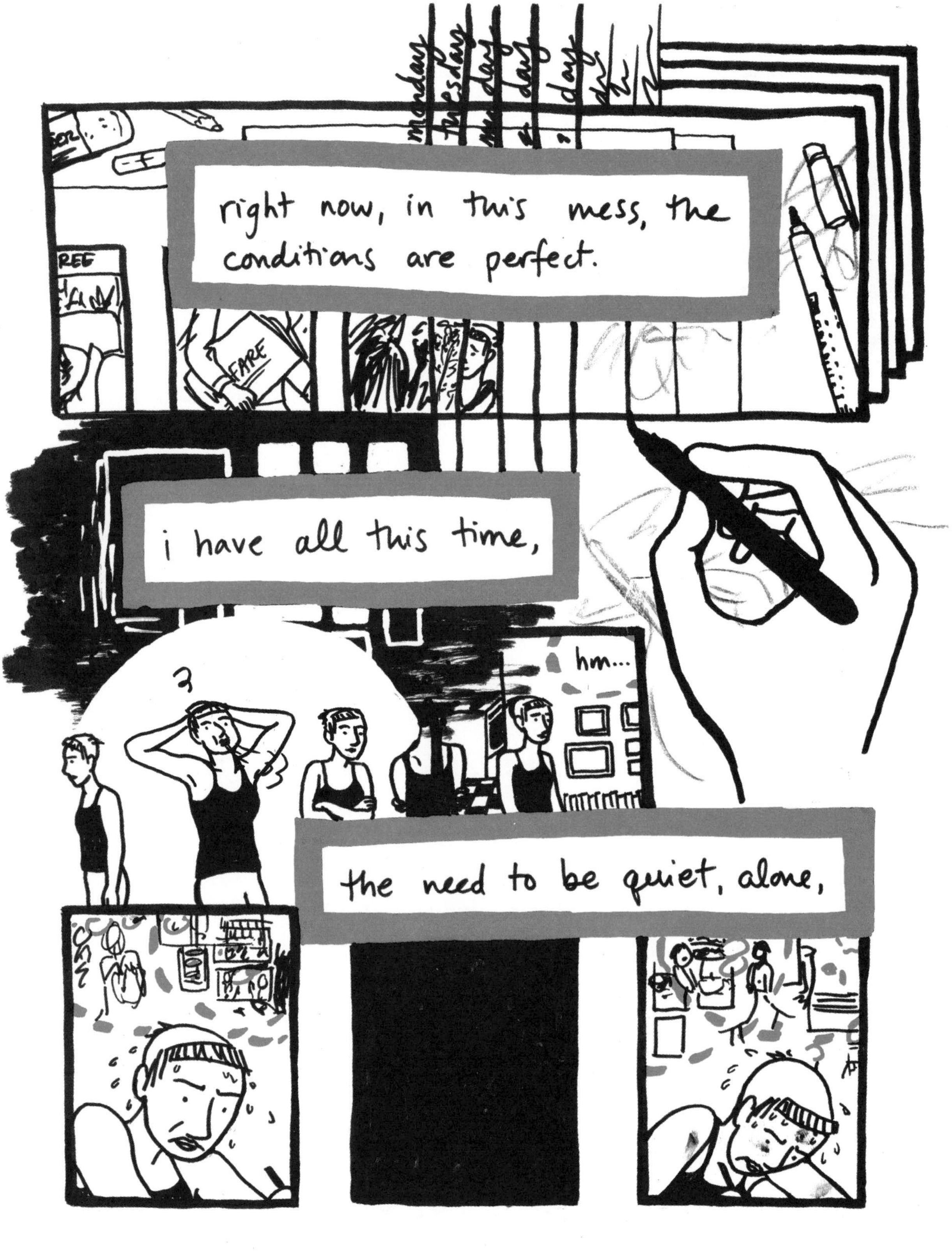
monday
tuesday
right now, in this mess, the conditions are perfect.
FARE
i have all this time,
?
hm...
the need to be quiet, alone,

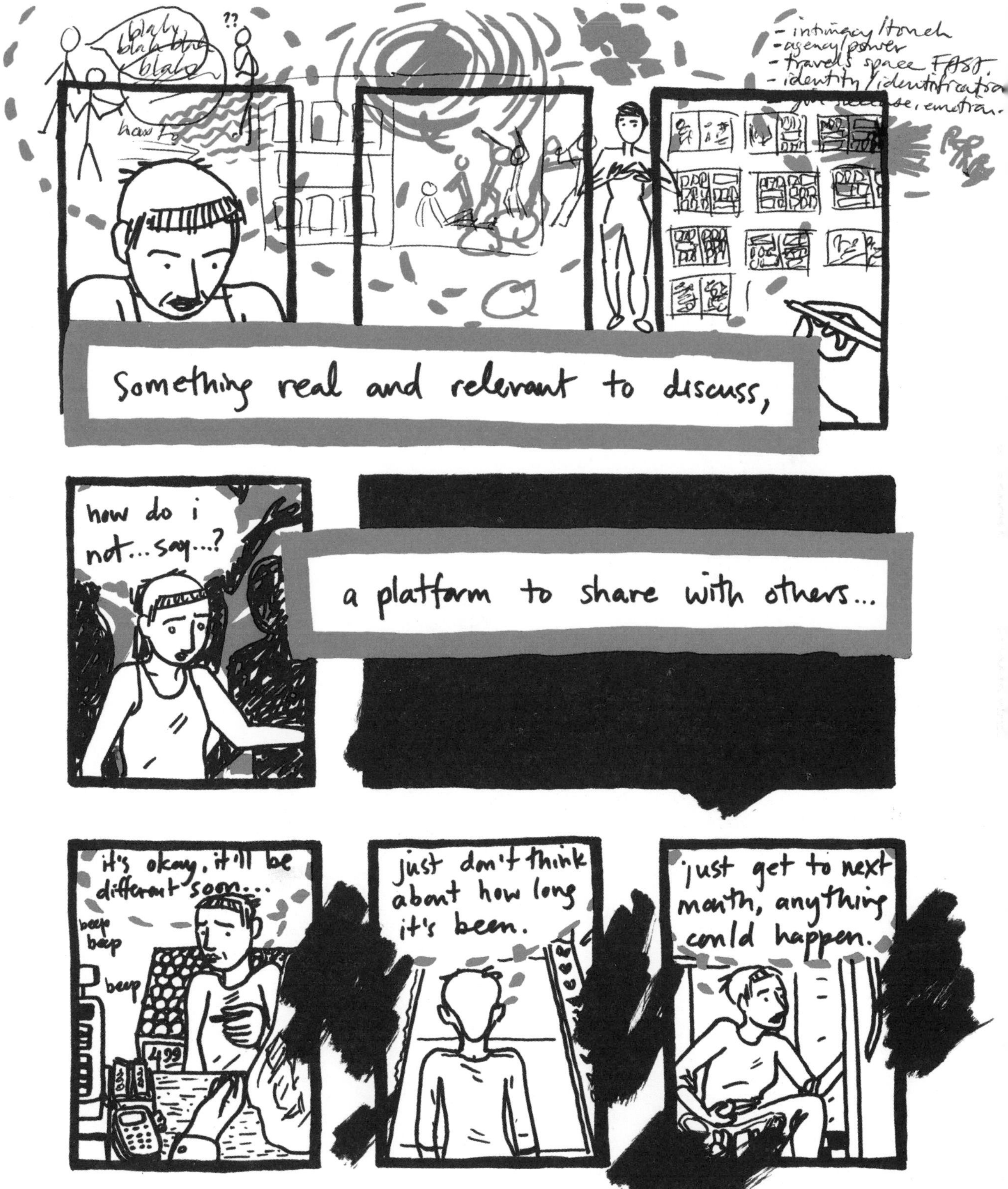

- intimacy/touch
- agency/power
- travels space FAST.
- identity/identification
Something real and relevant to discuss,
how do i not... say...?
a platform to share with others...
it's okay, it'll be different soon...
beep beep
beep
4.99
just don't think about how long it's been.
just get to next month, anything could happen.

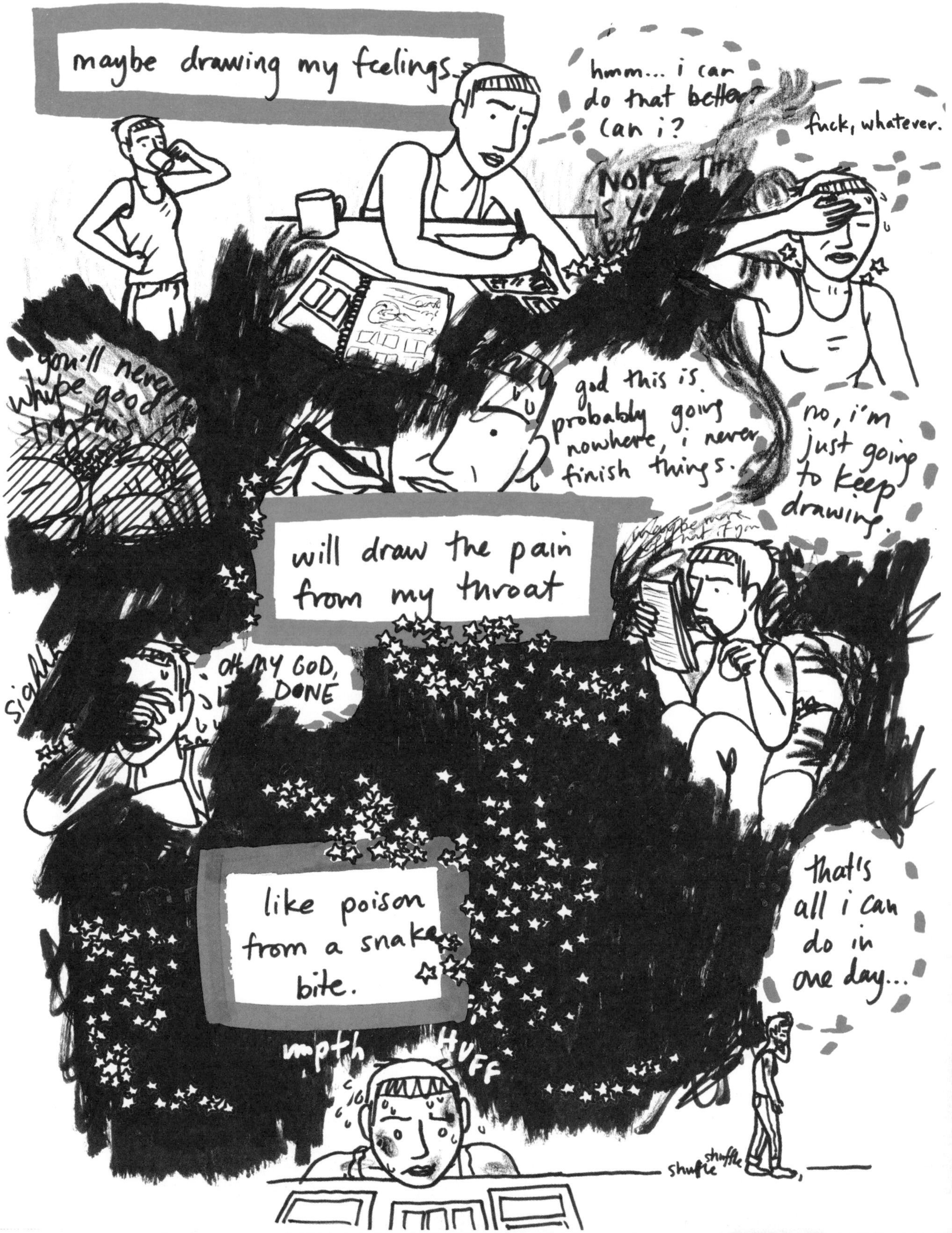
maybe drawing my feelings
hmm... i can do that better? can i?
fuck, whatever.
god this is probably going nowhere, i never finish things.
no, i'm just going to keep drawing.
will draw the pain from my throat
sigh
OH MY GOD,
DONE
like poison from a snake bite.
that's all i can do in one day...
umpth
HUFF
shuffle shuffle

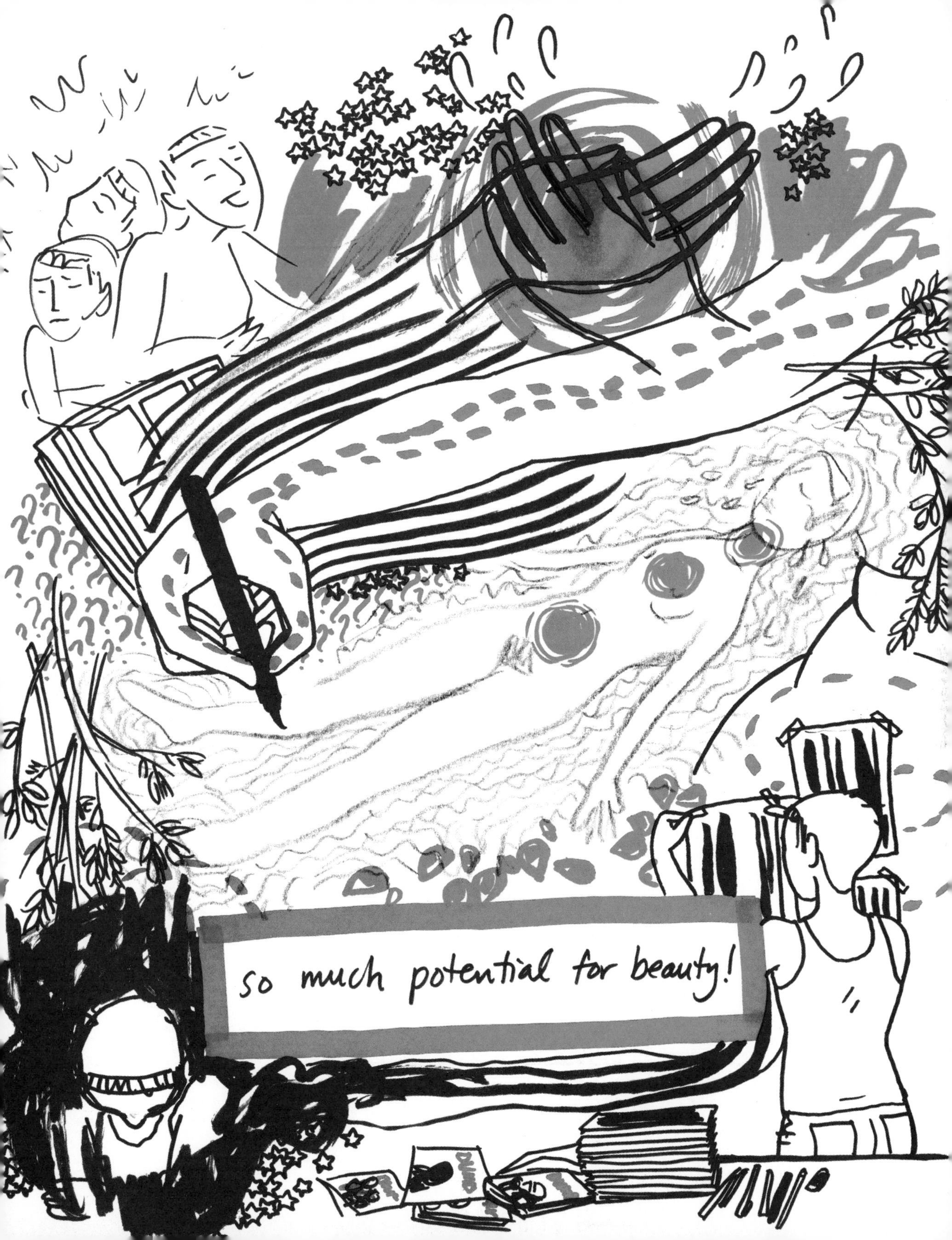
so much potential for beauty!

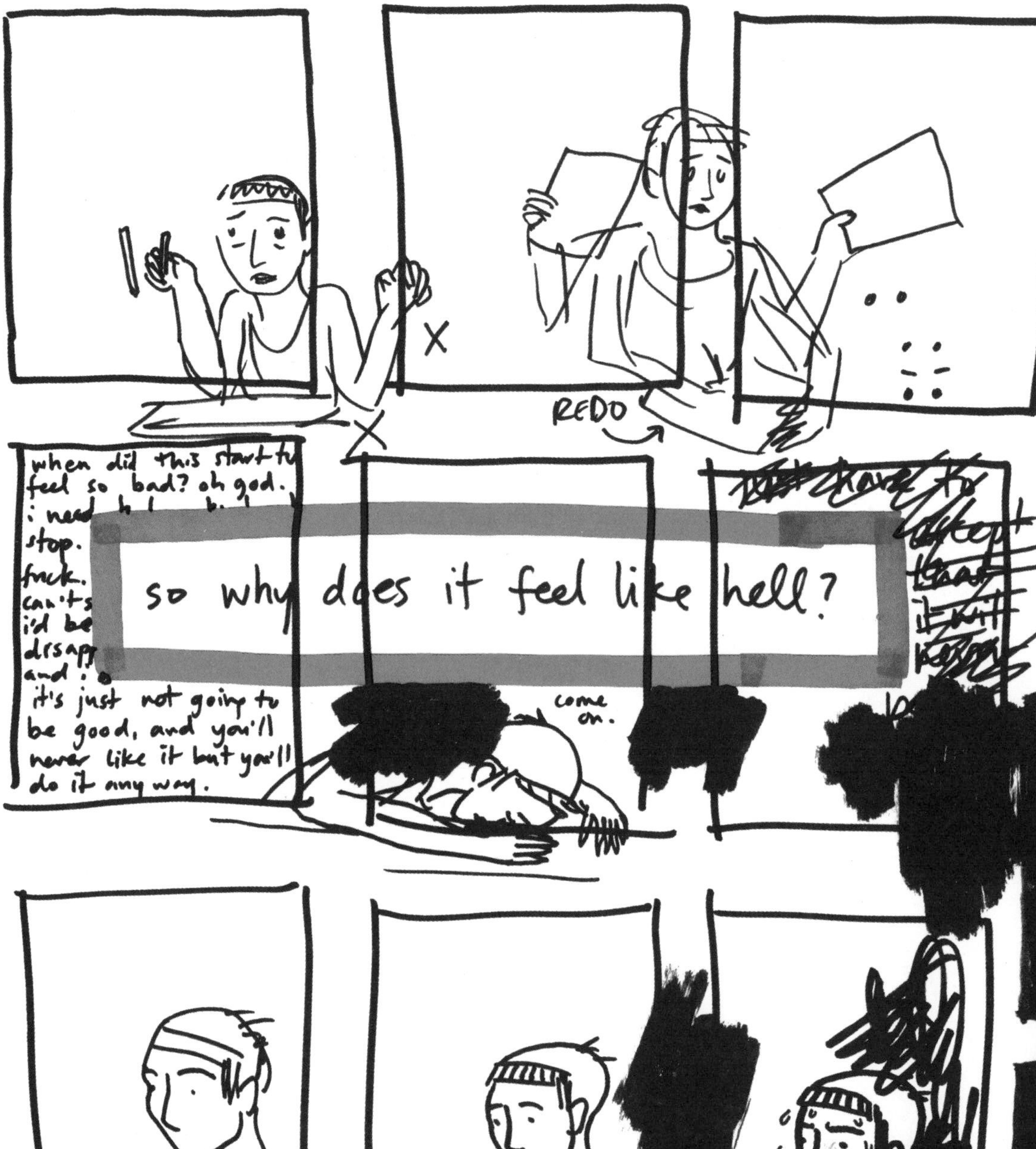
REDO
when did this start to feel so bad? oh god.
stop.
fuck.
it's just not going to be good, and you'll never like it but you'll do it anyway.
so why does it feel like hell?
come on.

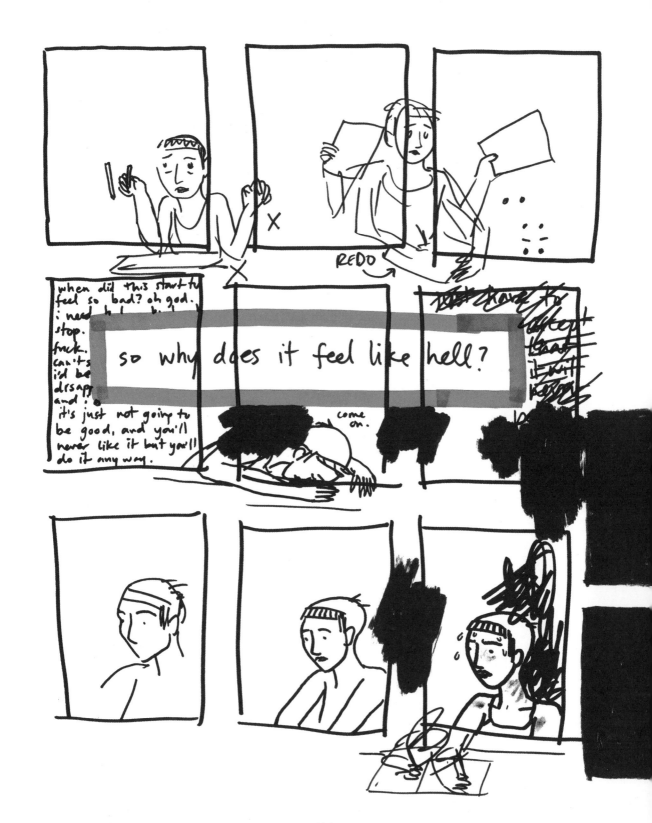

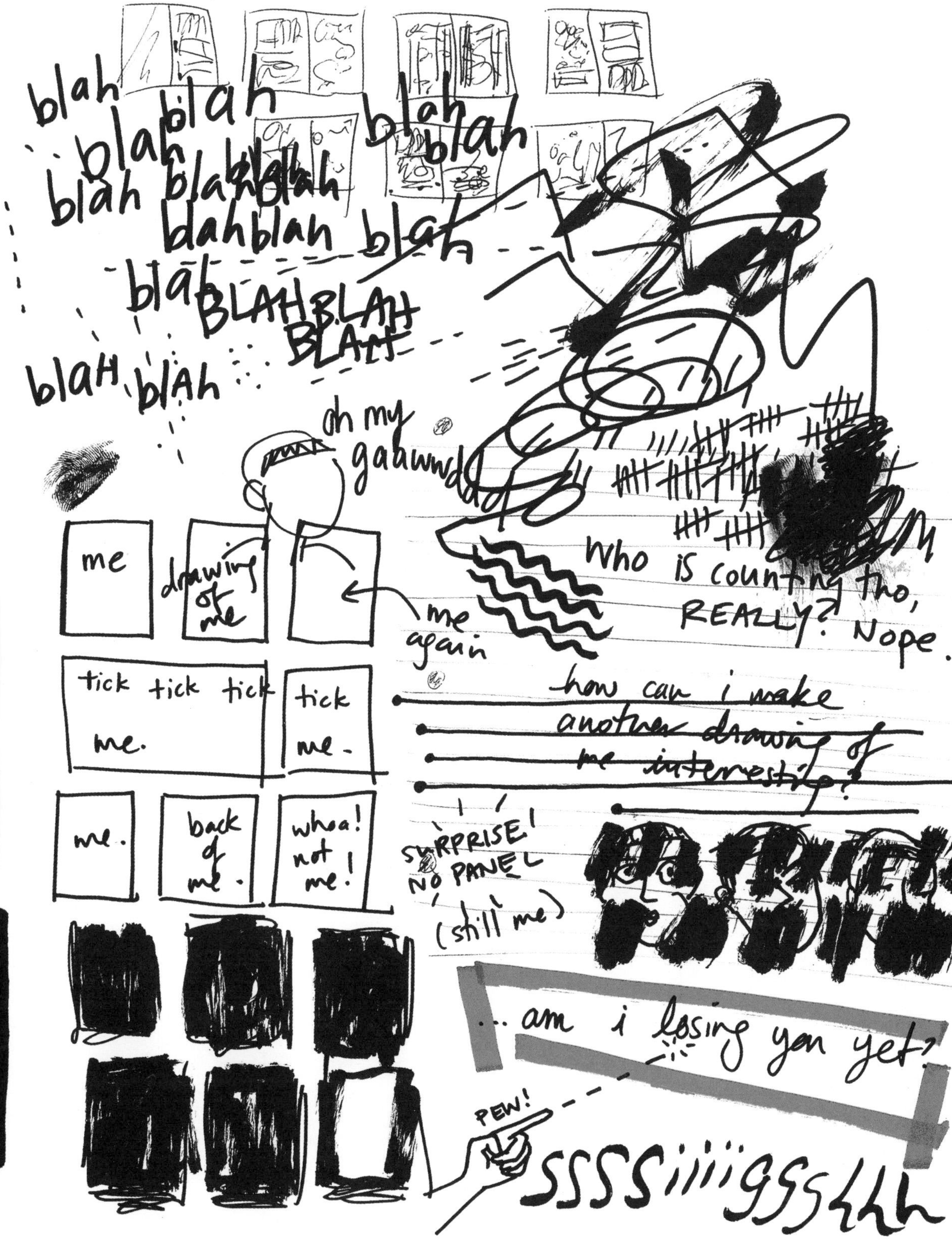
blah blah blah blah blah blah blah blah blah blah blah blah blah blah
BLAH BLAH BLAH
blah blah
oh my gaawwd
me
drawing of me
me again
Who is counting tho, REALLY? Nope.
how can i make another drawing of me interesting?
tick tick tick me.
tick me.
me.
back of me.
whoa! not me!
SURPRISE! NO PANEL (still me)
... am i losing you yet?
PEW!
SSSSiiiiggSShhh

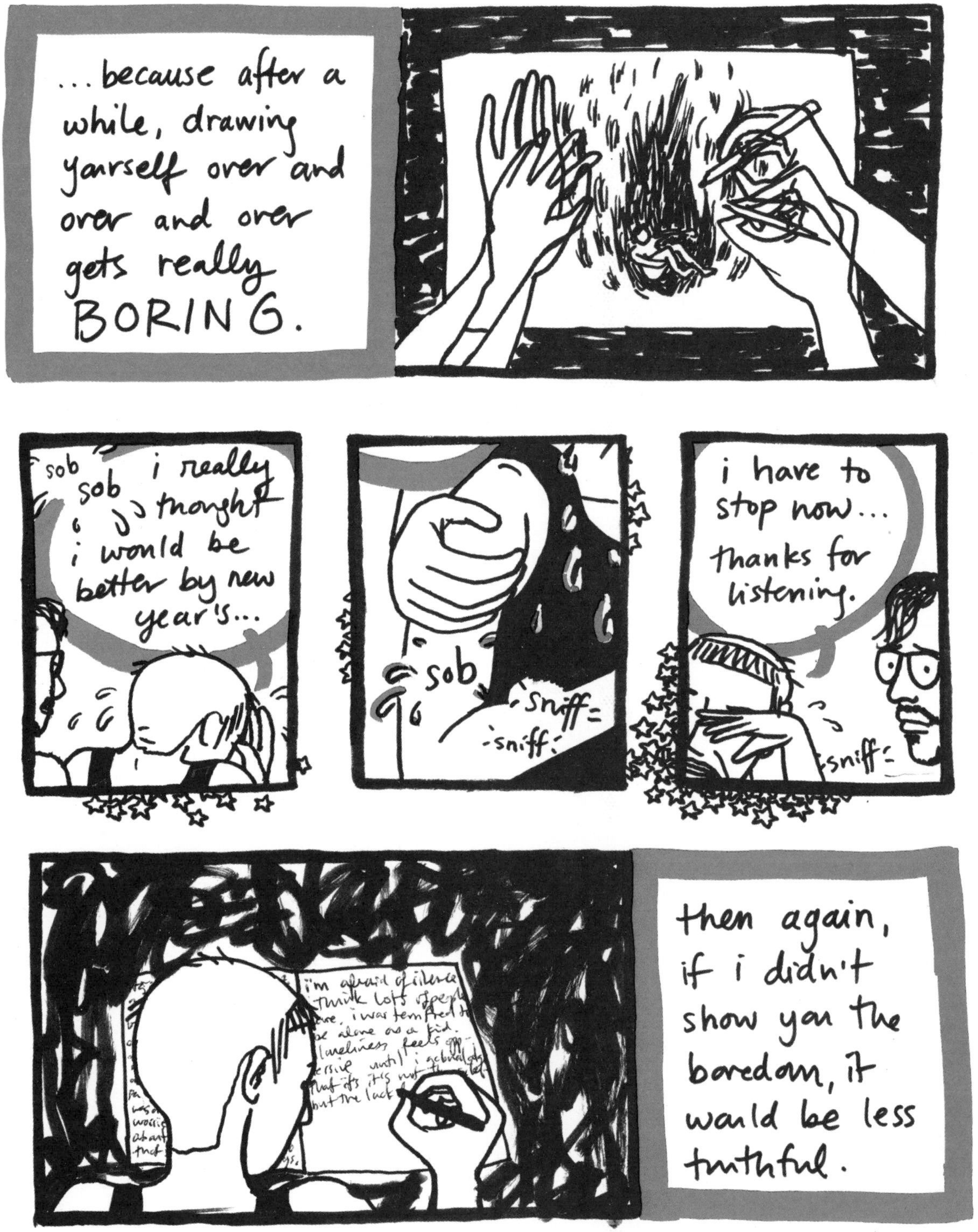
...because after a while, drawing yourself over and over and over gets really BORING.
sob sob i really thought i would be better by new year's...
sob
sniff
sniff
i have to stop now... thanks for listening.
sniff
then again, if i didn't show you the boredom, it would be less truthful.

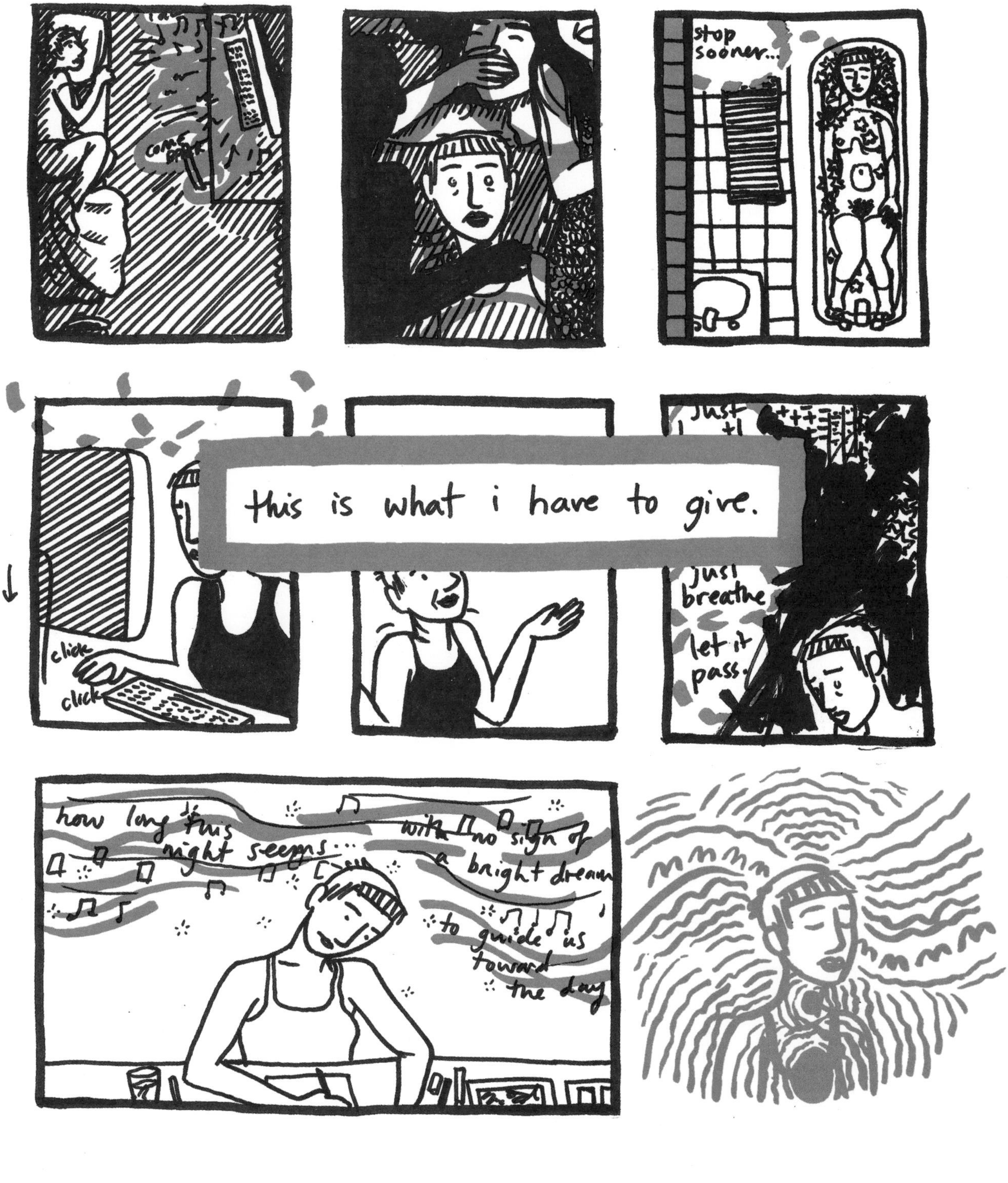

come back
stop sooner...
this is what i have to give.
click
click
just breathe
let it pass.
how long this night seems...
with no sign of a bright dream
to guide us toward the day
mmmm
mmmm

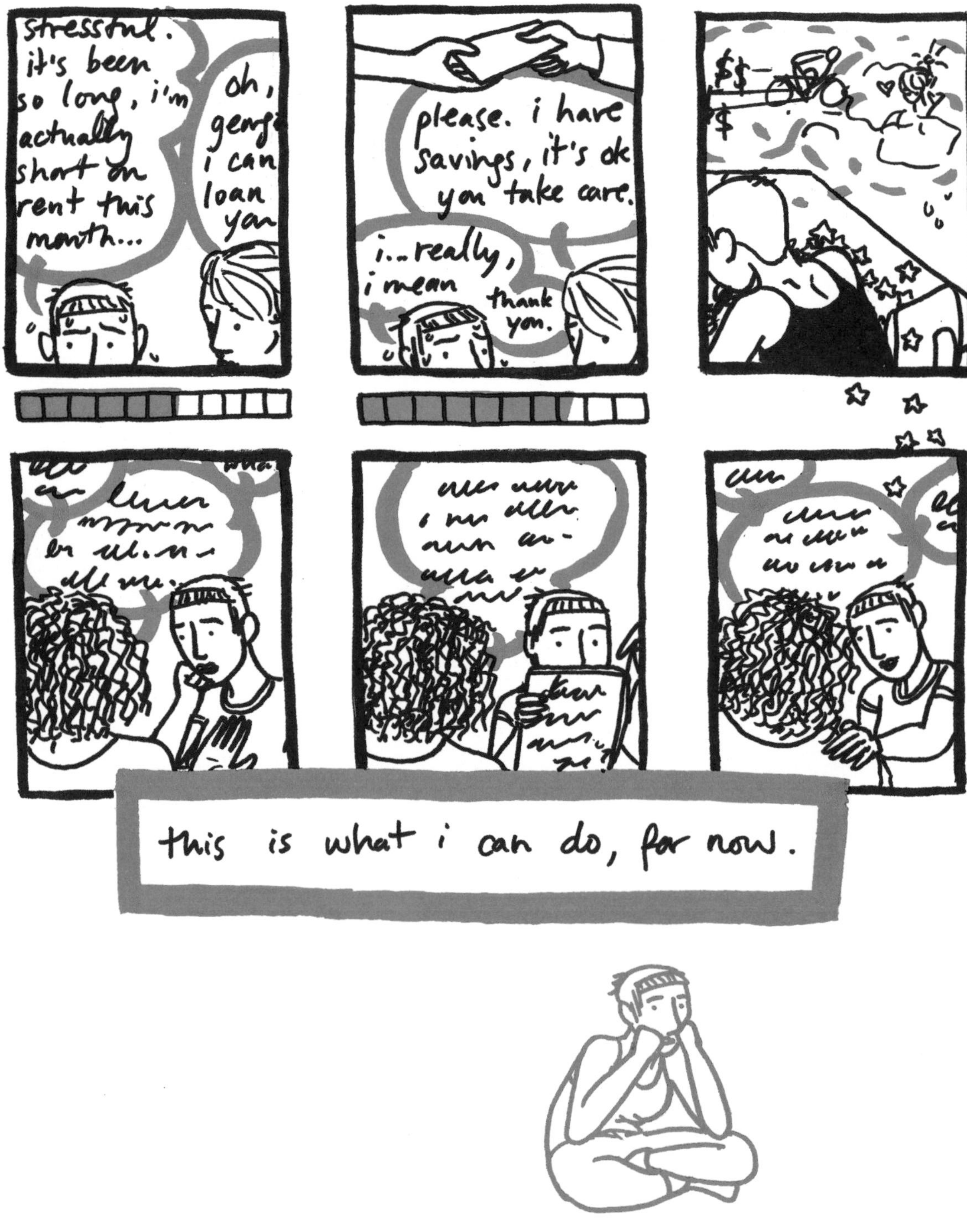
stressful. it's been so long, i'm actually short on rent this month...
oh, i can loan
please. i have savings, it's ok you take care.
i...really, i mean
thank you.
$$
$
this is what i can do, for now.

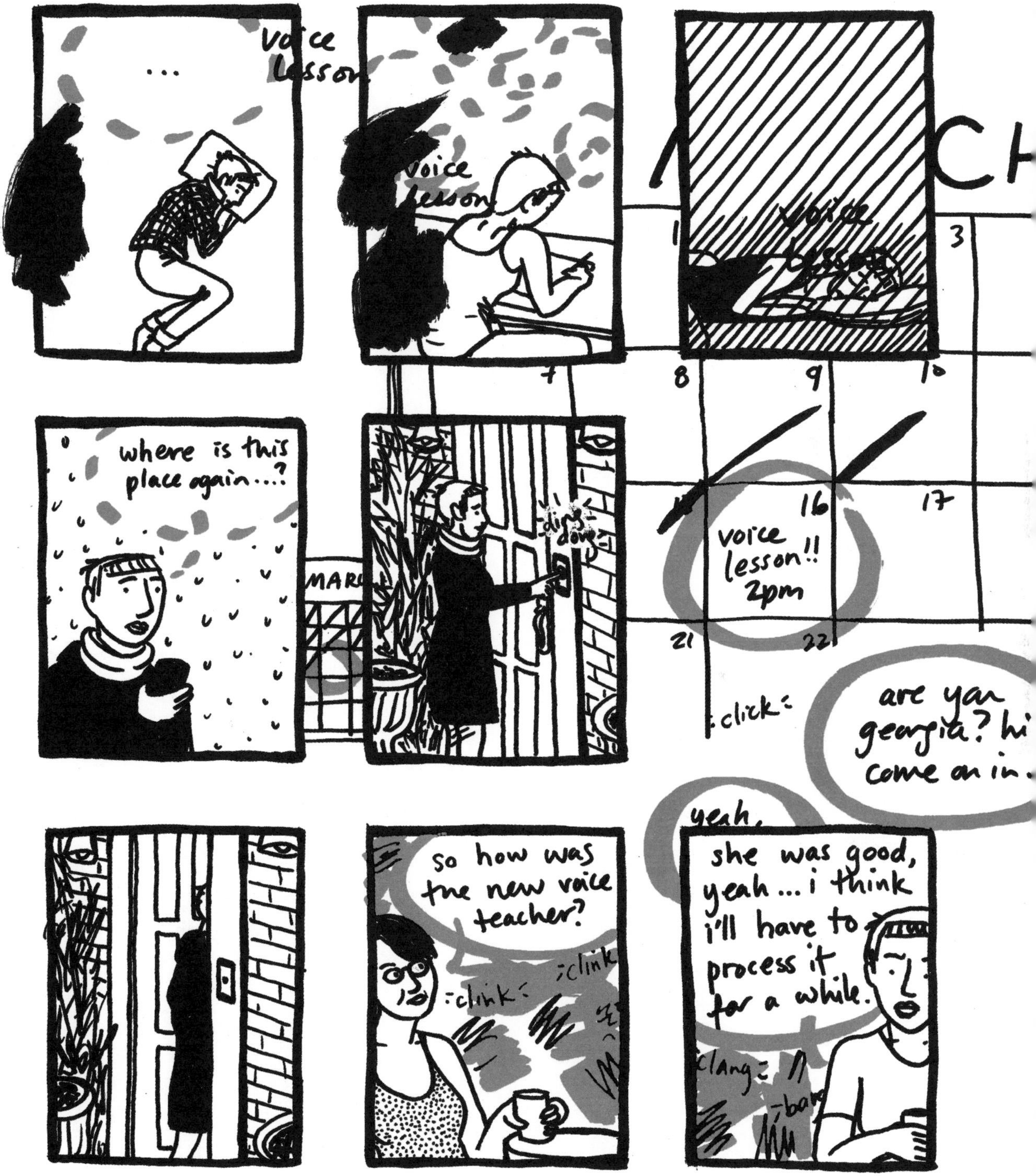

...
voice lesson
voice lesson
voice lesson
where is this place again...?
ding dong
:click:
are you georgia? hi come on in...
yeah.
so how was the new voice teacher?
:clink:
:clink:
she was good, yeah... i think i'll have to process it for a while.
clang:

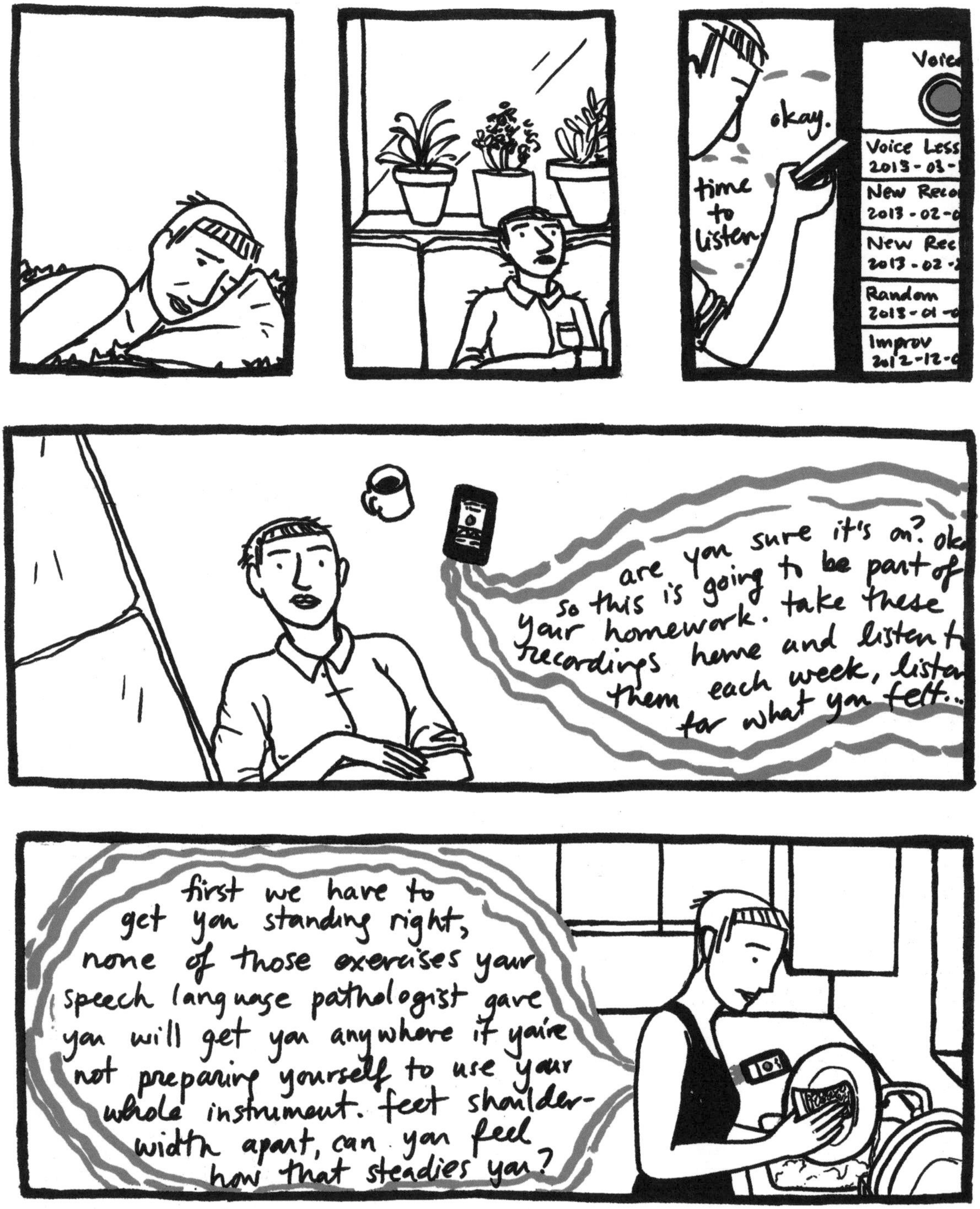
okay.
time to listen.
Voice Less
2013-03-
New Reco
2013-02-
New Rec
2013-02-
Random
2013-01-
Improv
2012-12-
are you sure it's on? ok so this is going to be part of your homework. take these recordings home and listen to them each week, listen for what you felt...
first we have to get you standing right, none of those exercises your speech language pathologist gave you will get you anywhere if you're not preparing yourself to use your whole instrument. feet shoulder-width apart, can you feel how that steadies you?

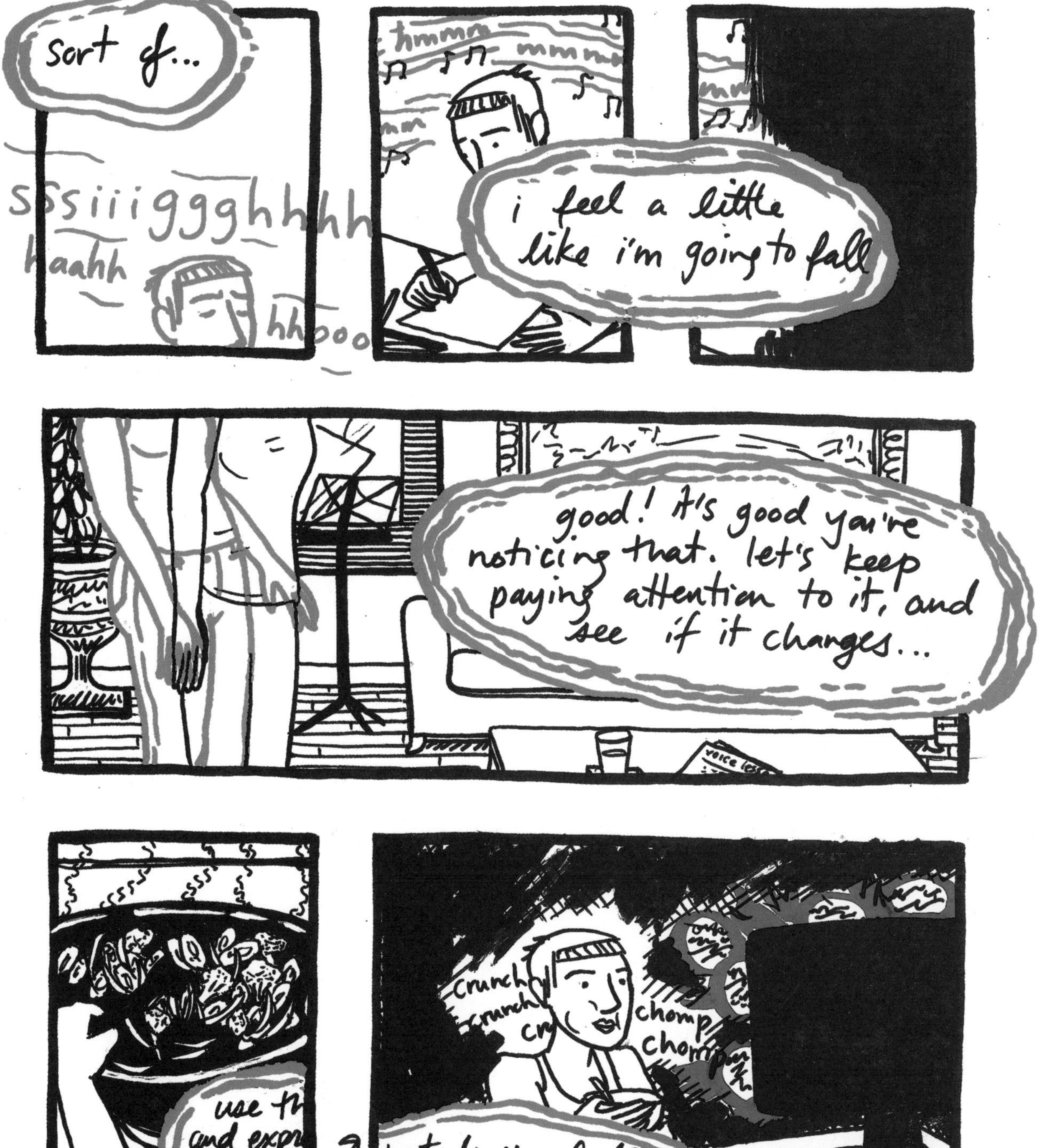
sort of...
ssiiiggghhhh
haahh
hhooo
hmmm
mmmm
i feel a little like i'm going to fall
good! it's good you're noticing that. let's keep paying attention to it, and see if it changes...
use th
and expr
crunch
crunch
cr
chomp
chomp
hat do you feel?
← probably redraw these?

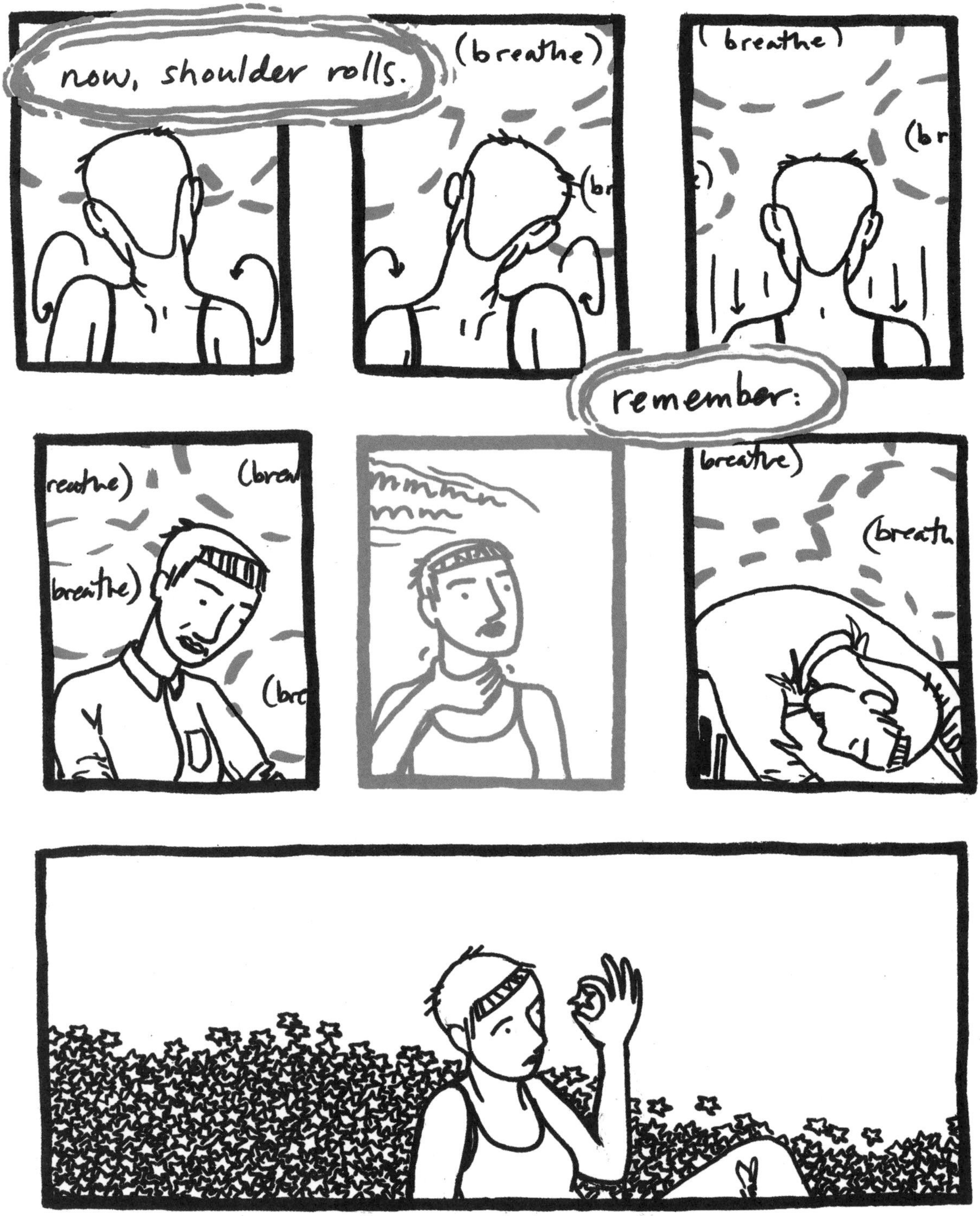
now, shoulder rolls.
(breathe)
(breathe)
remember:
(breathe)
(breathe)
(breathe)
(breath

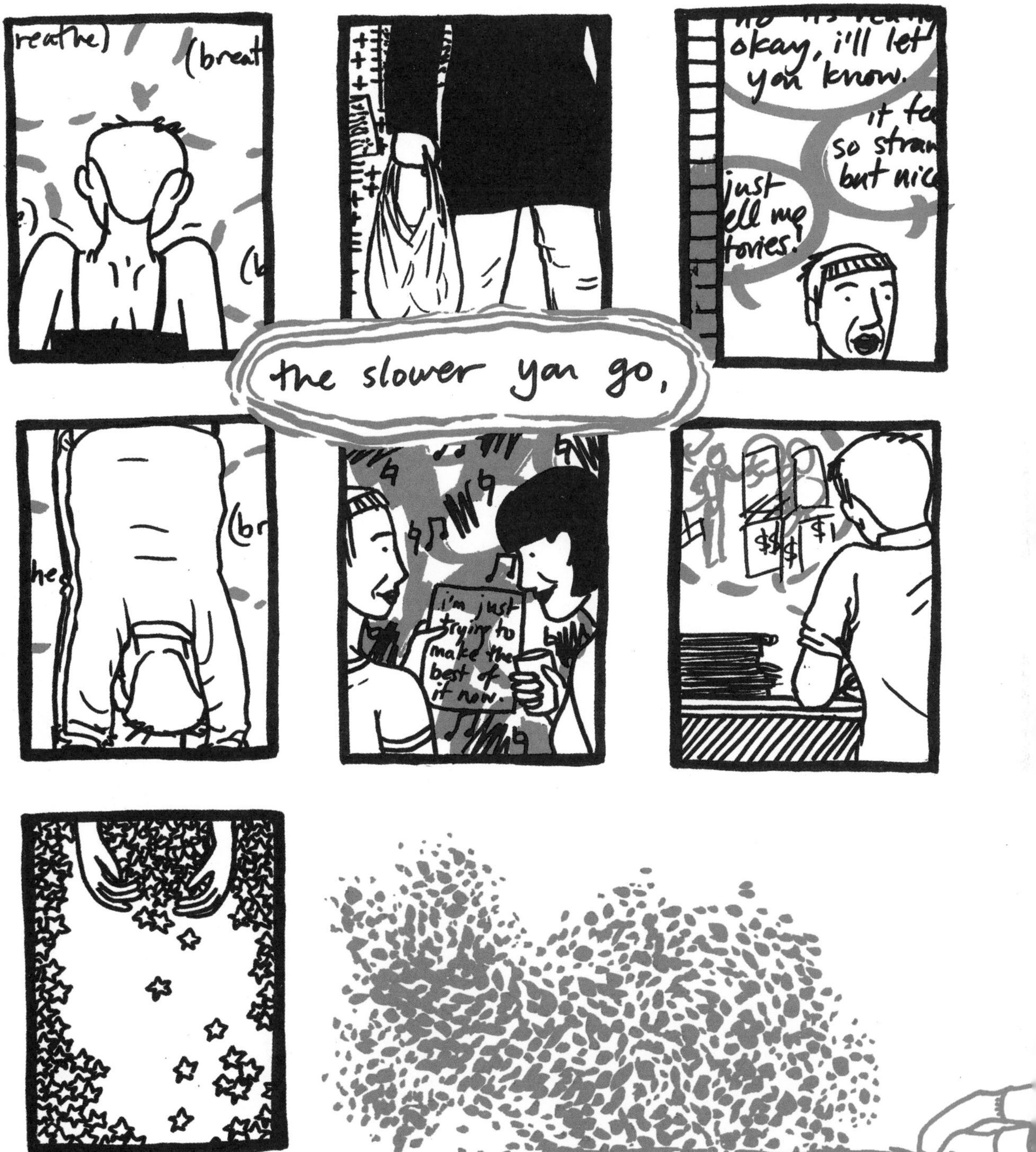
okay, i'll let you know.
the slower you go,
i'm just tryin' to make the best of it now.
the more you'll feel.

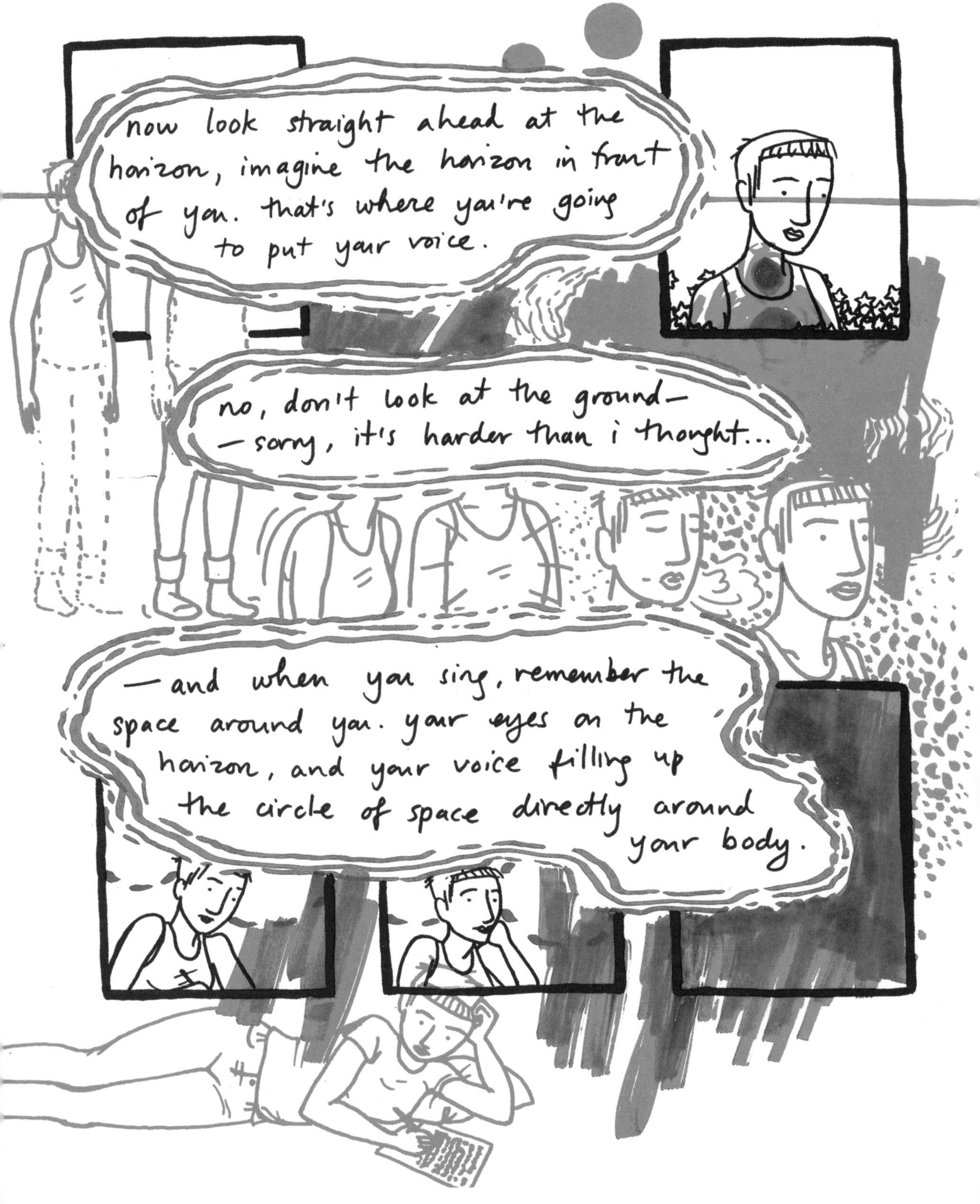
now look straight ahead at the horizon, imagine the horizon in front of you. that's where you're going to put your voice.
no, don't look at the ground— —sorry, it's harder than i thought...
—and when you sing, remember the space around you. your eyes on the horizon, and your voice filling up the circle of space directly around your body.

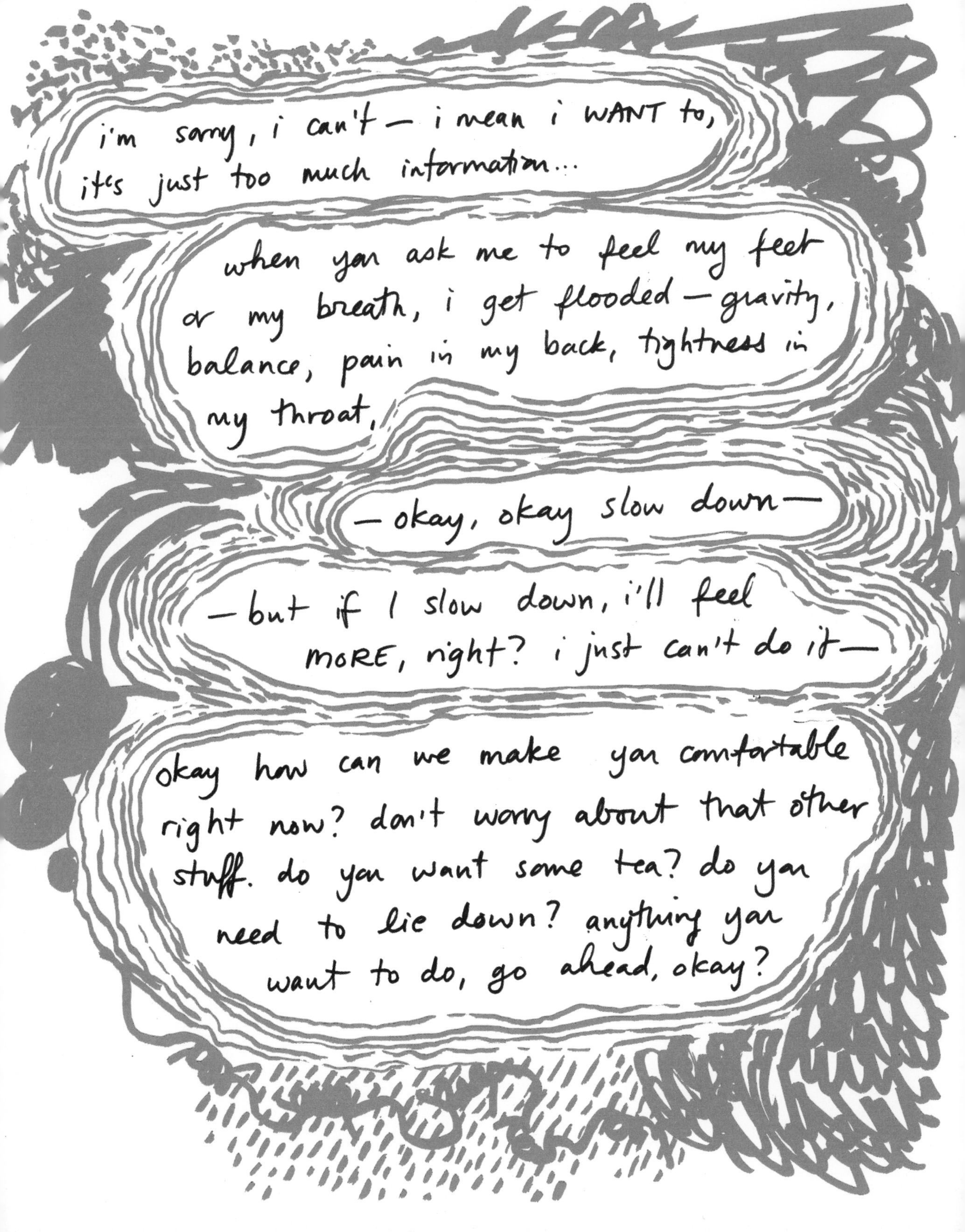
i'm sorry, i can't — i mean i WANT to, it's just too much information...
when you ask me to feel my feet or my breath, i get flooded — gravity, balance, pain in my back, tightness in my throat,
— okay, okay slow down —
— but if I slow down, i'll feel MORE, right? i just can't do it —
okay how can we make you comfortable right now? don't worry about that other stuff. do you want some tea? do you need to lie down? anything you want to do, go ahead, okay?

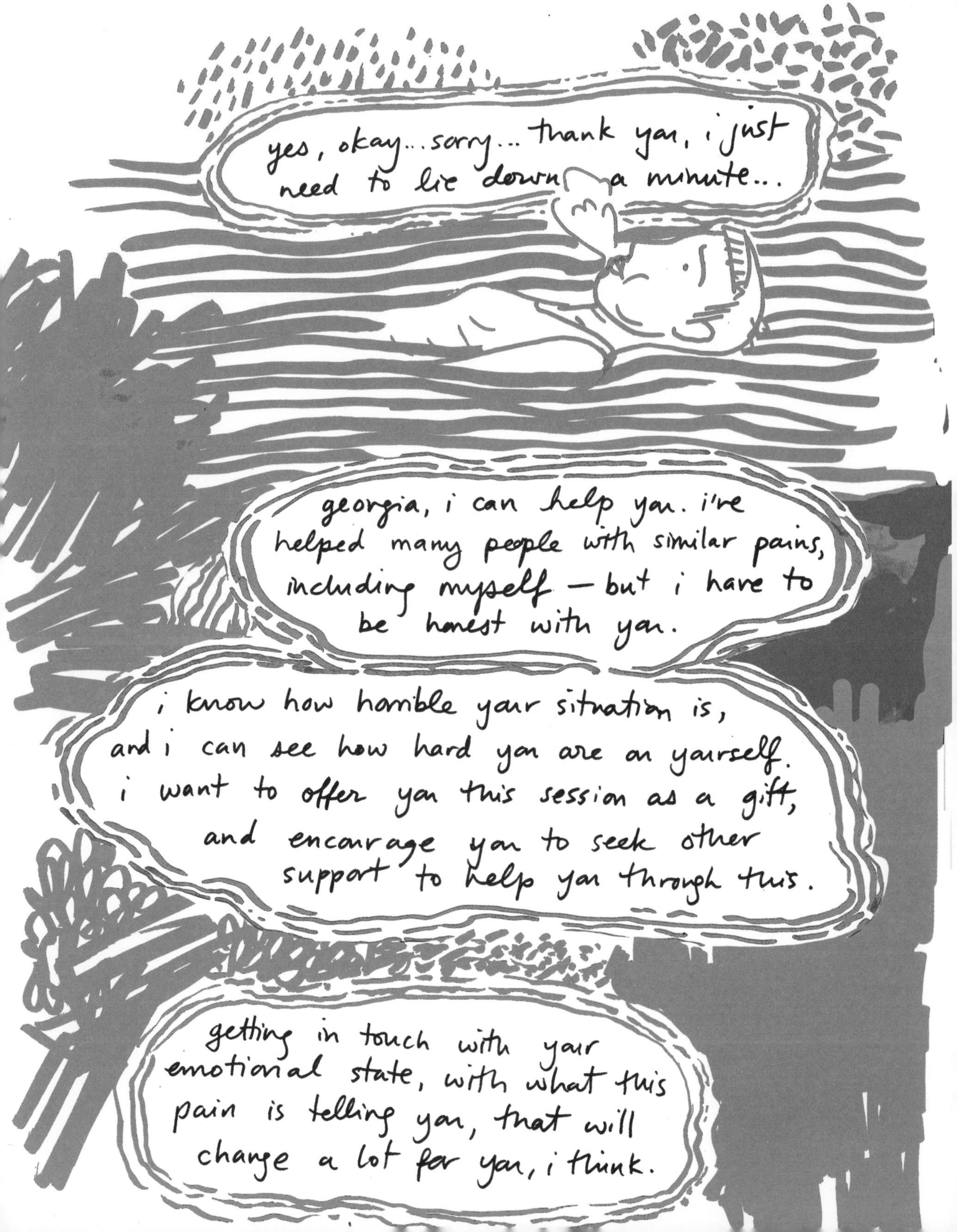
yes, okay... sorry... thank you, i just need to lie down a minute...
georgia, i can help you. i've helped many people with similar pains, including myself — but i have to be honest with you.
i know how horrible your situation is, and i can see how hard you are on yourself. i want to offer you this session as a gift, and encourage you to seek other support to help you through this.
getting in touch with your emotional state, with what this pain is telling you, that will change a lot for you, i think.

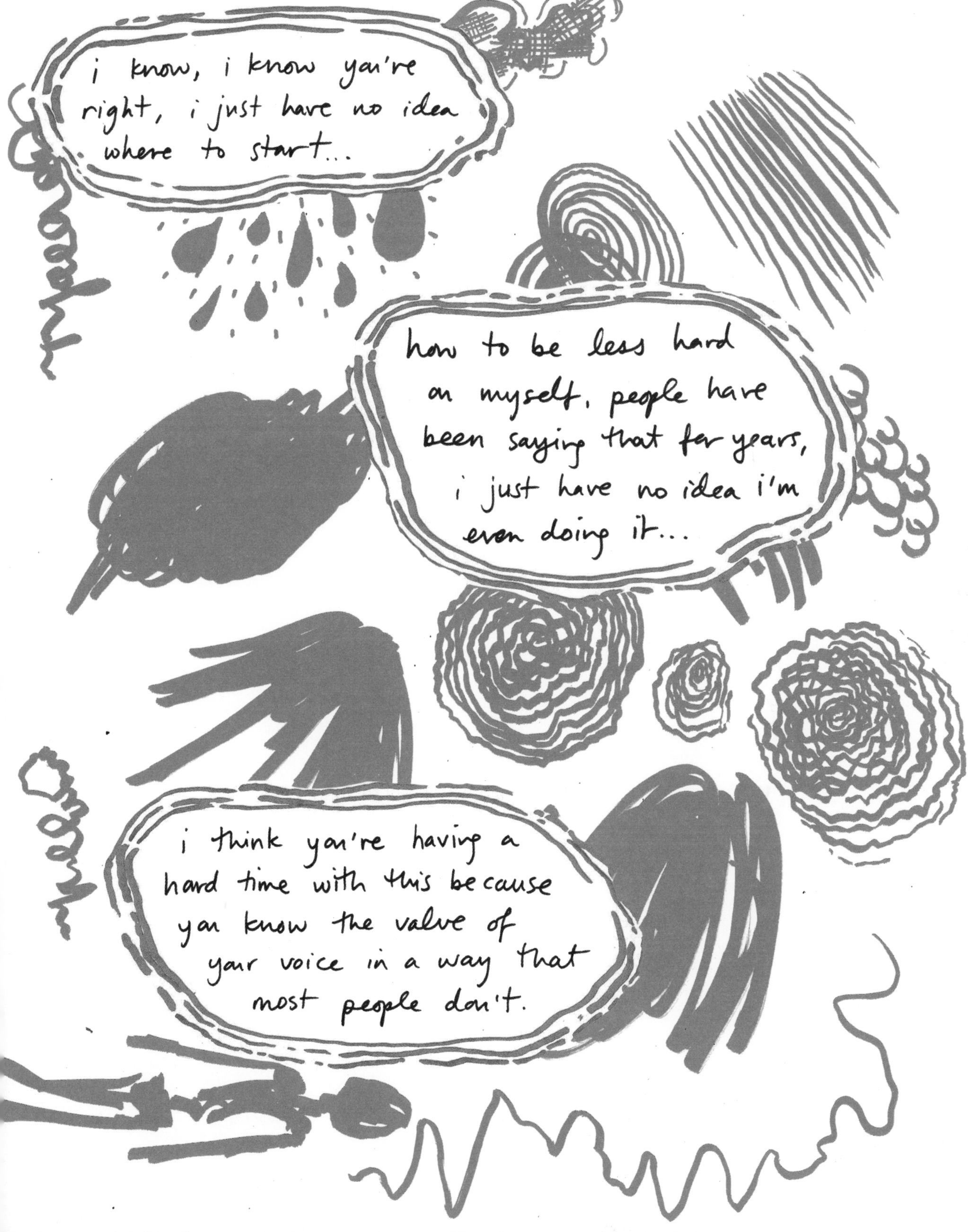
i know, i know you're right, i just have no idea where to start...
how to be less hard on myself. people have been saying that for years, i just have no idea i'm even doing it...
i think you're having a hard time with this because you know the value of your voice in a way that most people don't.

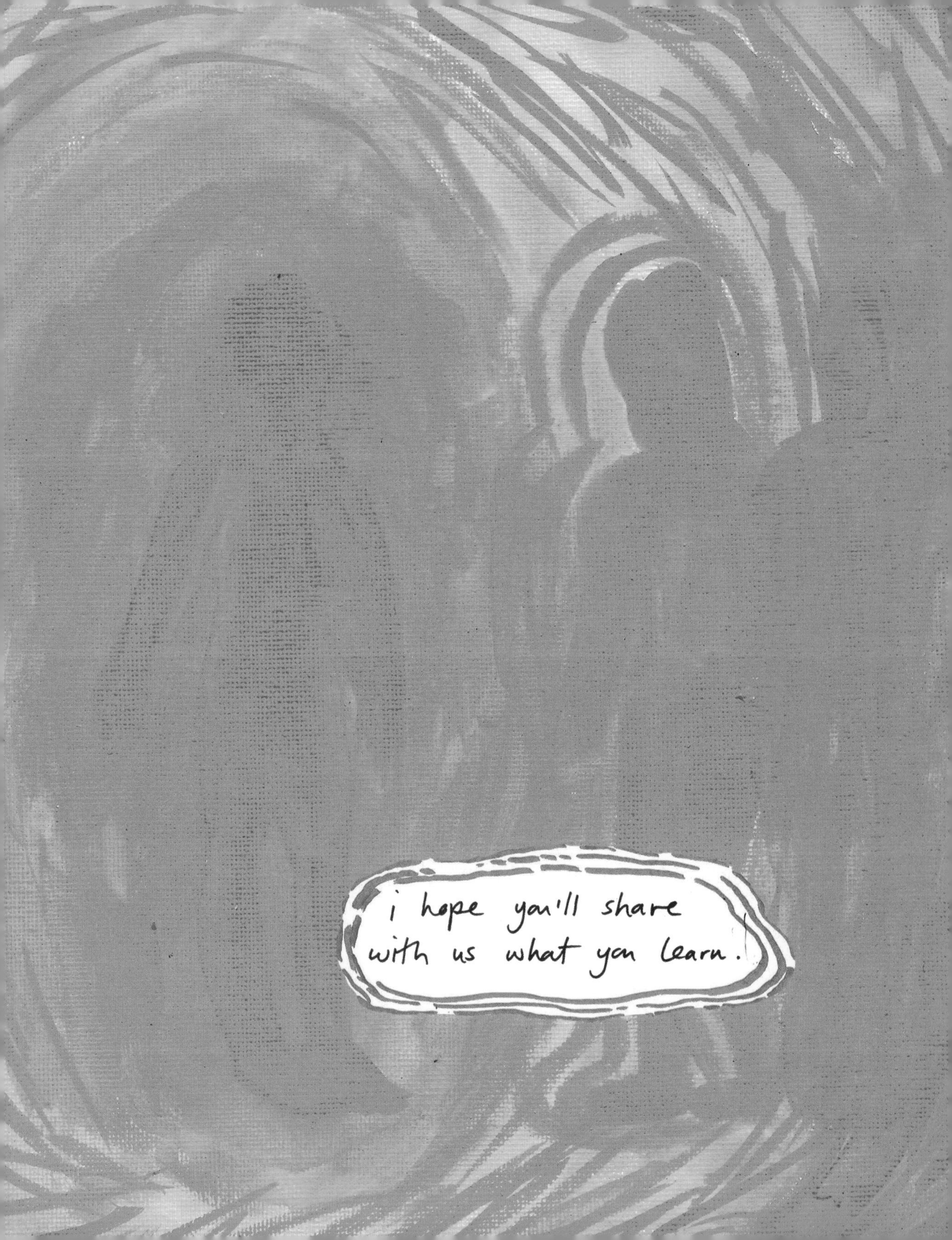
i hope you'll share with us what you learn.

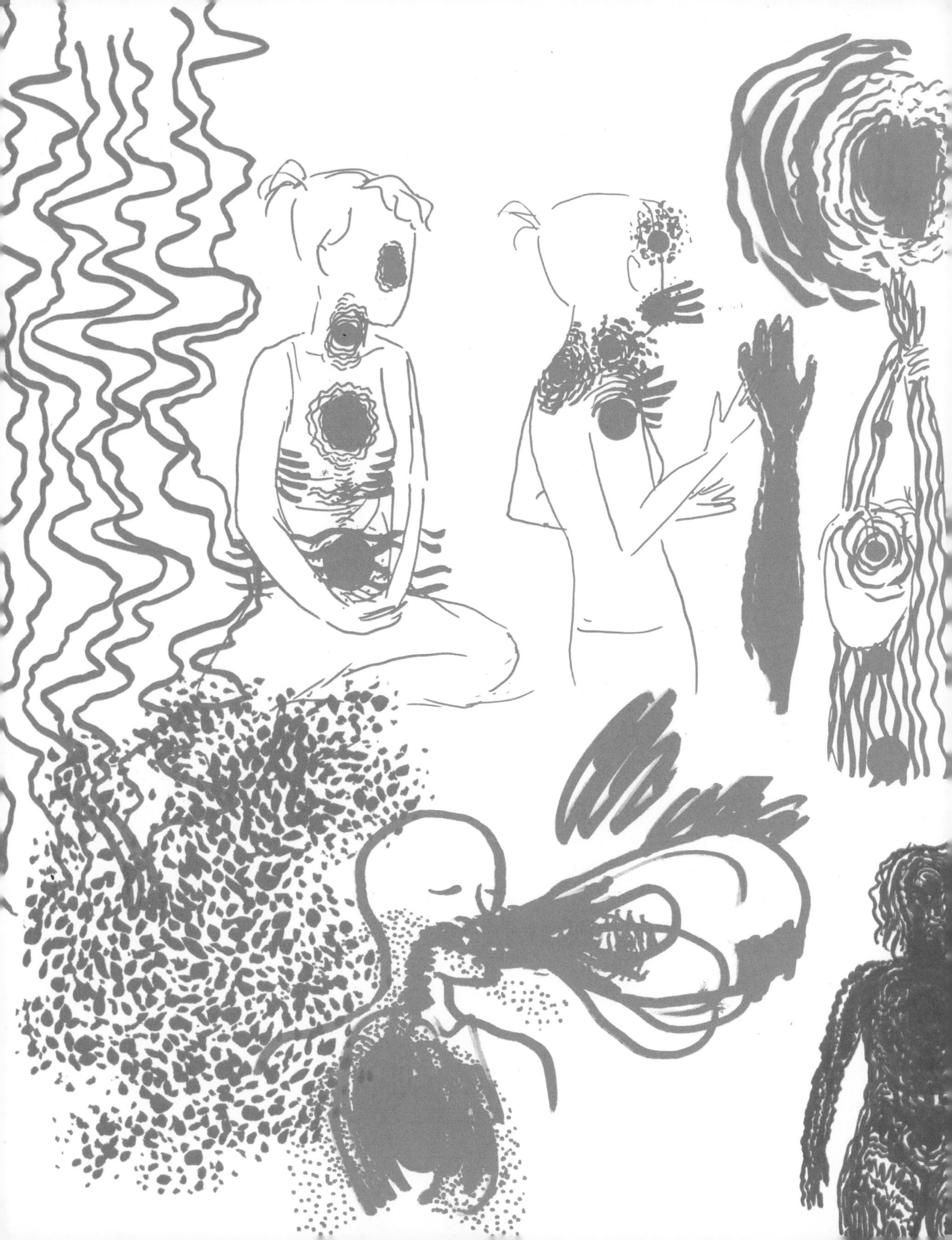

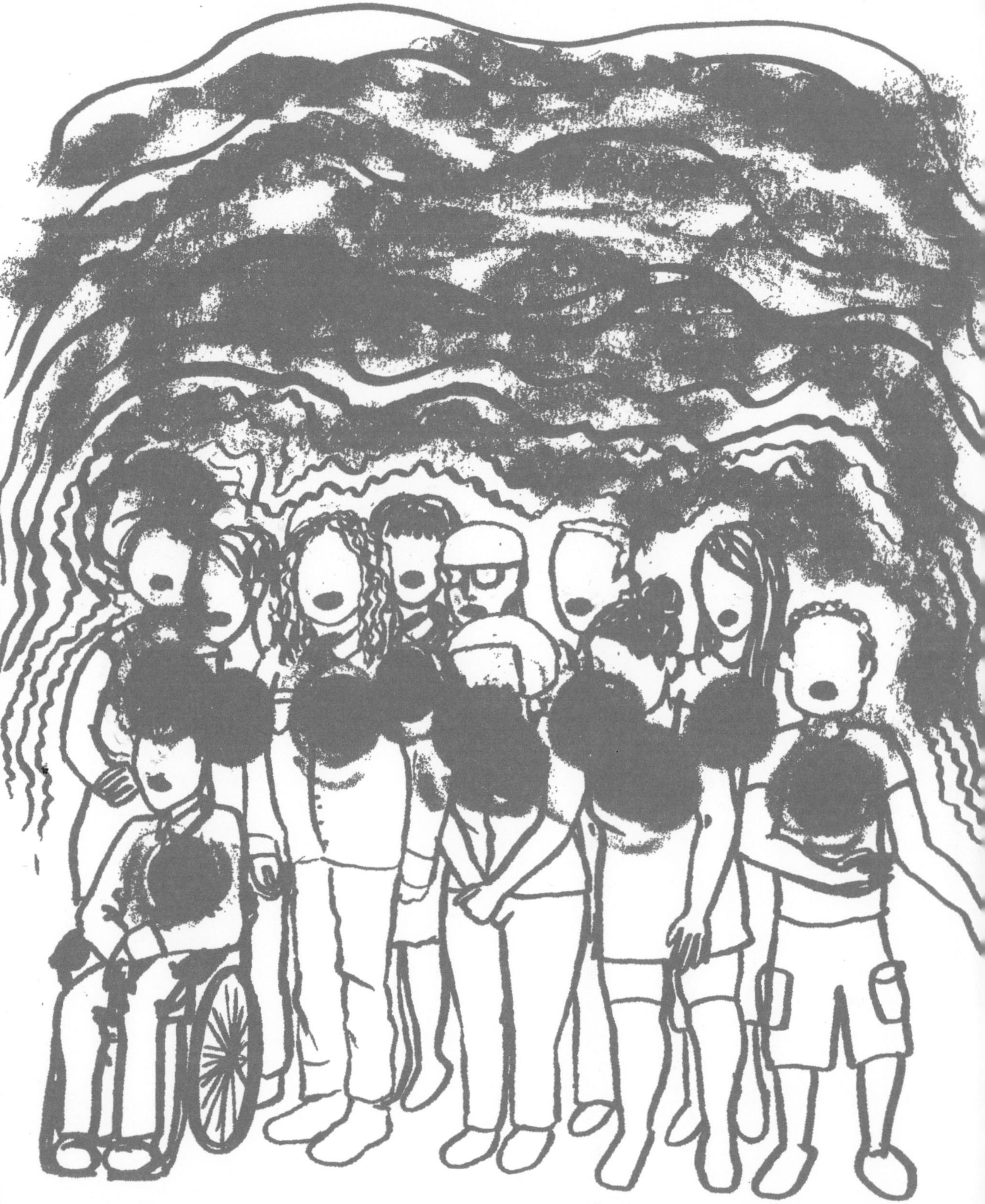

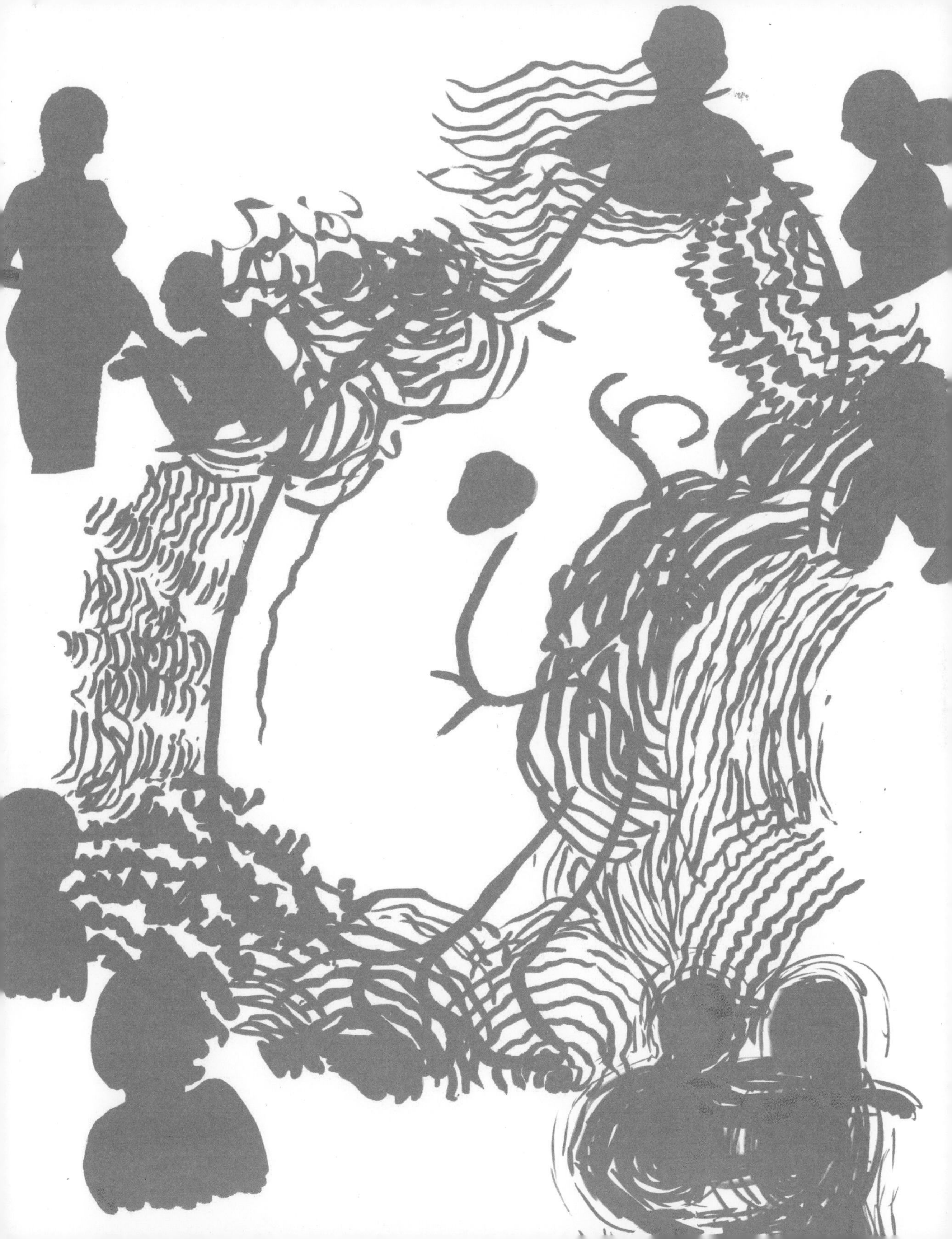

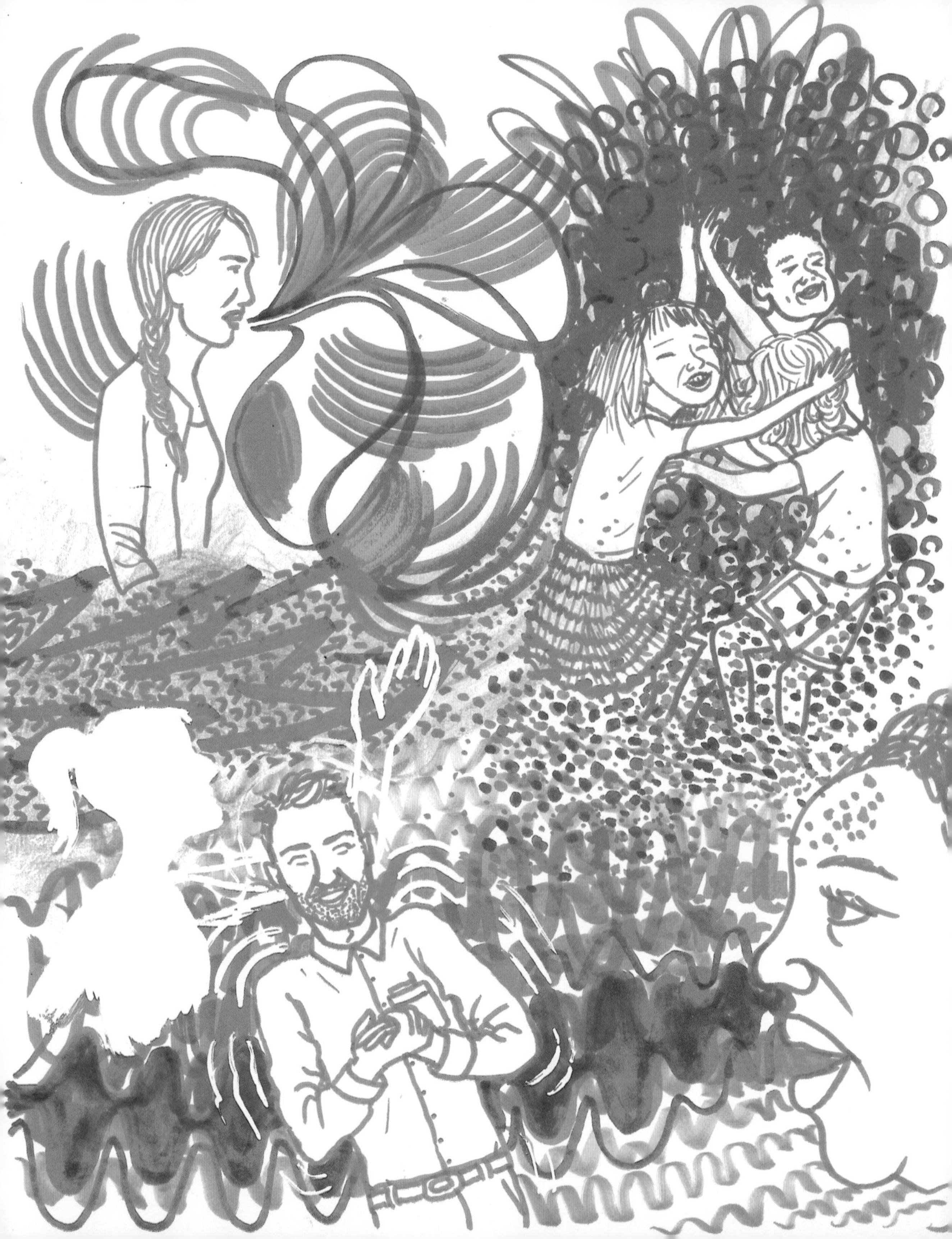

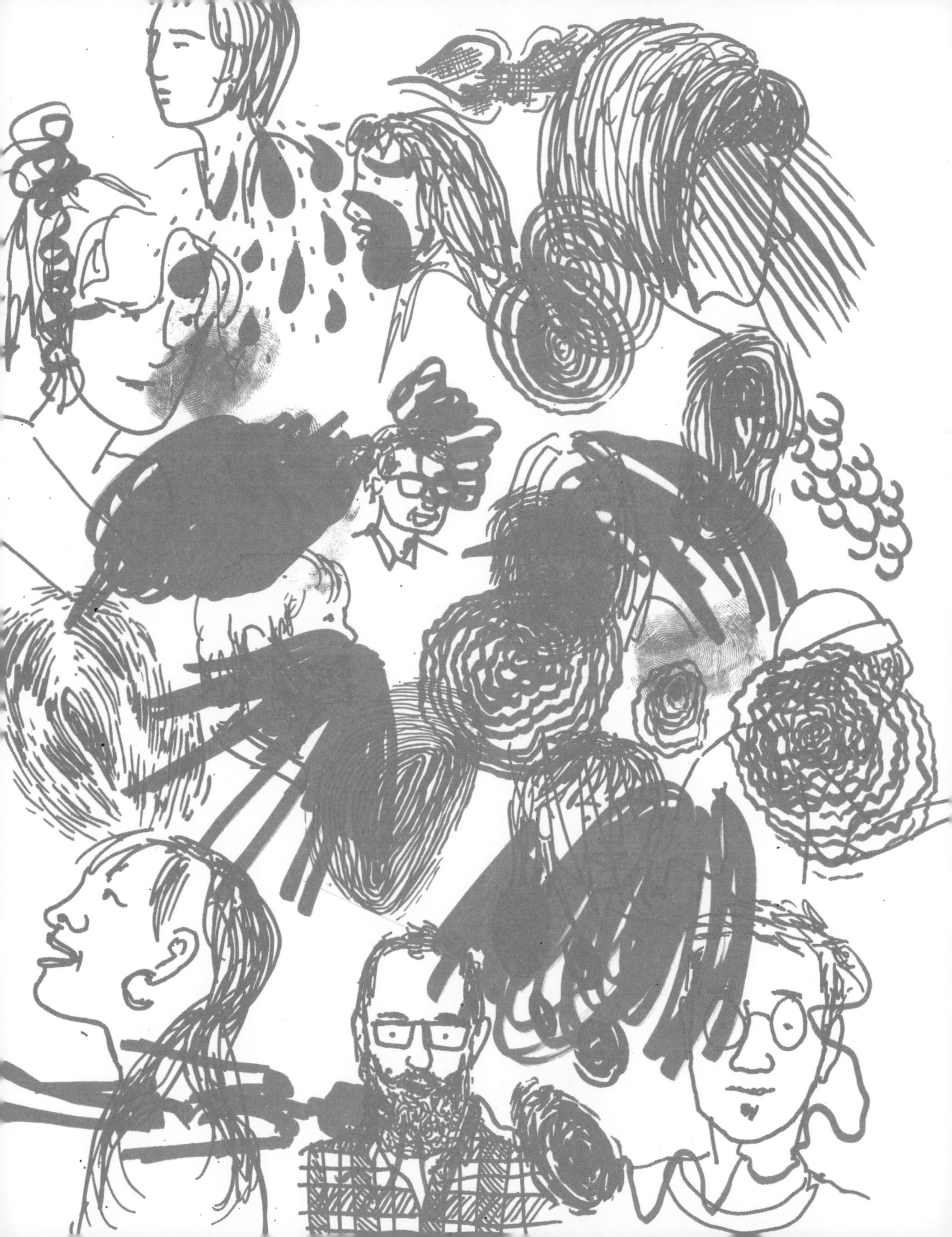

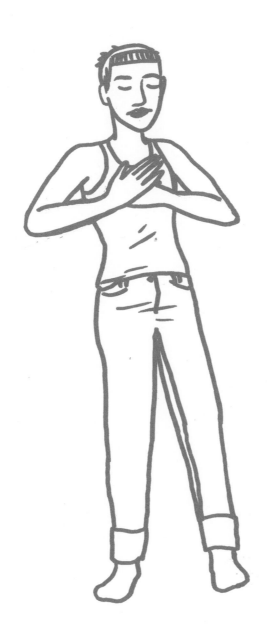